Ethics of Sport
and Athletics:

Theory, Issues, and Application

Ethics of Sport and Athletics:

Theory, Issues, and Application

ROBERT C. SCHNEIDER, EdD, MAT

Associate Professor, Sport Management
The Department of Physical Education & Sport
The College at Brockport, State University of New York
Brockport, New York

 Wolters Kluwer | Lippincott Williams & Wilkins
Health

Philadelphia • Baltimore • New York • London
Buenos Aires • Hong Kong • Sydney • Tokyo

r: Emily J. Lupash
or: Karen M. Ruppert
anager: Christen D. Murphy
Editor: Paula C. Williams
Doug Smock
ion Services: International Typesetting and Composition
er: R. R. Donnelley and Sons Crawfordsville

351 West Camden Street
Baltimore, MD 21201

530 Walnut Street
Philadelphia, PA 19106

Printed in United States of America

9 8 7 6 5 4 3 2 1

Library of Congress Cataloging-in-Publication Data

Schneider, Robert C.
  Ethics of sport and athletics : theory, issues, and application / Robert C. Schneider.—1st ed.
    p. cm.
  Includes bibliographical references and index.
  ISBN-13: 978-0-7817-8791-8
  ISBN-10: 0-7817-8791-2
  1. Sports—Moral and ethical aspects.   I. Title.
  GV706.3.S34 2009
  174′.9796—dc22

                                                    2008014958

DISCLAIMER

Care has been taken to confirm the accuracy of the information present and to describe generally accepted practices. However, the authors, editors, and publisher are not responsible for errors or omissions or for any consequences from application of the information in this book and make no warranty, expressed or implied, with respect to the currency, completeness, or accuracy of the contents of the publication. Application of this information in a particular situation remains the professional responsibility of the practitioner; the clinical treatments described and recommended may not be considered absolute and universal recommendations.

The authors, editors, and publisher have exerted every effort to ensure that drug selection and dosage set forth in this text are in accordance with the current recommendations and practice at the time of publication. However, in view of ongoing research, changes in government regulations, and the constant flow of information relating to drug therapy and drug reactions, the reader is urged to check the package insert for each drug for any change in indications and dosage and for added warnings and precautions. This is particularly important when the recommended agent is a new or infrequently employed drug.

Some drugs and medical devices presented in this publication have Food and Drug Administration (FDA) clearance for limited use in restricted research settings. It is the responsibility of the health care provider to ascertain the FDA status of each drug or device planned for use in their clinical practice.

To purchase additional copies of this book, call our customer service department at (800) 638-3030 or fax orders to (301) 223-2320. International customers should call (301) 223-2300.

Visit Lippincott Williams & Wilkins on the Internet: http://www.lww.com. Lippincott Williams & Wilkins customer service representatives are available from 8:30 am to 6:00 pm, EST.

I would like to dedicate this book to my parents, Bob and Dorothy, for instilling both an understanding of morality and a sense of discipline in me that have served me well throughout my professional accomplishments, not the least of which is the completion of this book.

I would also like to dedicate this book to my high school cross country coach, Mr. Larry Rader. To gain a full understanding of good and morally right actions in sport and beyond, I had to look no further than Coach Rader. Coach Rader served as our cross country team's foundation of moral guidance. When confronted with moral dilemmas, Coach Rader's athletes and students had to do nothing more than ask themselves: "What would Coach Rader do, or what would Coach Rader approve of?"

REVIEWERS

Jennifer M. Beller, PhD
Associate Professor
Washington State University
Pullman, WA

Lawrence P. Bestmann, PhD
Professor Emeritus
United States Sports Academy
Daphne, AL

Patrick J. Clemens, MSS
Instructor
Cardinal Stritch University
Milwaukee, WI

Craig A. Dyer, MBA, ATC
Assistant Professor
Indiana Tech
Fort Wayne, IN

Edward Etzel, EdD
Psychologist/Associate Professor
West Virginia University
Morgantown, WV

Kathryn Paxton George, PhD
Professor Emerita of Philosophy
University of Idaho
Moscow, ID

Douglas Hochstetler, PhD
Associate Professor of Kinesiology
Penn State University, Lehigh Valley
Fogelsville, PA

Russell Medbery, PhD
Associate Professor
Colby-Sawyer College
New London, NH

Duane Millslagle, EdD
Associate Professor
University of Minnesota Duluth
Duluth, MN

Michael Mondello, PhD
Associate Professor
The Florida State University
Tallahassee, FL

Susan P. Mullane, PhD
Associate Professor
University of Miami
Coral Gables, FL

Ronald W. Quinn, EdD
Associate Professor, Sport Studies
Xavier University
Cincinnati, OH

Bob Rinehart, PhD
Associate Professor
Washington State University
Pullman, WA

Brian A. Sather, PhD
Associate Professor
Eastern Oregon University
La Grande, OR

ABOUT THE AUTHOR

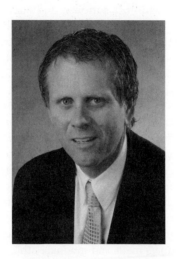

ROBERT C. SCHNEIDER, EdD, MAT

Associate Professor, Sport Management
The College at Brockport, State University of New York

Dr. Robert C. Schneider is an associate professor of sport management in The Department of Physical Education & Sport at The College at Brockport, State University of New York, located in Brockport, New York. He earned an EdD in Sport Management at Temple University, an MA in Teaching from the University of West Alabama, and a BS in Physical Education from the Ohio State University. From 1994 to 1997, Dr. Schneider served on the sport management faculty at Salem-Teikyo University in Salem, West Virginia, where he started and coordinated the sport management program while also serving as the athletic department's faculty athletics representative.

Since his arrival at Brockport in the fall of 1997, Dr. Schneider has established a reputation as a prolific scholar. In addition to *Ethics of Sport and Athletics: Theory, Issues, and Application*, he is also the sole author of *Basketball for all Levels* (American Press, 2008) and has authored or coauthored over 40 peer-reviewed publications, primarily in international and national sport management–related journals. This list of journals includes but is not limited to the following: *Journal of Physical Education, Recreation, and Dance; Journal of the International Council for Health, Physical Education, Recreation, Sport, and Dance; Recreational Sports Journal; Strategies; The Sport Journal; Journal for the Study of Sports and Athletics in Education; Sport Management and Related Topics Journal; Applied Research in Coaching and Athletics; The Physical Educator; International Sports Journal;* and *The Mid-Atlantic Journal of Business.*

Dr. Schneider has also conducted over 65 professional presentations, including but not limited to international, national, and state conferences in sport management, coaching, and related fields. Dr. Schneider's commitment to scholarly, peer-reviewed writing is further demonstrated by his editorial board membership on the following four professional journals: *International Journal of Sport Management; Applied Research in Coaching and Athletics Annual; Strategies; and Journal of the International Council for Health, Physical Education, Recreation, Sport, and Dance.*

Active in numerous professional organizations, Dr. Schneider holds memberships in the following: *North American Society for Sport Management; International Council for Health, Physical Education, Recreation, Sport, and Dance; National Intramural Recreational Sports Association; American Alliance of Health, Physical Education, Recreation, and Dance; National Association of Basketball Coaches;* and *Sports Lawyers Association.*

A hands-on teacher who actively engages students in the learning process, Dr. Schneider has taught a wide range of undergraduate, graduate, and activity courses since he began teaching in 1986. Dr. Schneider teaches in The College at Brockport's undergraduate sport management and graduate athletic administration programs. His teaching schedule currently consists of Coaching Sports; Budget, Finance, and Facility Management in Physical Education and Sport; Research in Sport Management; Administration and Supervision of Physical Education and Athletics; and Administrative Practices in Sport Management. An ethics of sport and moral values component is incorporated into each of these courses.

PREFACE

Morality in Sport

Sport continues to make its presence known throughout the world as it prospers at all levels. Amazingly, there is no end in sight to the popularity and growth of sport. Essential to sport's continued prosperity, growth, and overall livelihood is the sustenance of a firm moral base. It is the goal and hope of the author that you find this textbook to be a useful guide in helping you maintain and build upon the foundation of moral good that is required for sport to exist now and in the future.

The need to make good moral decisions in sport is constant. And, although opportunities to make such decisions in sport are seemingly endless, what is "moral" can be somewhat unclear. Given the various perspectives on morality and the lack of clear-cut distinctions between moral and immoral actions, disagreements regarding moral behavior and sport are likely to always exist. However, having a *blatant* disregard for good moral behavior in sport is difficult to defend from most any position.

Perhaps no incident better exemplifies a blatant disregard for good moral behavior in sport than the videotaping incident that occurred on September 9, 2007 during a game between the National Football League's (NFL's) New England Patriots and the New York Jets. NFL policy clearly states that no video recording devices of any kind are permitted on the field. Yet, a Patriots' cameraman, in clear view of everyone, was aiming his camera at and recording the Jets' defensive coaches, who were sending signals to their defensive team on the field. The commissioner of the NFL, Roger Goodell, acted swiftly with his punishment. Commissioner Goodell fined Patriots' head coach Bill Belichick $500,000 and the Patriots organization $250,000, while also requiring the forfeiture of the Patriots' top draft choices during the following year's draft.

Acting immorally to gain an edge that will be helpful in winning can be tempting in sporting organizations such as the NFL, which are centered on and reward winning. However, the challenge of choosing and remaining on the moral high road while involved in sport is not limited to competitive elite sport such as professional, Olympic, and major college organizations. Participants in all levels of sport, including youth, recreation, and intramural, face the many temptations to veer from the straight and narrow and must make a sustained effort to act morally. Aspects of sport that lure one into making immoral choices can be many and are addressed throughout this book.

Goals of This Text

Those involved in sport face a two-fold ethical challenge: (a) putting forth a constant effort to purify sport and (b) maintaining a strong, healthy emphasis on winning as a desired component of sport. A general goal of *Ethics of Sport and Athletics: Theory, Issues, and Application* is that it serve as a guide for constantly cleansing sport of moral impurities without diminishing its competitive element.

Pedagogy is an underlying theme of the book, and one of its primary goals is to provide the reader with the ability to act in ways that reinforce the moral foundation necessary for sport to function effectively. Arguably, the morality surrounding sport is no better or worse today than in the past. The challenge of maintaining the integrity of sport in the midst of such things as the strong emphasis placed on winning, along with performance-based prizes and recognitions, must continually be addressed. Simply stated, sport has been, is, and will continue to be susceptible to acts of immorality, which if left unchecked could shake the foundation of and possibly topple sport. Included in the teachings of this book, and necessary for preservation of sport's integrity, is how to apply moral reasoning skills to sport-related dilemmas.

Often, those confronted with dilemmas in sport want to make good moral choices but are not sure how to do so. This book provides guidance for making good moral decisions related to seemingly complicated, controversial, and confusing dilemmas in sport. To make good moral choices, frequently one must simplify dilemmas to their core components. What initially appear to be complicated problems are sometimes found to be quite simple after separating and dismissing unessential parts of the issue. This book provides the reader with the know-how to successfully engage in such a process.

Another goal of this book is to enlighten those closely involved in sport, including athletes, coaches, and sport managers, to the fact that the practice of good moral actions is central to the effective function of sport. The expectation is that, after accepting the notion that good moral actions are vital to the effective function of sport, those involved in sport will not only practice morally good actions but also point out the importance of doing so to others. Practicing and spreading the word of good moral behavior in sport will strengthen the foundation of sport.

Controversial sport matters that surface as dilemmas to be resolved by athletes, coaches, and sport managers are discussed in this book. Issues in the world of sport that require choices to be made are presented and supported by real sport examples. For instance, discussions related to hazing are supplemented by real examples in which those faced with the dilemma arrived at real decisions.

Organization

This book consists of two parts, totaling nine chapters. Part I contains the first three chapters, which primarily include the various theories and mechanics of moral reasoning, ethical and unethical behavior in sport, and the development of moral education through sport. Part II is made up of the final six chapters, which address real-world controversial sports issues, are application oriented, and present a variety of actual dilemmas in the form of case studies, ranging from simple to complex. The case studies are reflective of the sport issues presented in Part II, which include performance enhancement, violence, race, gender equity, and Title IX, along with issues relevant to interscholastic and intercollegiate sport, as well as sport managers.

Decision-Making Models

From the perspective of learning, a vital aspect of this book is the inclusion of four decision-making models. Three of the models are based on moral reasoning theory and the other on principles of strategic reasoning. These models provide the reader with a system to assist him or her in arriving at good moral resolutions to the case studies and, more importantly, to real dilemmas in the world of sport. Instead of guessing what the appropriate moral action may be to resolve a dilemma, the reader will be equipped with the three moral theory-based decision-making models—consequentialism, teleology, and deontology—which will provide him or her with a systematic and logical approach to theoretically grounded, morally appropriate actions. Although not morally based, the strategic reasoning model will provide an understanding of how decisions are often arrived at in sport without moral guidance.

Case Studies

The case studies are numerous, vary in level of complexity, and are intended to assist the reader in gaining experiences in making real-world ethical decisions without being exposed to the real-world consequences that come from such decisions. Questions related to the case studies follow and are separated into two sets. The first set is to be answered from a common-sense perspective, without necessarily applying a formal decision-making procedure. The second set requires the reader to analyze the case and arrive at a decision by applying one or a combination of the three moral theory-based decision-making models. After having reasoned through the case studies, readers will be better prepared to confidently make good moral decisions.

Other Features

Further serving as pedagogical tools are "mini" case studies, cartoons, and text boxes of ethical terms that are embedded in each chapter. The mini case studies provide students with the opportunity to practice and reinforce the process necessary to arrive at good moral decisions. The cartoons, in a lighthearted manner, reinforce key moral concepts and decision-making skills presented in the text. Also assisting the readers in their focus on ethical concepts are text boxes that feature important ethical terms and their definitions.

Additional Resources

Ethics of Sport and Athletics: Theory, Issues, and Application includes additional resources for both instructors and students that are available on the book's companion website at http://thePoint.lww.com/Schneider.

Instructors

Approved adopting instructors will be given access to the following additional resources:

- PowerPoint presentations
- Brownstone Test Generator
- Image bank
- WebCT and Blackboard Ready Cartridge

Students

Purchasers of the text can access the searchable Full Text On-line by going to the Ethics of Sport and Athletics: Theory, Issues, and Application website at http://thePoint.lww.com. See the inside front cover of this text for more details, including the passcode you will need to gain access to the website.

Summary

With practice, students will become acquainted with and eventually master the ability to effectively apply the moral theory-based decision-making models to the case studies in this book. After having repeatedly practiced the effective application of the moral decision-making models to the case studies, students will be prepared to apply the moral decision-making models to real-world dilemmas that take place in the competitive world of sport.

Understanding morality and good moral behavior is only the very beginning of "doing the right thing." The importance lies not in understanding *how* to act in good ways but to actually *act* in good ways. This book will provide you with an understanding of moral good and how to make good decisions in sport. It will be left to you, the reader, however, to actually make good decisions in and outside of sport. Information in this book will serve as a moral compass, but it is up to you as a holder of the compass to navigate the correct path when confronted with dilemmas in sport and beyond.

ACKNOWLEDGMENTS

There are many who deserve to be acknowledged, as the quality of this book was dependent on them. The reviewers, experts in sport ethics, and Lippincott Williams & Wilkins employees are just a few who deserve to be recognized.

The many reviewers deserve recognition, as I absolutely relied on their feedback on the first three chapters to ensure the formation of the strong theoretical foundation on which this book is based. The reviewers' feedback also guided the substance and delivery of the final six chapters, which include current issues in the form of moral dilemmas.

As an expert in sport philosophy, my friend and colleague Dr. Peter Hager deserves special acknowledgement for his philosophically grounded insights that were used to shape and create the moral theory decision-making models.

Emily Lupash's involvement from the beginning to end and complete knowledge of the whole process was instrumental in that I could pick up the phone and get an answer to any question with one call. As the managing editor, Karen Ruppert matched her superior skills with an unending positive energy and fun-natured approach that was contagious and helped make the process enjoyable. Gail Schoonmaker's brilliant artistic talent of transforming my text descriptions into the actual pictorials that I envisioned was nothing less than astonishing. Ann Seitz and David Payne deserve special acknowledgment for being able to enter and apply their superior editing skills in midstream without missing a beat. My thanks go out to Christen Murphy (marketing manager), Paula Williams (production editor), and Doug Smock (designer) for applying their expertise in their respective roles which contributed immensely to the quality of this textbook. I would also like to thank Arushi Chawla, project manager of the typesetting process for providing yet another layer of proofreading and editing. Finally, I would be remiss if I did not offer my thanks to the many persons who I did not communicate with directly but served vital roles in various aspects throughout the process of completing *Ethics of Sport and Athletics: Theory, Issues, and Application.*

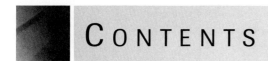

CONTENTS

Part II   Moral Application in Sport and Athletics

4. Performance Enhancement Issues in Sport 135

PART 1

Moral Theory in Sport and Athletics

1 Moral Reasoning: An Introduction

Learning Outcomes

After reading Chapter 1, the student will be able to:

1. Differentiate between moral reasoning and non-moral reasoning in sport.

2. Describe the components necessary to maintain a moral balance in sport.

3. Describe actions that foster the morality of sport.

4. Explain the importance of moral reasoning in competitive sport.

5. Apply the strategic reasoning decision-making model in solving moral dilemmas.

6. Identify ways to cultivate habits of action that will result in moral excellence.

7. Identify and differentiate between moral and social values.

8. Understand and be able to explain the roles that moral values and principles play in the process of moral reasoning.

9. Use the three decision-making models of moral reasoning—consequentialist, teleological, and deontological—in solving moral dilemmas.

With the tremendous focus on winning and advantage-seeking in modern sports, often there is little time to think about what is morally right, or to make sure that your on-field and off-field actions are in sync with your values and principles. Who has time to discuss issues related to fair play and good sporting behavior when so much preparation is necessary for the next event or season? How can coaches and administrators worry about whether athletes are learning good moral values from sport or displaying good moral character, when their jobs often depend on their teams' performances?

Morals are the beliefs and ideas a person has about what it is right or wrong to do. These beliefs are developed over time. Some are learned from parents, caregivers, family members, teachers, and friends; others are developed from observations of a person's culture and the world. Morals can take the form of rules or principles (the Golden Rule for example, discussed later in this chapter), or of particular traits or characteristics (moral values) that help you act well toward others.

Ethics is the area of philosophy that deals with questions about morality and assesses the rightness or wrongness of actions and decisions. Thus, ethics can help to mediate disagreements between moralities by employing moral theories and methods of reasoning to determine what is morally best under the circumstances.

This first chapter focuses on helping athletes, coaches, and administrators recognize and understand moral issues or dilemmas, and on helping the reader develop a clear distinction between the moral reasoning called for in different situations and the strategic reasoning that dominates the world of sport.

Understanding Moral Issues and Problems

morality: a system of norms, values, and rules that regulates the manner in which human beings treat one another.

When our morals are viewed as a set, they form a **morality**—a system of norms, values, and rules of action that govern our relationship with other human beings—that guides us when questions of right and wrong arise. According to Loland, such systems "prescribe how we should act so as to do good to others, how significant goods and burdens should be allocated, and how people should relate to one another in matters of promises and contracts."[1(p18)] Moralities can belong to individuals or to groups, cultures, or societies. Moralities differ according to time and place. Different cultures have differing views about what is right and wrong, and these views change over time as people's ideas about the world and other human beings change. In sport and athletics, teams, sporting communities, individual athletes, coaches, and administrators develop moralities to guide their conduct on and off of the field. The practice of analyzing issues related to morality that seeks to assess the rightness or wrongness of human decisions and actions is the branch of philosophy called **ethics.**

ethics: the area of philosophy that deals with questions about morality and assesses the rightness or wrongness of actions and decisions.

According to Frankena, ethics "is moral philosophy or philosophical thinking about morality, moral problems, and moral judgments."[2(p4)] Ethical inquiries are those in which the rightness and wrongness of human moral actions are assessed. Ethics is thus a normative brand of inquiry; it goes beyond describing how human beings act toward one another and asks and examines how they *should* act toward one another.[3] "In ethics," Loland notes, "we do not just seek empirical descriptions of the moral norms and values of a given group of people but attempt to reflect critically and systematically upon their nature."[1(p18)] A discussion of ethics thus requires us to not only evaluate moral beliefs, decisions, and actions but also carefully analyze their moral value using sound methods of moral reasoning.

> **moral reasoning:** a decision-making process that requires persons to use criteria such as moral values, moral principles, and/or the anticipated moral consequences of actions to determine whether a particular action is right or wrong, or whether we have a moral obligation to act in a particular manner toward others.

Moral reasoning is a decision-making process that requires individuals to use criteria such as moral values, moral principles, and/or the anticipated moral consequences to determine whether a particular action is right or wrong, or whether we have a moral obligation to act in a particular manner toward others. Non-moral reasoning does not require that you decide between actions that are morally good or bad, or ethically right or wrong. **Strategic reasoning** is also a decision-making process and has the objective of acting based on what will reward or bring the greatest advantage to a person or to that person's team, school, or organization.

> **strategic reasoning:** a decision-making process in which the decision made/action taken is based on that which will bring the greatest advantage or reward to an individual or that individual's 'in-group' (e.g., team, school, organization).

Moral Reasoning

When dealing with questions of moral right and wrong, you must consider how individual actions affect others within the sporting environment. Hence, moral dilemmas, issues, and questions require that you use moral reasoning, an **altruistic** form of reasoning that makes a person look beyond his/her own good in determining the right action to take in a certain situation. For example, a coach may be confronted with enforcing a mandatory suspension penalty against a player who has broken a curfew rule. When looking at this dilemma from a perspective of providing good for the *coach,* the coach may prefer to not enforce the suspension, since winning the game would then be more difficult. However, when looking at the long-term good that a suspension might provide for the *player,* the right choice might be to carry out the suspension. The suspended player may learn the importance of responsibility and punctuality, two behaviors that will serve the player well in his or her professional and personal future.

> **altruistic:** looking beyond one's own good in determining the right action to take in a certain situation; living for the good of others; doing good and not expecting anything in return.

Many theories of moral reasoning have been developed over time. These theories are based on what particular ethical theorists reasoned were the most important factors in determining the ethical acceptability or unacceptability of an action. Three such theories are examined later in this chapter. First it is necessary to further examine the difference between moral and strategic reasoning by working through an example. In doing so, arguments will be defined in a manner that explains how they can be used in different ways to present different types of reasoning.

Non-moral Dilemmas Faced by Sport Personnel

Sport personnel make many decisions on a daily basis. These decisions generally are non-moral ones and do not require what we call moral reasoning. "Moral reasoning is defined as the decision process in which a person determines the rightness or wrongness of a course of action."[4(p544)] **Non-moral reasoning** does not require that you decide between actions that are morally good or bad, or ethically right or wrong.

> **non-moral reasoning:** does not require that you decide between actions that are morally good or bad, or ethically right or wrong.

Human beings make many judgments every day. Some of these judgments have little or nothing to do with how we treat other people and do not call into question the moral value of their motives, intentions, and character traits. These judgments are non-moral judgments, and they are made through a process of decision making (non-moral reasoning) that uses various criteria to determine the value (goodness or badness) of items, experiences, and conditions that do not directly affect relationships with or actions toward others. For example, when deciding whether a material item such as a sandwich or a house is 'good' or 'bad,' a person will use subjective criteria (taste) or empirical criteria (building standards), respectively, in reasoning and coming to a judgment as to their non-moral value.[2(p62)]

From a sport perspective, athletes must decide, for example, what type of conditioning exercises will best prepare them for an upcoming game, whether or not to devote more time to psychological skills training, and what foods to include in their diets. Some hockey players emphasize strength training, while others train in a way that increases their speed, quickness, and reaction time. Some baseball players carefully follow a specific pre-game routine, while others make a conscious effort not to follow a routine before games. Generally, these are considered examples of non-moral reasoning. For, when choosing between various pre-existing methods of training endorsed by the sporting community, the reasoning is based on which training method is most appropriate for a sport and not on relationships or actions toward others.

Coaches also make non-moral decisions. They must decide which athletes should start games, how to spend their practice time with players, and what strategies will work best against an upcoming opponent. One youth soccer coach may determine starters based on who puts forth the most effort in practice, whereas the criteria for other coaches may be strictly based on performance outcomes such as who can score the most goals or defend most effectively. Some football coaches may decide to monopolize their preseason practices with conditioning drills, while others may work on fundamentals. Non-moral decisions made by basketball coaches include choosing among different offensive styles, such as a slow-down style or an up-tempo style.

Sport managers make non-moral decisions about such things as how to hire staff, how to best negotiate salaries for professional players, or what promotions to offer during a season. For instance, a college athletic director looking to hire coaches may hire from within his/her own organization, while another athletic

decision maker: person who settles an issue; person who arrives at a judgment or makes a choice; that is, athletes, coaches, and sport managers who are confronted with difficult decisions that call for adherence to a reasoning process or decision-making model to make the right choice.

moral value(s): particular traits or characteristics that help people act well toward others, including honesty, justice, kindness, respect, beneficence, and compassion; moral values consist of dispositions that influence one to do what is morally right and carry out one's moral responsibilities to others.

honesty (moral value): telling the truth; not lying; upright; faithful.

justice (moral value): fairness; equity; founded on fact.

beneficence: being kind to others; doing good; not harming others.

compassion (moral value): merciful; suffering with another; being able to understand another's position, ideas, problems, etc.; being able to understand the injustices or moral problems other persons are facing; a compassionate person is one who sees how cheating hurts and feels badly for those who have had illegal tactics used against them.

director may prefer to hire persons from the outside. Some Major League Soccer general managers choose to renegotiate player contracts while a player is still under contract, whereas others will only renegotiate when a player's contract ends. When deciding on promotional philosophies, one arena football marketing director may gear hers toward a demographic of 18- to 34-year-old males, whereas another may have a broad promotional strategy, targeting all youth, irrespective of gender.

As you can see, athletic personnel make numerous non-moral decisions throughout a season. Although it might be an exaggeration to refer to these decisions as routine, they usually do not require that the **decision maker** have an understanding of right and wrong. Players deciding how to improve their performance, coaches deciding how to improve individual players and teams, and sport managers deciding how to best manage their organization generally do not test the decision maker's scruples. Non-moral decisions such as these can be made without placing a primary emphasis on **moral values.** Moral values, according to Kretchmar, are character traits and motives that help make up a morally good person.[5] Moral values consist of dispositions that influence one to do what is morally right and carry out one's moral responsibilities to others. Examples of moral values are **honesty, justice, beneficence,** and **compassion.** Instead of basing decisions on moral values, non-moral decisions are often based on non-moral values that, according to Kretchmar, are items, experiences, and conditions that people desire such as wealth, pleasure, excellence, knowledge, and security.[5]

Moral Dilemmas Faced by Sport Personnel

The process of moral reasoning includes sorting out right from wrong, which provides the decision maker with the proper guidance when arriving at a decision. The anticipated good as well as bad that comes from the decision, and how many people benefit from the good and suffer from the bad, must also be considered. According to Frankena, "The sorts of things that may be morally good or bad are persons, groups of persons, traits of character, dispositions, emotions, motives, and intentions."[2(p62)] He refers to judgments pertaining to the **moral goodness** or badness of people, groups, or "elements of personality" as "judgments of moral value."[2(p9)] These differ from "judgments of moral obligation," in which "we say that a certain action or kind of action is morally right, wrong, obligatory, a duty, or ought or ought not to be done."[2(p9)] In short, actions are the kinds of thing that can be morally right or wrong; persons, groups, character traits, motives, and intentions are the kinds of things that can be morally good or bad.

moral goodness: condition of virtuousness; relates to persons and their character traits.

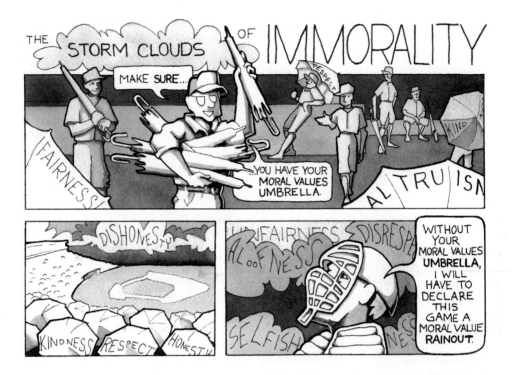

Decision makers such as athletes, coaches, and sport managers are constantly confronted with difficult decisions that call for adherence to a reasoning process or decision-making model to make the right choice. For example, what if an athlete must decide between increasing strength through proper nutrition and weight training, or through the use of illegal performance-enhancing substances like anabolic steroids or human growth hormone? Former Major League Baseball player Jose Canseco and current player Jason Giambi both admitted—Canseco through a self-authored book[6] and Giambi through federal grand jury testimony[7]—to making the choice to use steroids. In choosing to use steroids, did these players consider both the good and the bad that might come from their choice? Do others, such as players and coaches who were around Canseco and Giambi on a daily basis, hold some responsibility for not attempting to prevent them from using steroids? If players and coaches believe that players who use steroids are bad for the game overall, should those players and coaches have intervened and done what was necessary to stop Canseco and Giambi (and others) from using steroids?

What about the coach who must decide whether to allow an injured athlete to compete in a championship game when this action could increase the athlete's risk of more serious injury? When Willis Reed of the New York Knicks played with a torn thigh muscle in Game 7 of the 1970 National Basketball Association (NBA) championship game, it gave his team a tremendous mental lift but was risky to Reed's physical health. To protect Reed from further injury, should someone with the authority, such as the Knick's head coach, have insisted he not play? More recently, Terrell Owens of the Philadelphia Eagles insisted on playing in the 2005 Super Bowl despite not being 100% recovered from a broken bone in his leg. Should someone from the Eagles organization have prohibited Owens from playing to prevent further injury?

What if a sport manager/athletic director must decide whether to report the playing of an ineligible athlete, an action that would result in forfeiting regular season wins and a playoff spot? If left unreported it is possible that no one would find out, but by not reporting the infraction, does the athletic director run the risk of causing harm to coaches, players, and even fans? If the athletic director does report the ineligibility, what good and what bad will result from that decision, and how many people will be affected by both the good and the bad?

The above-mentioned scenarios are examples of **moral dilemmas.** They call for actions to determine which option is morally best. If Jason Giambi weighed his options and based his decision to take steroids on what he thought to be morally best, he approached the dilemma of whether or not to take steroids as a moral one. If Giambi did not attempt to try and determine whether the action of taking steroids was right or wrong, he did not fulfill a **moral obligation** to reason morally prior to taking the action. If the coaches of Willis Reed and Terrell Owens reasoned morally and arrived at an understanding of whether the action to play in the championship games was right or wrong, they fulfilled a moral obligation to base their actions on morals. In deciding whether or not to report the ineligible player, if the athletic director based the decision on what was best for all parties involved, the decision was a moral one. If he considered only himself and not the other players, coaches, or fans, the decision was not morally based.

To reiterate, the primary characteristic that separates moral questions from other kinds of questions is whether or not actions are based on what is determined, through a process of reasoning, to be morally best. Non-moral actions are not driven by what is morally best. When dealing with questions of right or wrong, human beings are faced with having to consider not only their own good but also the good of others. Considering the good of others complicates the decision-making process but is an important component of arriving at the right choice when confronted with a moral dilemma.

> **moral dilemma(s):** a situation that calls for actions to determine which option is morally best.

> **moral obligation:** moral obligations include moral judgments that people make that affect people's relationships and dealings with one another, and that bring the moral value of their motives, intentions, and character traits under scrutiny.

> **strategic obligation:** the type of judgment that is arrived at through a process of strategic reasoning that requires people to examine the possible consequences of actions to determine which action will bring the greatest advantage to them personally or to the group they represent (e.g., their team, school, or organization).

> **consequences of actions:** that which naturally follows an action; a result; moral theories contending that the consequences of actions are the primary element in determining the right action to take in a given situation are consequentialist moral theories; actions taken within the consequentialist moral theory are based on the consequences that will follow.

Shifting From Strategic Reasoning To Moral Reasoning

Judgments concerning moral obligation must be further distinguished from judgments of **strategic obligation.** This latter type of judgment is arrived at through a process of reasoning (strategic reasoning) that requires people to examine the possible **consequences of actions** to determine which action will bring the greatest advantage to them personally or to the group they represent (e.g., their team, school, or organization). Moral obligations, conversely, include judgments that people make that affect people's relationships and dealings with one another, and do bring the moral value of their motives, intentions, and character traits under scrutiny. These are moral judgments and they are developed through a decision-making process (moral reasoning) that requires the use of criteria such as moral values, moral principles, and/or the potential moral consequences of actions, to determine the rightness or wrongness of actions, or the goodness or badness of persons or their motives, traits, or intentions. Judgments regarding the rightness or wrongness of actions or the moral duties, responsibilities, or obligations of people, are "judgments of moral obligation"[2(p9)]; judgments concerning the goodness or badness of people, groups of people, or their motives or traits are "judgments of moral value."[2(pp9,62)]

In sport, considering the good of others and what is morally best requires a shift from the everyday type of strategic thinking on which many sports personnel such as players and coaches tend to rely. In everyday morality, you would not necessarily attempt to defeat your opponents for the sole purpose of defeating them, as is often the goal in sport. Typical strategic thinking in a non-sport context usually is less extreme. In non-sport contexts, in which people are not directly competing against one another, strategic thinking exists but not to the extent it does in a sport context, in which athletes and coaches are strategizing directly against their opponents. For example, when an employee of a business seeks to advance within the company, he or she can usually do so by performing and producing better than other employees, as opposed to defeating them. In doing so, the atmosphere can be one that is more morally oriented. In sport, the goal of players is to strategize a way to defeat their opponents.

In the everyday life of students, they may strategize to schedule classes, take tests, and ultimately graduate. Given that, in most all cases, success is not based on head-to-head competition with other students (as it is in sport), the degree of strategic reasoning is not as intense as it is in sport. Shields and Bredemeier[8] referred to the context in which sport operates as a **bracketed morality.** Bracketed morality is a morality that grants sport participants greater moral freedom when involved in a sporting contest than is expected outside of sporting contests. Bracketed morality allows sport participants to emphasize self-interest, related to the goals of sport, more than does everyday morality. Furthermore, bracketed morality may be used as a justification by players and coaches to support behaviors within sport that may be perceived as questionable by those not operating within its realm. Among sport participants there seems to be a collective agreement and acceptance of a more loosely defined set of moral expectations when compared with the moral expectations of everyday living. Those participating in sports, however, are not granted full deferment of morality; they are still required to uphold basic aspects of the broader morality relating to **fairness, equal opportunity,** and **safety.**

Regarding this concept, Jones and McNamee[9] stated that the bracketed nature of moral reasoning in sport is separate from, less mature than, and therefore inconsistent with reasoning about real life. Stuntz and Weiss added to the understanding of how those in sport

bracketed morality: a morality that grants sport participants additional moral freedom when involved in a sporting contest than what is expected outside of sporting contests; allows sport participants to emphasize self-interest, related to the goals of sport, more than everyday morality; may be used as a justification by players and coaches to support behaviors within sport that may be perceived as questionable by those not operating within its realm.

fairness (moral value): just; impartial; straightforward justice; being objective.

equal opportunity: the same chance; participants who compete under the same conditions have equal opportunity to succeed.

safety: protection from harm.

reason by pointing out that the form of morality that takes place allows contestants and those assisting them to think more egoistically.[10] In other words, sport culture is accepting of participants who put their own interests and the interests of their teams ahead of the interests of others.

"Major League Tantrum Thrown by Little League Pitcher"

Interested in inserting his 'closer' into game 4 of the Little League best-of-seven championship series to get the final two outs, the head coach decides to remove his star pitcher from the game. The star pitcher had only allowed three hits in six and two-thirds innings, and he demonstrated his outrage with the decision by throwing a Major League tantrum. While walking from the pitcher's mound to the dugout, the youngster aimlessly kicked dirt and shouted four-letter word after four-letter word. Making matters worse, the opposing fans began to chant, "loooooser," "loooooser," "loooooser." Having now reached a level of complete infuriation, the out-of-control star pitcher turned to the opposing crowd and gave them the middle finger while simultaneously screaming "F*&$ all of you!" Knowing full well that his star pitcher's next scheduled start would be the final game of the championship series, the head coach, nevertheless, immediately announced that his star pitcher would be suspended for game seven. Now that game seven is just a day away, however, the head coach is beginning to second guess his decision.

Questions
1. Does this dilemma call for moral reasoning?
2. What factors should the head coach consider if he is basing his decision on the best interests of his star pitcher?
3. What factors should the head coach consider if he is basing his decision on strategic reasoning?
4. How might strategic reasoning become part of the decision-making process?

> **winning at all costs:** placing winning ahead of all else; compromising moral values and sportsmanship in the interest of winning.

The phrase **winning at all costs** is representative of putting one's own interests and the interests of the team ahead of others. Another phrase, nice guys finish last, is somewhat symbolic of bracketed morality in that it suggests that beneficent or altruistic sporting behavior cannot lead to success in sport. As coaches and players establish strategies to win, moral reasoning is often not a consideration. For example, if it is known that a football quarterback is prone to concussions, it may actually be a strategy of an opposing team to hit the quarterback 'hard and high' in an attempt to knock him out of the game. This is an extreme example of a team placing its own interests ahead of the interests of others. The opposing team's interest is in winning, and to that end they have consciously established a strategy to exploit the quarterback's vulnerability to hard hits above the shoulders.

This strategy to 'knock the quarterback out' is placed ahead of the interest of the quarterback to perform and remain healthy. In this example, behaving in a morally correct way is not a consideration. Establishing and implementing a strategy to win supersedes the process of reasoning in a way that is morally best.

Another example of placing one's own interests and the team's interests ahead of others is when a pitcher in baseball puts foreign substances on a baseball to make the ball move in an unpredictable manner as it approaches home plate. When attempting to hit this pitch, which is more commonly known as a 'spitball,' the batter is at a distinct disadvantage. Baseball's rule makers have determined this disadvantage to be an unfair one and have thus established a rule making the spitball illegal. When a pitcher chooses to throw a spitball, he is making a conscious decision to place his interest in personal statistics and his team's interest in winning ahead of the officials' interest in maintaining fair competition and the game's interest in maintaining a structured competitive balance between the offense and defense (pitcher and batter).

moral egocentrism: in sport, the tendency to interpret the sporting world in terms of self. Putting one's own interests or the team's interest ahead of others, often times to a non-moral end.

These two examples support the claim by Shields and Bredemeir that sport is, in part, shaped by **moral egocentrism.**[11] Moral egocentrism is a phrase that describes putting one's own interests or the team's interest ahead of others. Moral egocentrism allows for others involved in sport (i.e., opponents, officials, and even the game itself) to take a backseat as athletes, coaches, and administrators focus their attention on what is best for themselves and for their teams. The knocking out the quarterback and spitball cases are clear examples of how the interests of the opponents, officials, and the game itself took a backseat to the interests of the players and teams. As Shields points out, however, even the bracketed morality of sport will disintegrate if those involved fail to consider certain factors that help to maintain a moral balance within it.[12] Conditions of equal competition, equal opportunity, and overall fairness, along with safety, must be maintained within a sporting context if that con-

integrity (moral value): uprightness of character; being honest.

text is to keep its **integrity** in relation to athletic excellence. If the outcomes of sporting contests and tournaments are to mean something, actions that betray the integrity of the sport by jeopardizing its moral balance must be minimized, and actions that foster its morality must be emphasized.

For sport to function effectively, its integrity must be maintained. Behaviors in sport must be honest, honorable, upright, and decent. When behaviors are not honest, honorable, upright, and decent, measures must be taken to help ensure that the integrity of sport will remain. If acts that are dishonest, dishonorable, and indecent are allowed to take place within sport, sport will lose its ability to function effectively and lose its appeal for fans. Fans, players, coaches, and others affiliated with sport appreciate and expect the integrity of sport to be maintained. For example, during the 2005 season, Major League Baseball (MLB) commissioner Bud Selig suspended Texas Rangers pitcher Kenny Rogers for repeatedly shoving the camera held by a field reporter. In suspending Rogers, Selig was attempting to deter or eliminate future actions by players who might consider engaging in future similar actions. Rogers' actions were inappropriate, indecent, and unfitting, and, in Selig's view, betrayed the integrity of the game. During the 2004–2005 season, NBA commissioner David Stern also made an attempt to minimize actions that betray the integrity of professional basketball by suspending players from the Indiana Pacers and Detroit Pistons for their role in a brawl that broke out involving players and fans.[13] Stern realized the inappropriateness of players going into the stands to confront fans, and knew that he had to take action to help prevent such inappropriate acts from reoccurring, acts that could be detrimental to the game.

The National Collegiate Athletic Association (NCAA) rules enforcement body constantly attempts to minimize actions that betray the integrity of their sports by monitoring and punishing schools that commit rules infractions. For instance, to maintain conditions of equal competition among member schools, the NCAA has put in place and enforces recruiting guidelines. One such rule disallows NCAA schools from giving players money as a way to entice them to attend an NCAA school. If someone affiliated with an NCAA school provides a recruit with money, the NCAA rules enforcement body will impose punishments on the school committing the infraction. This is one attempt by the NCAA to provide all schools throughout the country with an equal opportunity to recruit players. If schools were allowed to 'buy' players, opportunities for all schools would not be equal since the richest schools would be able to recruit all of the best players.

"Mary Marginal"

Mary Marginal's father, Mr. Marginal, is the owner of the local sporting goods store. Mary Marginal is a marginal field hockey player. Mr. Budget is the athletic director. Mr. Budget is considering persuading/demanding that Mary's head coach name Mary as a starter so that the entire athletic department can receive discounted prices on all purchases at the store. Mary's coach does not know what to do since Mary is an average player and, if judged on her field hockey abilities, is not talented enough to be one of the starters.

Questions
1. As Mary's head coach, what decision would you make and does it foster morality?
2. Would naming or not naming Mary as a starter jeopardize the moral balance of the situation? Explain your answer.
3. Would naming or not naming Mary as a starter jeopardize equal competition, equal opportunity, or the integrity of the sport of field hockey?

Emphasizing Actions That Foster Morality

It is important to emphasize and reinforce actions that foster morality. Athletes, coaches, players, administrators, and even fans are in a position to not only act in a moral way, but also reinforce moral actions by others. For years, the National Hockey

League (NHL) has maintained a post-game handshake between teams. When the game ends, players line up on the ice and shake the hand of each opposing player. As part of a pre-game ceremony, Olympic athletes exchange gifts with players on the opposing team. During athletic contests, athletes, on occasion, congratulate opposing players for executing a good play.

Athletes who abide strictly by the rules of the game also foster morality. Fans often foster morality by demonstrating their genuine concern for the health of athletes. In the past, fans have shown their concern and caring for the health of an injured athlete—even if the injured athlete is on the opposing team—by applauding as the player walks or is carried off the field. Applauding, in this case, is an example of fans emphasizing morality.

> **egoistic:** self-interested; devoted to own interests and advancements.

The type of thinking required to maintain conditions of fairness, equality, and safety within sport differs greatly from that used to secure advantages within it. The **egoistic** or strategic thinking utilized in sport is primarily aimed at improving an individual's or team's odds of winning. Here the question being asked by the decision maker is: "How will this move benefit me (us)?" Kavussanu and Roberts note that when winning is at stake, the ego-oriented athlete will be tempted to chose a behavior that helps accomplish this goal, even if the behavior is not congruent with his or her moral ideals.[14] For example, a baseball player might choose to 'cork' the bat to give his team a better chance to win. Or a youth softball catcher's parent, someone normally morally responsible, might become obsessed with the desire to win and persuade his or her child to make contemptuous and mean-spirited comments to the opposing team's batters in an attempt to intimidate and gain an advantage. A lacrosse coach who, when not coaching, may be known to be moralistically pure, may behave immorally by teaching his players how to injure opposing players for the sake of winning.

Choosing Between Strategic and Moral Reasoning

An Example

The Explorers of East High School are leading their opponents, the Central High School Dragons, 2–0 late in the third period of an interscholastic hockey game. The Dragons mount an offensive charge and manage to set up their leading scorer, Randy, on a breakaway. If James, the Explorers' left defenseman, does not trip Randy, then Randy will be left one on one against the goaltender. But if James does trip Randy, James will be breaking the rules of hockey, and the Dragons will almost certainly be awarded a penalty shot. James knows his goalie has a better chance of stopping a penalty shot for which he is prepared than a shot off an unexpected breakaway. What should he do?

The Choice

How the word 'should' is interpreted here is crucial. If James reasons strategically in this case, he will take this 'should' to mean "What is the best thing I can do for my team?" This interpretation will lead him to consider the possible positive and negative

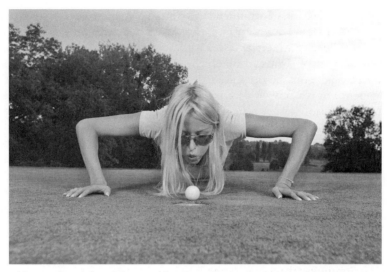

1-1 *Breaking rules violates the moral value of honesty and can hurt others.*

consequences of the trip. If he trips Randy, James knows the referee will almost definitely award the Dragons a penalty shot. This would seem to place James' team at a disadvantage. However, James also knows that if he does not trip Randy, there is an excellent chance that Randy will score, and that his goaltender's ability to stop penalty shots is strong enough to make it worth taking the penalty. There is a risk involved, but that risk is smaller than the risk of allowing James' goalie to face a breakaway shot from the opponent's best scorer. Hence, if James is reasoning strategically, he will decide that what he "should" do (i.e., what is best for his team) is trip Randy and accept the penalty and possible consequences that could result from that decision.

> **argument:** a form of reasoning; a set of statements explaining what a person believes is true and why he or she believes it is true; the content of an argument (its premises and conclusion) must be true if the argument is to be strong.

> **premises:** statements explaining why someone believes something; part of the content of an argument; if the premises of an argument do not firmly support its conclusion, the argument will be a weak one; premises make up a set of claims from which a conclusion is drawn.

> **conclusions:** statements asserting what someone believes; conclusions are only as strong as the premises upon which they are grounded.

Statements, Premises, Arguments, and Conclusions

James' reasoning can be captured in the form of an **argument.** An argument is a form of reasoning, a set of statements explaining what a person believes is true and why he or she believes it is true. Statements are sentences that are either true or false. The statements explaining why someone believes something are called **premises** (P). These clearly state the reasoning or rationale behind a certain action. Statements asserting what someone believes are **conclusions** (C). Arguments and their conclusions are only as strong as their premises. If the premises of an argument do not firmly support its conclusion, the argument will be a weak one.

"In order for an argument to be sound, it must be so with respect to its matter (its content) and to its form."[15(p60)] The content of an argument (its premises and conclusion) must be true if the argument is to be strong. Since the premises "compose the set of claims from which the conclusion is drawn," it is essential that evidence or reasons be presented that demonstrate their truth.[16(p3)] The stronger the evidence or reasons for accepting the premises, the greater the support they lend to the conclusion; that is, the greater the support for the conclusion, the stronger the argument.

We must also be aware, however, that a conclusion is "the product and result of a chain of inference."[16(p3)] Hence, the premises of a sound argument must not only be true, they must also be ordered in such a way as to clearly lead you to the conclusion. When the truth of a conclusion can be clearly inferred from its premises, the structure of the argument is strong. When an argument is well structured, and strong evidence or reasons are offered that display the truth of its premises, that argument is a sound argument.[15]

The Strategic Argument

In a strategic argument, a conclusion is firmly supported if the premises of the argument clearly explain why a particular action is advantageous to the person presenting the argument or the group they represent. Returning to the hockey example, the argument will be strategically sound if it demonstrates that tripping the Dragons' leading scorer on a breakaway is the action that is best for the Explorers under the circumstances. James' reasoning is captured in the following argument:

(P1) Tripping the opponent's leading scorer on a breakaway will result in a penalty shot.

(P2) Our goaltender has a better chance of stopping a penalty shot than a shot on a breakaway.

Therefore,

(C) I should trip the opponent's leading scorer.

While this strategic argument is probabilistically and strategically sound, it is morally questionable.

The Moral Argument

In the initial statement of the example, it was pointed out that if James trips Randy, he will be breaking the rules of hockey and, thus, will be playing unfairly and in an unsporting manner. The action is drawn further into question because if James trips Randy, he will be using an illegal tactic to negate an advantage that Randy and his Dragons teammates earned fairly against the Explorers. If James emphasizes these factors in his reasoning rather than those related only to his own team's interests, he will be using moral reasoning since he is considering the interests of others in his reasoning. The moral argument he might develop could look something like this:

(P1) If I trip Randy, I will be using an illegal tactic to take away an advantage Randy and his team earned fairly.

(P2) Using illegal tactics such as tripping is against the rules of hockey and, therefore, is unfair and unsporting.

Therefore,

(C) I should not trip Randy.

In this example of moral reasoning, the focus of the argument turns from the advantage that James can gain for his team to the moral value of fairness or **fair play** and **respect** for his opponent. Randy and his Dragons teammates earned their breakaway through their clean, hard work on the boards and well-executed passes. To use an illegal tactic (tripping) to attempt to reduce or negate a fairly earned advantage of this kind is to show disrespect for those whose efforts and skills have earned it. Furthermore, it can be argued that if a player uses illegal tactics, he or she shows disrespect toward the rules that partially constitute the sport and, thus, displays disrespect for the sport itself.

This example also emphasizes the importance of the moral value of justice or fairness. As will be discussed in Chapter 2, fairness is one of the essential values of moral sport competition. Fairness makes it possible for meaningful comparisons to be made between teams and individuals, and for the outcomes of contests to be accurate representations of the levels of excellence displayed by contestants during a particular game. Without an emphasis on fairness, sport can become a free-for-all in which players do whatever they believe is necessary to win. Hence, it is important that the value of fairness be recognized by athletes, coaches, and administrators, and utilized by them in their reasoning and decision making if sports are to be strong moral enterprises.

Clarifying the Differences Between Strategic and Moral Reasoning

James' dilemma has been helpful in providing an understanding of the differences between the strategic reasoning that is prevalent in sport and tends to dominate sporting contexts, and the moral reasoning that is often ignored or downplayed within such contexts. Strategic reasoning is egoistic in nature; it emphasizes identifying the action that will be most advantageous for a particular individual or group. Moral reasoning requires that individuals consider the good or interests of others in sport, such as opponents, officials, and fans, and emphasizes moral values such as fair play and respect in their reasoning.

Now that a clearer idea of moral reasoning has been established, different ways in which people reason morally must be discussed. To this end, we will consider three different moral theories that identify different elements as being the most important in helping individuals make moral decisions and act morally. We begin with a strategic decision-making model that many in sport seem to utilize when analyzing moral dilemmas.

STRATEGIC REASONING DECISION-MAKING MODEL

Model Stated in the Form of Directives
Step 1: Describe the moral problem in detail.
Step 2: Determine your possible options given the circumstances.
Step 3: Determine which option serves your own interests best.
Step 4: Engage in the action that best serves your own interests.

Model Presented Using Questions
Step 1: What is the moral problem with which you are faced?
Step 2: What are your possible options given the circumstances?
Step 3: Which option will best serve your own interests?
Step 4: Did you engage in the action you determined would best serve your own interests?

The strategic decision-making model above is grounded in the theories of psychological hedonism and psychological egoism. **Psychological hedonism** is "the theory that claims that all we ever desire for its own sake is pleasure and the avoidance of pain."[17(p67)] Psychological hedonists believe that it is the nature of human beings to seek out actions that will bring them pleasure or that at least will help them elude painful consequences. With this view, when persons are "faced with a choice between two courses of action, they will always choose the one they believe will provide the greater balance of pleasure over pain."[18(p26)]

> **psychological hedonism:** the theory claiming that human beings will seek out actions bringing them the most pleasure and absence of pain.

In sport, there are cases in which athletes, coaches, and administrators do not seek pleasure but do seek what is in their own best interests. Athletes, for example, may be willing to accept the negative side effects of performance-enhancing substances if they believe taking these substances will increase their status within a sport. The broader theory of psychological egoism applies in such cases. Almond defines **psychological egoism** as "the rather wider view that, while people do indeed act only in order to promote some interest of their own, this self-interest need not be a matter of physical pleasure—it could be happiness in some wider sense, or even an ideal like self-perfection."[18(p26)]

> **psychological egoism:** the view that the ultimate aim of each person is his or her own self-interest.

Almond further noted that both of these egoistic theories deny that altruistic thought and action are possible for human beings. It is this claim that separates egoistic theories from utilitarian, teleological, and deontological moral theories, all of which emphasize altruistic thinking in some manner. The strategic decision-making process below is one that could be utilized by individuals adopting an egoistic stance toward moral situations.

THE STRATEGIC DECISION-MAKING PROCESS

Step 1: Describe the moral problem in detail.

Before trying to make a decision, examine the situation in which you find yourself. Establish the facts of the situation, and make sure that you take note of factors that may affect your interests or bring you pleasure or pain.

Step 2: Determine your possible options given the circumstances.

After examining the situation, determine what courses of action are available to you. Be careful not to overlook possible options that may have positive consequences for you.

Step 3: Determine which option best serves your own interests.

Once possible actions are established, you need to reason out which of these will bring you the results you desire, whether these are the ones that will bring you the most pleasure or the ones you believe are in your own best interests. When assessing your interests, do not forget to consider long-term interests as well as short-term ones. Failure to do so may lead you to a drastically different conclusion that may not maximize pleasure, minimize pain, or serve your interests in the best way possible.

Step 4: Engage in the action that best serves your own interests.

Once you determine which action will give you what you want, engage in that action.

Moral Theories and Sport

Consequentialism

Moral theories contending that the consequences of actions are the primary element in determining the right action to take in a given situation are consequentialist ethi-

> **consequentialism:** contending that the consequences of actions are the primary element in determining the right action to take in a given situation.

cal theories. Portmore explains that **consequentialism** has persevered over the years because of its simple and seductive idea that it can never be wrong to produce the best available state of affairs.[19] In consequentialist theories, actions are judged according to how they affect oneself or others, rather than on the principles or values upon which the actions are based. Holowchak goes so far as to say that elite sport is in a "crisis state," susceptible to insidious consequences that come from the ethical judging of right and wrong not by intentions but by consequences.[20] In other words, actions in sport are often justified and perceived to be okay even if they are not grounded in moral values—as long as the consequences do not end up being immediately hurtful to others. The consequentialist perceives the means by which he or she arrives at the end to be okay as long as the outcome is perceived as positive to those involved and not hurtful to others.

Several examples exist in elite sport whereby actions are based on the consequences that will follow and not on values that drive the actions. The consequences of winning the Super Bowl Most Valuable Player (MVP) Award is winning a new car. Certainly one cannot assume that the only reason players strive to win awards are for the consequences that follow, but consequences that make one feel good are factors that have an influence on the willingness and desire to achieve. If, however, players only strive to achieve for the purpose of gaining the consequences that follow, in the form of awards, moral values may be overshadowed, de-emphasized, or even dismissed in favor of 'feel good' consequences.

Conversely, playing the game within the framework of moral values that fosters a greater good often, at least on the surface, seems to be inconsequential. What recognition does the respectful player who loses at Wimbledon truly receive? What does the fifth-place competitor who displays honesty at the X Games receive? How is the beneficent swimmer who does not make the Olympic team reinforced to continue to behave altruistically? Athletic personnel must have an innate realization of the good they are spreading by acting morally in sport contests. Elite sport reinforces winning with positive consequences as described above, making it a challenge for athletes, coaches, and administrators to ground their actions in moral values and principles instead of in consequences that are sure to follow the action.

"The Offering of a Bribe to Coach Pandemonium"

The national economy's recession is finally having a real effect on local interscholastic athletic programs. The athletic director at high school #45 has announced a 30% budget cut for the softball team. The head coach, Coach Pandemonium, upon hearing the news has been in a constant state of panic. With a 30% budget cut, Coach Pandemonium has calculated that at least two away games will have to be eliminated, umpires will not be able to be paid for at least five games, necessary equipment will not be purchased, and the end-of-the-year banquet will have to be cancelled. Melissa Mundane's father sees this as an opportunity to get his daughter, who has always wanted to be on the softball team but was and is not good enough, a spot on the team. Mr. Mundane approaches Coach Pandemonium and offers to provide the coach/program with the entire 30% of the money that was recently cut from the budget. Mr. Mundane explicitly states that he will only give the program the money if his daughter Melissa is guaranteed a spot on the roster. Coach Pandemonium is caught off guard with the request and states that he needs 24 hours before responding.

Questions
1. Make some true statements that are descriptive of the essential elements in this dilemma.
2. Based on the statements, can you establish a premise on which a moral argument might be based?

"The Offering of a Bribe to Coach Pandemonium" (*Continued*)

3. On what premise(s) (what is your rationale?) would you base your decision to accept or not accept the money from Mr. Mundane?
4. What argument could you make for accepting the money or not accepting the money from Mr. Mundane?
5. What conclusions can be drawn from your moral argument?

Hedonism

A variety of consequentialist ethical theories have been developed over time. These

hedonism: the doctrine that pleasure is the most important pursuit in life.

happiness: as described by John Stuart Mill, the intended pleasure and the absence of pain.

include different types of **hedonism,** a theory holding that you should do whatever brings you the greatest amount of **happiness.** The problem with such a theory is that it is essentially based on strategic reasoning. It requires that people attempt to figure out what will make them happiest, but does not require them to weigh the interests of others in their reasoning.

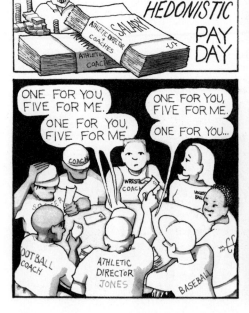

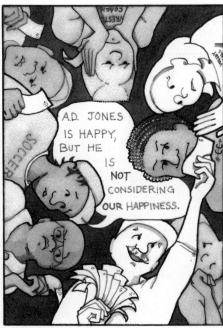

When decisions are made based on what can bring oneself the greatest amount of happiness, oftentimes that happiness is not shared by others. Take for example the talented starting pitcher who has made a commitment to play for his local high school team, then in mid-season decides to take advantage of an offer to pitch for the local powerhouse team across town. In doing so, the pitcher makes himself happy but is not considering the happiness of his current coaches, teammates, or fans. The coaches are unhappy because they had developed team strategies under the assumption that this pitcher was going to uphold his commitment to play the entire season. Teammates are unhappy because the anticipated successful season now seems unlikely. Fans were also looking forward to a successful season, and some had even purchased season tickets based on the 'ace' pitcher's season-long commitment.

Utilitarianism

Utilitarianism, a universal form of hedonism, was developed by philosopher John Stuart Mill and his predecessor, Jeremy Bentham. This consequentialist theory states that when you are faced with a moral decision, you should choose the act that will bring the greatest amount of happiness to the greatest number of people. In *Utilitarianism,* Mill discusses his **greatest happiness principle.**[21] Mill stated, "The creed which accepts as the foundation of morals 'utility' or the 'greatest happiness principle' holds that actions are right in proportion as they tend to promote happiness; wrong as they tend to procedure the reverse of happiness."[21(p36)]

> **greatest happiness principle:** actions are right based on their creation and promotion of the greatest amount of happiness.

In describing Mill's greatest happiness principle, Burton stated: "That is useful which, taking all times and all persons into consideration, leaves a balance of

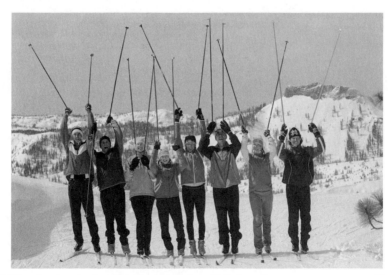

1-2 *Utilitarianism is choosing the act that will bring the greatest amount of happiness to the greatest number of people.*

happiness; and the creation of the largest possible balance of happiness became Jeremy Bentham's description of the right end of human actions."[22(pp17-18)] In sport organizations, it becomes nearly impossible to make decisions that will make everyone happy. Bentham's greatest happiness principle might serve as a guide to assist in making decisions. As the Executive Director of the NCAA, Miles Brand must sometimes make decisions that will have an effect on hundreds of NCAA member institutions. If Dr. Brand uses Mill's greatest happiness principle as a guide in making decisions, the majority of schools affected by his decisions should end up happy, or at least with a certain level of satisfaction. In maintaining this balance of happiness among NCAA member institutions, the NCAA stands a better chance of functioning effectively as an organization.

Utilitarianism does emphasize the good of others instead of the good of the individual decision maker. As Mill explains in *Utilitarianism*:

> "The utilitarian standard is not the agent's own greatest happiness, but the greatest amount of happiness together . . . there can be no doubt that it makes other people happier, and that the world in general is immensely a gainer by it."[23 (p173)]

In today's sports world, the person who makes decisions takes on the role of the agent of whom Mill speaks. The agent or decision maker might be the athlete, the coach, or the sport manager. An athletic director who allocates a disproportionately large sum of money to her favorite sport of ice hockey might make herself and persons affiliated with the hockey program happy, but make unhappy all of the other sports personnel in the athletic department. In making such a decision, the agent (i.e., athletic director) weighed only her own interests in her pursuit of her own greatest happiness and did not consider what it would take to make others in the department happy. The athletic department most likely did not gain immensely by the athletic director's action. Although the hockey program did happen to gain happiness, this happiness was not necessarily intended by the athletic director, but instead a by-product of her attempt to gain individual happiness. In other words, the athletic director took only her own interests into consideration and the hockey program happened to be a beneficiary of her interests.

One might point out here that utilitarianism frames 'the good' in terms of happiness or pleasure, and it is questionable whether this is the best way to conceptualize goodness. Mill cautioned that utilitarianism is not meant to be interpreted as referring everything to pleasure or as mere pleasures of the moment.[23] With this caveat in mind, Mill's claim does seem to fit well in the reasoning of North American society, including sport. In North America, people often think of 'the good' in terms of what brings happiness to themselves and others. But sometimes, in sport and in society, it is difficult to view goodness in this way.

Returning to the interscholastic hockey example presented earlier in the chapter, it would be ridiculous for James to trip Randy for the purpose of making a larger number of people happy, since East High School has more fans than Central High School does, or because East has a greater student population. An East win would make the school's supporters happy and the trip would increase the likelihood of an

Explorers victory, but this reasoning is not grounded in strong moral reasoning. It is somewhat strategic in nature, but its primary weakness is that it simply does not make sense to determine right and wrong in this manner since it involves breaking a rule and could cause harm. It is not ethically acceptable for the most popular teams or the least popular teams to break rules, and it certainly is not fair or sportsmanlike. Hence, to strengthen the consequentialist viewpoint, we will need to consider other ways to conceptualize 'the good.'

Best Interests of All

One possible alternative to framing good solely in terms of happiness and pleasure is to define good in terms of **best interests;** that is, define it as what will be best for the individuals affected by a moral decision. When a coach sets up a practice for his players, he does so with not just the idea of the coach knows his players will have to work hard and be disciplined r conditioning, skills, and performance. Even with creative, challeng- n emphasis on fun, the coach knows his players will not enjoy every- of them in practice. Some things like running wind sprints, weight her conditioning and performance drills are not fun for many athletes. e primary objective for players is to play up to their potential in each may know that such drills and sacrifice are necessary and, thus, in the erests. Normally, both coaches and players desire to make sacrifices to ighest level possible.

Tennis greats Venus and Serena Williams have undergone these types of best-interest sacrifices. Both sisters experienced challenging tennis workouts that their father coached them through during their youth. The girls' father understood that even though at times his daughters did not enjoy every moment of their childhood workouts, the rigorous workouts, ultimately, would be in their long-term best interests. In the end, the training seems to have served the Williams sisters well, in that both have won several major championships and earned substantial amounts of prize and endorsement money.

Although the above examples are not moral ones, they may be helpful in providing a better understanding as to how the term 'good' may be framed relative to the best interests of those participating in a sport setting. Returning to the hockey example, certainly the Explorers might be happier with a win, but is it in either team's best interest if James tries to improve his team's chances of winning by violating the rules of hockey and tripping Randy? Does he want to be viewed as someone who would do anything for a win? Do his teammates and coach want to be perceived in this way? James knows his coach and teammates spent time before and during the season discussing sportsmanship and its importance to the team. Does James now wish to win at the expense of sportsmanship? Is it in the best interest of players from either team to use illegal tactics in seeking an advantage for his team?

"Skipping Weight Training to Study for the Big Test"

Donald Diamond has a major biology test scheduled for 8:00 a.m. tomorrow morning. As a starter on his high school baseball team, Donald has worked hard to excel on the field and in the classroom. Although able to achieve his athletic goals with relative ease, Donald has had to work hard, on a daily basis, to remain in good academic standing. Today is no different. Baseball practice is scheduled from 6:00 to 8:00 p.m., followed by a two-hour weight and individual training session. Aware of the lack of time available to study for his major biology test the next morning at 8:00 a.m., Donald has decided to ask his coach to be excused from the two-hour training session so that he can study for his test.

Questions
1. As Donald's coach, how would you consider the best interests of all in deciding whether or not to excuse Donald from the training session?
2. Describe some of your past habits of action linked with moral excellence that will help you make this decision.

It does not appear to be in the best interests of the team, the opponent, and the sport to engage in the illegal act of tripping. To do so would be to act in an unsporting manner; it would be unfair to the Dragons, disrespectful to them and to the sport of hockey, and would call into question the moral integrity of the Explorers. By playing fairly and not using illegal tactics, James would be protecting the Explorers' integrity by acting in a sporting manner toward his opponent and respecting the rules of hockey. Thus, when the utilitarian maxim "do the act that brings the greatest amount of good to the greatest number of people" is framed in terms of the best interests of the people involved in the sport and of the sport itself, a stronger version of consequentialist moral theory is established that can be used effectively within sport settings. Below is a brief description of the consequentialist decision-making model.

CONSEQUENTIALIST DECISION-MAKING MODEL

Model Stated in the Form of Directives
Step 1: Describe the moral problem in detail.
Step 2: Determine your possible options given the circumstances.
Step 3: Determine who will be affected by each option, and how they will be affected.
Step 4: Determine which option will bring the greatest amount of good to the greatest number of people.
Step 5: Engage in the action that brings the greatest good to the greatest number of people.

Model Presented Using Questions
Step 1: What is the moral problem with which you are faced?
Step 2: What are your possible options given the circumstances?
Step 3: Who will be affected by each option? How will they be affected?
Step 4: Which option will bring the greatest amount of good to the greatest number of people?
Step 5: Did you engage in the action you determined would bring the greatest good to the greatest number of people?

In his work *Ethics and Morality in Sport and Physical Education: An Experiential Approach*, Earle Zeigler presents a "test of consequences," designed to determine the "total effects" of actions in a given situation, in his "triple play approach" to ethical decision making.[24(p50)] In describing the logical basis of this test, Zeigler uses the following sequence of moral reasoning:

1. The act that—on the basis of the best evidence available at the time of acting—produces the greatest good is right.
2. This act will produce the greatest total good.
3. Therefore, this act is right.[24(p51)]

Although Zeigler presents a logical basis for consequentialist decision making, he does not explicitly describe how to reason through moral dilemmas using consequences. To this end, consequentialist decision-making models are offered to help guide you in working through the real-life moral problems faced by athletes, coaches, and administrators. The model is grounded in the utilitarian consequentialist view. Recall that the act that produces the greatest good for the greatest number should be understood as the act that brings about the best interests for the most people, and is a cornerstone of the utilitarianism consequentialist view. Below is a brief description of the consequentialist decision-making process.

THE CONSEQUENTIALIST DECISION-MAKING PROCESS

Step 1: Describe the moral problem in detail.
Before attempting to make a decision, the decision maker needs to understand the moral scenario he or she is facing. Establish the facts of the case, making note of who is involved and of factors that may need to be accounted for in the moral decision-making process. For example, you should note what actions people took and how those actions affected other parties in the scenario.
Step 2: Determine your possible options given the circumstances.
After laying out the moral problem, map out the different possible actions related to a given situation. Be careful to examine the scenario thoroughly so as not to leave out potential options. These may be precisely the ones that will bring the most moral good given the situation.

Step 3: Determine who will be affected by each option, and how they will be affected. For each option, the decision maker needs to figure out which individuals or groups will be affected by the decision, and whether, and to what degree, they will be affected positively or negatively. For this step, it is important to make sure and establish the sphere of influence of each option. The decision maker needs to make sure not to ignore or forget people who will be affected by a decision in ways difficult to anticipate, and to take the long-term consequences of actions into account as well as the short-term consequences.

Step 4: Determine which option will bring the greatest amount of good to the greatest number of people.

Examine all the options and their possible effects. Which option will be in the best moral interests of the most people under the circumstances? Which one will help the most people or harm the fewest, given the situation? This is the option that you should act on according to consequentialism.

Step 5: Engage in the action that brings the greatest good to the greatest number of people.

Once it is determined which action will be in the best moral interest of the most people, engage in that action.

Teleological Moral Theory

What are the moral values that a good person should possess? What are the values that a good sports person should cultivate and display? These are questions that a teleological moral theorist would ask. *Telos* is an ancient Greek word meaning 'purpose.' Teleological ethical theorists require that you consider your purpose as a human being. By defining one's purpose, an understanding about what it is to be a good human being and determining the moral values that make up a morally good person can result. According to the classical Greek philosopher Aristotle in Book I, Chapter 8 of *Nicomachean Ethics*, happiness is "the best, noblest, and most pleasant thing."[25(p373)] In

> **virtues:** values; good qualities; characteristics, attitudes, and habits of action that help people do good things.

Book I, Chapter 3 of *Eudemian Ethics*, Aristotle presented the discussions of **virtues** that lead to happiness and stated that "happiness is there for those who cultivate a certain character in themselves and their actions."[26(p481)] Cultivating a certain character can be done by instilling and cultivating moral values in yourself and in others.

When applying teleology to sport, the questions that need to be asked center around the makings of good sport behavior. Certainly, a teleologist will ask what values will exude good sport behavior, but for this assessment to be meaningful and of practical use we must first understand the nature and purpose of sport. Once these questions are answered, it will be possible to develop a clear profile of the good sports person. Until then, however, such a profile risks inaccuracy. A thorough examination of sport's nature and purpose will be offered in Chapter 2. For now, we can accept Dixon's claim that "a central purpose of competitive sport is to provide a comparison . . . that *determines* which team or player is superior."[27(p10)]

Moral and Social Values

It is equally important to have a clear understanding of values and of the different types of values that make up the good sports person. Values or virtues (henceforth referred to as values) are characteristics, attitudes, and habits of action that help people do good things. For further understanding, it is necessary to distinguish between two types of values: moral values and **social values.** Moral values are those that are essential in the development of strong teleological moral reasoning. These are values such as justice or fairness, honesty, compassion, beneficence, and respect. These values can be distinguished from social values such as **teamwork, discipline, diligence,** and **leadership.** While the latter set can be important positive values in human life, they cannot morally stand on their own. For instance, the Nazi Third Reich and Al Qaeda terrorist organization are groups that demonstrated hard work, discipline, and teamwork and had strong leadership, but they used these values in the murder of innocent people in World War II and in the World Trade Center and Pentagon attacks of September 11, 2001, respectively.

social values: values such as teamwork, discipline, diligence, and leadership; the cultivation of social values alone is not enough to guarantee the fostering of moral reasoning or action.

teamwork (social value): working together; cooperation among members of a group.

discipline (social value): a systematic self-control directed toward accomplishment.

diligence (social value): hard working; industriousness.

leadership (social value): being able to guide; to persuade; having traits that make others want to follow you.

welfare: the best interests or well-being of a group or individual.

The cultivation of such social values alone is not enough to guarantee the fostering of moral reasoning or action. Social values must be grounded in moral values, which, when cultivated, influence individuals to consider the good, health, and **welfare** of others in their decisions. In sport, the social values of teamwork, discipline, diligence, and leadership can also be practiced to a non-moral end. The 1919 Black Sox gambling scandal serves as an historic sport example. It was discovered in 1920 that eight members of the American League champion Chicago White Sox had conspired with gamblers to fix the 1919 World Series.[28] The social value of leadership was demonstrated when some team members convinced others to participate in the 'fix.' Teamwork was evident as several of the White Sox worked collectively as a team to carry out the fix. Although you may not consider the fix as hard work, there was work involved to make sure it took place in a way that was not obvious to those who were not involved. And given that a plan had been devised to carry out the fix, the involved players had to practice discipline to effectively execute the plan.

Even though the 1919 White Sox practiced several social values, moral values were not evident, which, as mentioned previously, foster health, good, and the welfare of others. Players from the opposing Cincinnati Reds team would not be able to truly appreciate winning a game that was fixed and hence would not reach the level of happiness they deserve when winning a championship game. The White Sox players who were not involved in the fix experienced significant disappointment and unhappiness, and felt betrayed by their teammates who had chosen to corrupt the game and the sport as well. This example shows how the practice of social values alone does not necessarily lead to the good that will come from the practice of moral values.

Obviously, moral values are necessary for the development of the good sports person, but are some moral values more necessary than others? Since sport's primary purpose is a test of skills between two or more opponents, fairness is clearly one of these necessary values. If opponents unfairly seek an advantage, they change the contest for themselves and the others involved. This lessens the validity of the sport as a test of skills.

Off the field, fairness or justice also play an important role in moral reasoning. Similar to athletes on the field who test their playing skills against one another, coaches test their recruiting skills against one another when trying to persuade players to attend their school and play for their team. If recruiting rules are followed, the recruiting skills of the coaches are tested against each other and the coaches who successfully acquire the best players win the recruiting game. If, however, the recruiting rules are not followed, as is the case with the provision of cash to a player, the successful recruiting of a player is not the result of the coach's recruiting skills but simply the result of giving the player money. Unless all the other coaches are also 'buying' players, the coach's recruiting skills are not being tested.

Compassion and respect also play an important role in moral reasoning in sport. Compassion is suffering with another and the ability to empathetically put yourself into another's shoes and understand another's position, ideas, and problems. With compassion for others you are able to better understand the injustices or moral problems other people are facing. Compassion can help you see, for example, how discriminatory hiring practices hurt potential minority and female coaches and administrators. This is an example of compassion because when a person has cultivated and developed the moral value of compassion, he or she is better able to recognize when others are being harmed. A compassionate person is also one who sees how cheating hurts and feels badly for those whom illegal tactics are used against. An athletic director might base his or her actions on the value of compassion. A wrestler, after defeating an opponent, may console the losing athlete because in the past the winning wrestler experienced losing and the hurtful feelings that came with it.

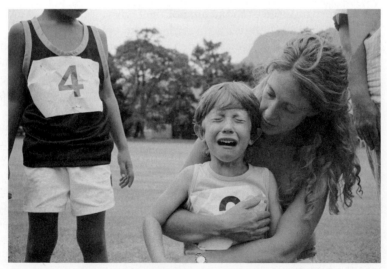

1-3 *Compassion is suffering with and being merciful toward another.*

Respect is recognizing others in sport as fellow human beings who deserve to be treated as such. Respectful treatment includes treating opponents, officials, fans, and others in sport as people, not as things, obstacles, or enemies. Whether others treat you well or not, it is necessary to recognize the humanity of these individuals and to treat them with the respect they are due as human beings. Respect is shown when a player congratulates his or her opponent for executing an outstanding play. Respect is *not* shown by taunting your opponent after making a great play against them. Humiliating an opponent is an example of disrespect.

Practicing Moral Values

Teleological ethical theory calls on individuals to cultivate values such as justice or fairness, honesty, compassion, beneficence, and respect in their lives, and to utilize these as guides to right conduct and action. In sport, teleologists will look to athletes, coaches, administrators, officials, and fans to consider their purposes within the sport setting and the purpose of sport itself in determining which values should influence their actions. In athletics, participants frequently must decide in a split second how to act. If you have thought about the right values for certain situations, you are more likely to act well in that situation. As Aristotle noted in Book II, Chapter 1, of *Nicomachean Ethics*, "Moral excellence comes about as a result of habit."[25(p376)] This is one of the strengths of teleological moral theories. When individuals prepare themselves by learning and practicing moral values, they may cultivate habits of action that help them to display strong moral character when they are called upon to do so.

"A Once-In-A-Lifetime Chance for Coach Longevity"

For the first time since the opening of the high school 36 years ago, the head football coach, Coach Longevity, might have the opportunity to take his team to the state tournament. No one can match Coach Longevity's long-standing dedication, hard work, and sacrifices he has made over the years for the betterment of the football program and the high school. Now 72 years old, Coach Longevity is planning to retire after this season. Finishing his career by competing in the state tournament would put an exclamation point on an already outstanding career. To get into the tournament, Coach Longevity has determined that he must not only win Friday's game, but win it by 63 points. Shrugging off his calculations, the coach comments to one of his assistants, "Against this team, I will be happy to win by just one point." As the game progressed, however, it became apparent that Coach Longevity's team was up for the challenge as they were dominating the game by a score of 44–0 going into the fourth quarter. Completely caught off guard by his starting team's annihilating performance through three quarters, Coach Longevity was torn between taking out his starters as an act of kindness to the opposition, or keeping them in for the purpose of running up the score to 63 points and getting into the playoffs.

"A Once-In-A-Lifetime Chance for Coach Longevity" (*Continued*)

Questions

1. Identify some social values in this case.
2. Identify some moral values in this case.
3. If you were Coach Longevity, using the teleological theory, how would you use moral values to decide whether or not to keep your starters in the game?
4. What role would anticipated consequences play in making your decision?

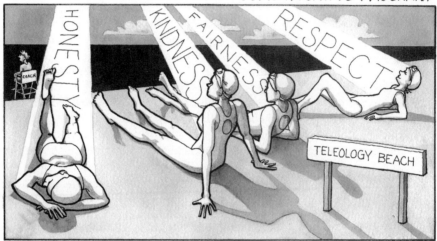

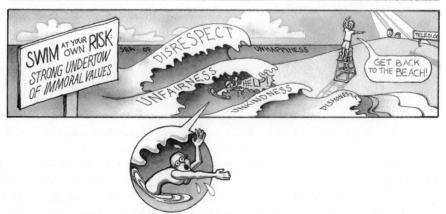

For example, if throughout a person's life, his parents, teachers, and coaches consistently instilled the moral value of honesty in him, the likelihood of that person practicing honesty in a sport situation is probable. In fact, the moral value of honesty might even become reflexive. In other words, honesty becomes a habit of action. A person who has been consistently exposed to situations calling for honesty often times does not need time to ponder or reason; he or she can simply react honestly when the situation calls for the moral value of honesty to be applied. In the example in the first sentence of this paragraph, years of mentoring by his parents, teachers, and coaches have provided that individual with the ability to expeditiously recognize when it is appropriate to apply the moral value of honesty.

The process required to arrive at good moral decisions must be practiced by the decision maker until it becomes second nature. After repeatedly applying an approach grounded in moral values to various moral dilemmas, the decision maker, with practiced decision-making experience, will be able to efficiently and quickly determine actions to be used relative to moral dilemmas. Guided by sound moral theory, practice is reinforced through the repetition of steps necessary to arrive at good moral decisions. At this point the teleological decision-making model will be introduced. It is a step-by-step guide to reaching decisions to moral dilemmas. Habits of good action can be established after repeatedly applying the teleological decision-making model to moral dilemmas.

TELEOLOGICAL DECISION-MAKING MODEL

Model Stated in the Form of Directives
Step 1: Describe the moral problem in detail.
Step 2: Determine the moral values that an individual in your capacity (as athlete, coach, sport manager, etc.) should possess.
Step 3: Determine how a person who has these moral values would act given the circumstances.
Step 4: Engage in the action that the morally good person in your capacity would engage in.

Model Presented Using Questions
Step 1: What is the moral problem with which you are faced?
Step 2: What moral values should a person in your capacity (as athlete, coach, sport manager, etc.) possess?
Step 3: How would a person who has these moral values act given the circumstances?
Step 4: Did you engage in the act in which the morally good person in your capacity would choose to engage?

---

teleological moral theory: driven by moral values such as justice or fairness, honesty, compassion, beneficence, and respect; rooted in the work of Aristotle; requires that you consider your purpose as a human being by determining the moral values that make up a morally good person.

As mentioned previously, **teleological moral theory** has its roots in the work of Aristotle (384–322 B.C.). In his *Nicomachean Ethics*, Aristotle contended that happiness is the ultimate good for human beings, and that "happiness is an activity of the soul in accordance with perfect virtue."[29(p950)] Moral values for Aristotle are habits of action developed through practice. It is through the cultivation of such virtues, then, that human beings attain happiness, their highest good, or *telos*.

In the 20th century, virtue theorist Alasdair MacIntyre developed a version of teleological moral theory based on the claim that virtuous activity is determined in relation to social practices.[30] From this theory, as indicated by Morgan, it may be implied that moral and immoral action within a sport is to some extent determined by the sport's purpose as a test of particular skills.[31] This being so, it is important that sport community members determine the values they need to cultivate as athletes, coaches, and sport managers for the good of their sport. Put another way, it is important that sport community members establish what values the morally good athlete, coach, or sport manager should possess so they can better determine how to act morally within their sport. The teleological decision-making process below represents how sport community members might use moral values to reason out the various moral dilemmas they encounter.

THE TELEOLOGICAL DECISION-MAKING PROCESS

Step 1: Describe the moral problem in detail.

In preparing to make a moral decision, you should take the time to carefully examine the situation with which you are faced. Be sure to establish your role in the scenario—to establish whether you are an athlete, coach, sport manager, etc.—and to note any moral values that seem important to the situation.

Step 2: Determine the moral values that an individual in your capacity (as athlete, coach, sport manager, etc.) should possess.

Think about your role. What moral values do you need to have to be a morally good athlete, coach, sport manager, etc.? Be thorough in your development of this profile of values; make sure you understand each value and why it is an important one for a person in your position to possess.

Step 3: Determine how a person who has these moral values would act given the circumstances.

Ask yourself how the morally good athlete, coach, or sport manager would act in the situation that you are facing. To help determine this, you will need to figure out which values are relevant in your particular case, and prioritize these according to their importance within the scenario. Sometimes fairness will be the most significant value in a situation; other times, respect, honesty, or compassion will have greater importance. Take care in prioritizing your values so that you make the right decision for the situation.

Step 4: Engage in the action in which the morally good person in your capacity would engage.

Once you have prioritized your values and determined what the morally good athlete, coach, sport manager, etc., would do if they were in your shoes, engage in the act that is recommended by your prioritized values.

Deontological Moral Theory

moral principles: statements prescribing or proscribing particular types of action.

Moral principles are statements prescribing or proscribing particular types of action. The most famous version of **deontological moral**

> **deontological moral theory:** a form of ethics that believes actions that are considered "good for me are good for all"; determines what is right by considering whether an action would be generally accepted if applied to all people; the Golden Rule is representative of deontological moral theory.

> **categorical imperatives:** universalizable principles that are good and under which one would want anyone to act.

theory was the one put forth by the 18th century philosopher Immanuel Kant, who stated in one version of his **categorical imperative** that you should, "Act only on the principle of which, then and there, you would be willing to make general law."[32(p182)] According to Kant, we should only act upon moral principles that we would want universalized. The Golden Rule—doing unto others as you would have them do unto you—is reflective of Kant's discussion related to acting only on principles that are good for not only you but also others and that you are willing to make general law. Universalizable principles, such as the kind called for by the categorical imperative, push decision makers to look beyond the consequences they want in a given situation. Following such principles will, according to Kant, lead you to act morally.[32]

The deontologically-based decision-making model described below is primarily grounded in the work of Immanuel Kant (1724–1804).[33] Kant believed that all actions of moral value are done out of duty, and that actions from duty derive their moral value from the principles upon which they are based. In his words, "an action from duty has its moral worth *not in the purpose* to be attained by it but in the maxim in accordance with which it is decided upon."[33(p13)] Kant argued that the only principles that were worthy of being acted upon were those that met the criterion of universalizability he established in his first formulation of the categorical imperative. In this formulation, he states that "I ought never to act except in such a way that I could also will that my maxim should become a universal law."[33(p15)]

> **hypothetical imperative:** principles calling for the action that leads to achievement of a desired state, consequence, or desire.

Principles meeting the criterion of universalizability are different from those stated as **hypothetical imperatives.** Kant defined hypothetical imperatives as principles that "represent the practical necessity of a possible action as a means to achieving something else that one wills."[33(p25)] A person seeking happiness or some other particular consequence (e.g., winning) will follow hypothetical imperatives that recommend what he or she should do to achieve the desired state. For example, some elite athletes believe that "If I am to win, I must take steroids." This conditional statement is a hypothetical imperative stating what the athlete must do to achieve victory.

Principles formulated as categorical imperatives, on the other hand, are principles upon which one would want anyone to act. Categorical imperatives are universalizable principles that recommend actions that are good in and of themselves. In contrast, according to Kant, hypothetical imperatives are principles that bring about actions that fulfill a specific desire or bring about certain consequences.[33]

Sport is a realm in which moral agents consistently act on Kant's hypothetical imperatives. According to Kant, when considering a hypothetical imperative, one never knows beforehand what it will contain until its condition is given.[32] In other words, it is the wants and desires of individuals that determine the content of hypothetical imperatives. When utilizing hypothetical imperatives, people figure out the consequences they want and act in a way they believe will give them their desired results. This type of reasoning is a form of strategic reasoning and does not produce sound moral reasoning.

For example, a high school athlete who wants to remain academically eligible but believes he lacks the skills to pass math might reason, "If I want to remain eligible, I must cheat on my math exams." This conditional statement telling us the state of affairs the athlete desires (maintaining eligibility) and the act in which he believes he must engage to achieve it (cheat on his math exams) is a hypothetical imperative.

The consequence of winning is one of the most common desires of persons affiliated with sport. Athletes, coaches, and sport managers act in ways to achieve victory. If they are guided exclusively by their desires to win, moral reasoning most likely will not be a part of the process involved in winning. Conversely, deontological moral theories are theories holding that it is the moral principles that you act upon that determine whether an action is morally right or wrong. Many people who consider themselves good moral individuals will tell you that it is important to 'stand on principle' to do what is right.

The firing of Bob Knight as the head men's basketball coach at Indiana University was controversial, to say the least. The legendary and all-time winningest coach of men's Division I basketball was fired in 2000 from Indiana University (IU) for a series of verbally and physically abusive incidents that involved not just players, but IU administrators and staff members as well. At the time of his firing, Knight had a 661–240 record, had won three NCAA championships, 11 Big Ten titles, and coached the 1984 men's U.S. Olympic team to a gold medal.[34] Knight began his college coaching career at the United States Military Academy at West Point in 1963, coached at Indiana University from 1971 to 2000, and then at Texas Tech beginning in 2001 before resigning in February of 2008 as the winningest coach in the history of basketball with 902 wins.

Knight's firing from Indiana University can be examined to determine whether or not deontological theory was a basis for the decision. Making the controversial decision to fire Knight were the president and Board of Trustees of Indiana University. The decision to fire the coach was grounded in the deontological theory if, and only if, those deciding to conduct the firing were willing to apply the same punishment to other coaches and themselves if the conditions were the same or nearly the same. If the decision makers, at the moment of Coach Knight's firing, were willing to make general law the principles under which they fired Coach Knight, then the decision has the makings of deontology and characteristics of Kant's categorical imperative.

When acting under the guidance of the categorical imperative to resolve moral dilemmas, the decision maker will base his or her decision on not only what is good for him or her but also what is good for others. If the decision maker is unwilling to universalize, or apply the decision to all persons, including self, then he or she should not make that decision. Under the categorical imperative of deontology the decision must be applicable in a satisfactory way across the populations that the decision may affect.

Conflicting Values and Principles

One problem deontologists face, however, is that even universalizable principles can conflict in certain situations. In such cases, we need to have some method of weighing out which of the conflicting principles to follow. To use a standard example,

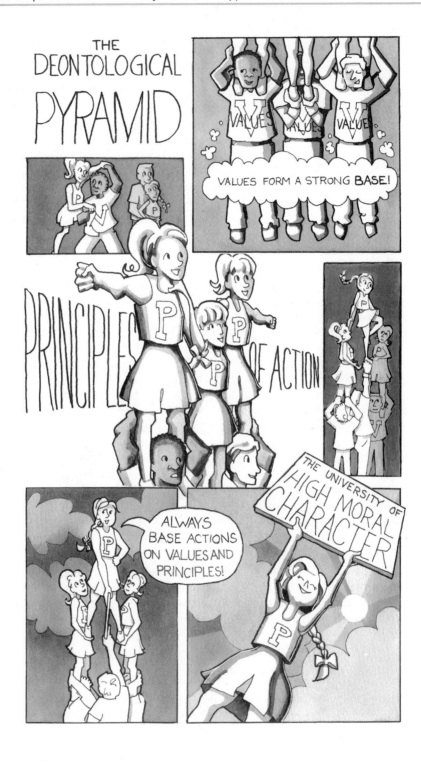

imagine yourself a German citizen during World War II. As a kind person who is opposed to torture and the murder of innocents, you have allowed a Jewish family to hide in your basement. German soldiers come to your door one night and ask whether you are harboring Jews in your house. You have always lived by the principle "Never tell a lie," but the truth will likely see you imprisoned and the Jewish family killed. You have also lived by the principle "Never harm a fellow human being," and choose to act upon this principle rather than the other in this case, since you believe the moral value of the lives on the line is greater than that attained through telling the truth.

Sometimes principles will conflict. In other words, to follow one principle, sometimes another may not be able to be followed. In sport, you will find that it is important to refer to the nature and purpose of sport when attempting to work out moral dilemmas in which principles conflict. After understanding the nature and purpose of sport, being able to effectively select between conflicting principles when confronted with a decision within the context of sport will become clearer. Recognize that moral principles are frequently developed from moral values. For example, Lumpkin, Beller, and Stoll's statement that "I should not cheat, lie or steal" is a principle that can be developed from a proper understanding of the importance of the moral value of honesty.[35] If you value honesty, you should not attempt to deceive opponents, officials, and fans by cheating; you should not lie to coaches when asked if you are taking steroids; and you should not steal from your team or school.

In the case of hiring a Division I head football coach, the values of fairness and responsibility may clash. There were only five African-American Division I-A football coaches during the 2006 season.[36] Although it may not appear to be fair to a qualified non-minority candidate to hire an equally qualified minority applicant for a Division I head football coaching position, it may be more responsible—responsible in the sense that, historically, minorities have not had equal educational and networking opportunities—to offer a qualified minority candidate the opportunity to learn the skills of and obtain employment as a Division I head football coach. In essence, the equally qualified minority candidate might be hired for the sake of equity. Thus, according to Lumpkin, Beller, and Stoll, deontological ethical theories can help you take the values you believe are important for moral action and develop them into guidelines or principles for action.[35] Of these principles, those that are universalizable are the strongest guidelines to moral reasoning and moral action. These may conflict at times, but, all things being equal, they will, if followed, help you to act morally well.

To effectively implement an approach to decision making based on the conversion of moral values into universalized principles, a systematic guide is useful. The deontologically-based decision-making model below serves as that guide. It outlines a step-by-step process to arrive at good moral decisions to moral problems. The deontologically-based decision-making model is based on acting only on values-based principles that can be universalized to all persons and circumstances.

DEONTOLOGICALLY BASED DECISION-MAKING MODEL

Model Stated in the Form of Directives

Step 1: Describe the moral problem in detail.

Step 2: Determine your options given the circumstances.

Step 3: Develop a general moral principle based upon each option.

Step 4: Determine which principles are universalizable.

Step 5: If only one principle is universalizable, go to Step 6.

If more than one principle is universalizable, prioritize the universalizable principles according to their moral importance given the circumstances.

Step 6: Act on the universalizable principle recommended by your moral reasoning.

Model Presented Using Questions

Step 1: What is the moral problem with which you are faced?

Step 2: What are your possible options given the circumstances?

Step 3: What general moral principle can be developed in relation to each option?

Step 4: Which of these general moral principles are universalizable?

Step 5: Is only one principle universalizable? If so, go to Step 6.

If more than one principle is universalizable, which one has greater moral significance given the circumstances?

Step 6: Did you act upon the principle recommended by your moral reasoning?

THE DEONTOLOGICALLY BASED DECISION-MAKING PROCESS

Step 1: Describe the moral problem in detail.

Before attempting to make a moral decision, survey the moral situation with which you are presented. Be sure to take note of factors that may assist you in developing moral principles in Step 3, such as the moral values emphasized in the situation.

Step 2: Determine your possible options given the circumstances.

After examining the moral problem, establish the courses of action that are available to you. Make sure you account for all your possible options given the conditions under which the decision must be made.

Step 3: Develop a general moral principle based upon each option.

Consider each possible action you might choose, and develop a general moral principle in relation to that action (e.g., "I should always tell the truth" or "I should never harm others").

Step 4: Determine which principles are universalizable.

Examine each principle and ask whether it is one upon which you would morally want everyone to act. One question that could help you in answering this question is if the action is one you would want done to you. If not, then, logically, it will not be one you want universalized.

Step 5: If only one principle is universalizable, go to Step 6.
If more than one principle is universalizable, prioritize the universalizable principles according to their moral importance given the circumstances.

If only one principle is universalizable, then you should act upon it. There are situations, however, in which more than one principle may be universalizable or universalizable principles may conflict. In such cases, determine which principle carries the most moral weight given the situation. For example, if your friends on your baseball team are physically and psychologically abusing new team members, the principle "Do not allow harm to others" will take precedent over the principle "Always be loyal to friends."

Step 6: Act on the universalizable principle recommended by your moral reasoning. Once you have established which moral principle is universalizable, or which of a set of universalizable principles has the greatest moral significance, act on that principle.

Conclusion

The importance of moral reasoning in sport is frequently underrated by the athletes, coaches, and administrators who make up sporting communities. It is often dismissed in favor of the strategic concerns of teams and individuals, and seldom is prioritized within sporting contests in which winning is strongly emphasized. This chapter has demonstrated the essential role that moral reasoning plays in sport, and the difference between the strategic reasoning individuals use in determining how to gain advantage, and the moral reasoning that stresses fair play, honesty, and sportsmanship—values often left behind in the pursuit of victory. In examining consequentialist, teleological, and deontological moral theories, three methods have been identified that athletes, coaches, and administrators can apply to ethical dilemmas to reason out the morally right action in particular instances. By recognizing the importance of moral reasoning and learning how to work out what is morally right in given situations, individuals take the first steps toward improving the moral conditions within sport and the sport experiences of its participants, officials, and fans.

References

1. Frankena WK. *Ethics.* 2nd ed. Englewood Cliffs, NJ: Prentice-Hall; 1973.
2. Loland S. *Fair Play In Sport.* London: Routledge; 2002.
3. Shields DLL, Bredemeier BJL. *Character Development and Physical Activity.* Champaign, IL: Human Kinetics; 1995.
4. Weinberg RS, Gould D. *Foundations of Sport and Exercise Psychology.* 4th ed. Champaign, IL: Human Kinetics; 2007.

5. Kretchmar RS. *Practical Philosophy of Sport and Physical Activity.* Champaign, IL: Human Kinetics; 2005.

6. Conseco J. *Juiced: Wild Times, Rampant 'Roids, Smash Hits, and How Baseball Got Big.* New York: Harper Collins; 2005.

7. Soja E. Two out? Decision on deck. *News Media & the Law.* 2006;30(4):16.

8. Shields DLL, Bredemeier BJL. *Character Development and Physical Activity.* Champaign, IL: Human Kinetics; 1995.

9. Jones C, McNamee M. Moral reasoning, moral action, and the moral atmosphere of sport. *Sport, Education and Society.* 2000;5(2):131–146.

10. Stuntz CP, Weiss MR. Influence of social goal orientations and peers of unsportsmanlike play. *Research Quarterly for Exercise and Sport.* 2003;74:421–435.

11. Shields DLL, Bredemeier BJL. Sport, militarism, and peace. *Peace and Conflict: Journal of Peace Psychology.* 1996;2(4):369–383.

12. Shields DL. *Opponents or enemies: Rethinking the nature of competition.* Paper presented at the Inaugural Conference of the Mendelson Center for Sport, Character and Culture. South Bend, IN; 2001:May.

13. Lage L. Pacers-Pistons game halted by brawl. *USA Today* website. Available at: http://www.usatoday.com/sports/basketball/games/2004–11–19–pacers-pistons_x.htm. Accessed March 2, 2007.

14. Kavussanu M, Roberts GC. Moral functioning in sport: An achievement goal perspective. *Journal of Sport & Exercise Psychology.* 2001;23(1):37–54.

15. McInerny DQ. *Being Logical: A Guide to Good Thinking.* New York: Random House; 2005.

16. Baggini J, Fosl PS. *The Philosopher's Toolkit: A Compendium of Philosophical Concepts and Methods.* Oxford: Blackwell Publishing; 2003.

17. Benn P. *Ethics.* Montreal: McGill-Queen's University Press; 1998.

18. Almond B. *Exploring Ethics: A Traveller's Tale.* Oxford: Blackwell Publishers; 1998.

19. Portmore DW. Combining teleological ethics with evaluator relativism: A promising result. *Pacific Philosophical Quarterly.* 2005;86(1):95–113.

20. Holowchak MA. "Fascistoid" heroism revisited: A deontological twist to a recent debate. *Journal of the Philosophy of Sport.* 2005;32:96–104.

21. Mill JS. Utilitarianism. In: Smith JM, Sosa E, eds. *Mill's Utilitarianism: Text and Criticism.* Belmont, CA: Wadsworth Publishing Co. Inc.; 1969:31–88. Original work published in 1861.

22. Burton JH. Introduction to the study of the works of Jeremy Bentham. In: Bowering J, ed. *The Works of Jeremy Bentham.* Vol. 1. New York: Russell and Russell; 1962:1–83.

23. Mill JS. Utilitarianism. In: Plamenatz J, ed. *Mill's Utilitarianism: Reprinted with a Study of the English Utilitarians.* Oxford: Basil Blackwell; 1949:161–228. Original work published in 1861.

24. Zeigler EF. *Ethics and Morality in Sport and Physical Education: An Experiential Approach.* Champaign, IL: Stipes Publishing Company; 1984.

25. Aristotle. Nicomachean ethics. Ross WJ, Urmson JO, trans. In: Ackrill JL, ed. *A New Aristotle Reader.* Princeton, NJ: Princeton University Press; 1987:363–478.

26. Aristotle. Eudemian ethics. Woods MJ, trans. In: Ackrill JL, ed. *A New Aristotle Reader.* Princeton, NJ: Princeton University Press; 1987:479–506.

27. Dixon N. On winning and athletic superiority. *Journal of the Philosophy of Sport.* 1999;26:10–26.

28. Fimrite R. His own biggest fan: Baseball's first commissioner, Kenesaw Mountain Landis, was part hero, all ego. *Sports Illustrated.* 1993;79(3):76–80.

29. Aristotle. Nicomachean ethics. Ross WD, trans. In: McKeon R, ed. *The Basic Works of Aristotle.* New York: Random House; 1941:927–1112.

30. MacIntyre A. *After Virtue.* 2nd ed. South Bend, IN: University of Notre Dame Press; 1984.

31. Morgan WJ. The logical incompatibility thesis and rules: A reconsideration of formalism as an account of games. *Journal of the Philosophy of Sport.* 1987;14:1–20.

32. Kant I. The metaphysical foundations of morals. In: Blakney RB, ed. & trans. *An Immanuel Kant Reader.* New York: Harper & Brothers; 1960:163–200. Original work published in 1785.

33. Kant I. *Groundwork of the Metaphysics of Morals.* Gregor M, trans. Cambridge: Cambridge University Press; 1997. Original work published in 1785.

34. *Indianapolis Star* [serial online]. 2007. Bob Knight former Indiana University basketball coach. Available at: http://www2.indystar.com/library/factfiles/people/k/knight_bob/knight.html. Accessed March 2, 2007.

35. Lumpkin A, Stoll SK, Beller JM. *Sport Ethics: Applications for Fair Play.* 3rd ed. New York: McGraw-Hill; 2003.

36. Binnette C. College sports receive mixed marks for diversity in latest UCF report card. *University of Central Florida* website. Available at: http://news.ucf.edu/UCFnews/index?page=article&id=0024004105bd60439010c0c76ce2f003cf8&mode=news. Accessed March 2, 2007.

Concussion After the Whistle

In a competitively played game, the Hickory High School varsity football team was leading Neptune High School by one touchdown with just under three minutes left in the game. With this victory, Hickory would position itself to make the playoffs with a win in their final regular-season game next week.

Hickory's star quarterback, Jeff, could clinch this game with the conversion of just one more first down. Jeff needed only two yards to run out the clock and win the game. Head coach, Bob Bruiser, called a quarterback sneak. With a good push from the offensive line, Jeff gained just enough for the first down. After the play had been blown dead, however, Jeff received a vicious helmet-to-helmet hit from Neptune's middle linebacker, Fred. The intensity of the hit was such that Jeff was knocked unconscious and remained so as he was carried off the field by the athletic trainers.

Jeff regained consciousness on the sideline several minutes later, but was still disoriented, unaware of where he was or what had happened. The head athletic trainer, Lee, told Jeff that he probably had a severe concussion and that more tests would be necessary during the week to determine the extent of the injury.

After the game, Fred realized the ferocity of his hit and publicly apologized during an interview. Fred apologized to Jeff, as well as to Jeff's teammates, coaches, and family members. "I was upset about the way we played out there today," he said, "and took it out on Jeff after the play. It was wrong of me and I feel terrible about what happened, and for that I sincerely apologize." Although a 15-yard penalty was assessed for unnecessary roughness, it essentially served no purpose, since for all intents and purposes the game was already over. The league did decide, however, to review the play and vote on whether or not Fred should be eligible to play the final game of the season.

A couple days later, CT scan results revealed that the hit was more damaging than originally believed. Jeff had a minor case of temporary memory loss from the concussion. Most things he could remember, but other things were a little fuzzy. As the head athletic trainer, Lee informed Jeff, his parents, and the coaches of the seriousness of the situation: "Presently Jeff is fine, but if he were to receive another hit to the head in Saturday's game, there is a slight chance he could incur permanent brain damage."

Coach Bruiser, being from the old school, told Lee, "I played with concussions and broken bones when I was in high school. Everyone did! Some teams did not even have pads. Football is not a game for crybabies." Lee tried to explain the risks, but felt threatened by Coach Bruiser. Being young and inexperienced, Lee was worried about losing his job if he did not give Jeff clearance to play on Saturday.

Jeff's teammates and classmates were urging him to play because they knew it would be difficult to make the playoffs without him. Even with all the risks involved, Jeff was begging the coach to let him play. His family, on the other hand, was distraught over the possibility that Jeff might play. Only a couple of days remained to make a decision.

Critical Thinking: Finding Common-Sense Solutions

1. Do you believe a 15-yard penalty is strict enough to deter helmet-to-helmet hits such as this from taking place in the future? Elaborate. If not, what types of penalties or actions might sufficiently deter such illegal hits?

2. Do you believe that Fred's genuine apology is sufficient recompense for the helmet-to-helmet hit on Jeff after the whistle? Why or why not?

3. If you were the commissioner of the league, would you allow Fred to play in the final game of the season? Why or why not?

4. If you were one of Jeff's parents, would you take further action to make sure Jeff does not play on Saturday? Why or why not? If yes, what would these actions be?

5. If you were, Lee would you allow Coach Bruiser's intimidation tactics to influence your decision concerning whether or not to clear Jeff to play? Explain your decision.

Critical Thinking: Moral Theory-Based Decision Making

6. Basing your decision on the *deontological theory,* if you were Lee, describe the thought process by which you would arrive at the decision of whether or not to allow Jeff to play.

7. Thinking egoistically, if you were Coach Bruiser, on what would you base your decision to play or not to play Jeff on Saturday?

8. If you were Jeff, how would you balance *your own good* along with the *good of others* when deciding whether or not to play on Saturday?

Pressure to Change Hakeem's Grade

Migraine High School is a school known for its sports programs, especially boys' basketball. This year, Migraine is off to an extraordinary start and has not lost a single game. Led by the 32 points per-game average of freshman sensation Hakeem Hops, Migraine is carrying a 22–0 regular season record into the tournament. Although a star basketball player, Hakeem struggles academically. A personal tutor was assigned to him and he was required to attend the athletes' study hall twice a week. Even with this extra help, Hakeem's academic performance is still poor, as evidenced by his failing of both algebra and English this past grading term.

The grading process at Migraine High School entails several steps. After the teachers submit grades to the school's office, the grades are forwarded to the district's central office where they are processed into report cards and mailed to each student's home. The central office also forwards the report cards of all student-athletes to their respective athletic departments, where athletic directors review them to determine athletic eligibility.

After glancing at Hakeem's grades, it was obvious to Migraine's athletic director that Hakeem was ineligible for the playoffs. Because he considered winning in the boys' basketball playoffs to be of the utmost importance, the athletic director decided to discuss Hakeem's academic situation with the teachers of the two classes that Hakeem failed. The athletic director asked both teachers to re-evaluate Hakeem's work in a way favorable to Hakeem. The athletic director also asked the two teachers if they could provide Hakeem the opportunity to complete make-up work to improve the failing grades. Throughout his plea, the athletic director explained the essential role that success in the boys' basketball playoffs would serve in promoting a positive image for Migraine High, and emphasized how unlikely success would be without Hakeem.

Hakeem's algebra teacher, Ms. Timorous, is a second-year teacher who has an interest in coaching girls' tennis in the spring. Ms. Timorous was well aware that the athletic director would be upset if she did not acquiesce to his request to find a way to justify changing Hakeem's "F" in algebra to a passing grade. She also knew that the athletic director would be the one deciding who would be hired to coach the girls' tennis team. Feeling pressured, Ms. Timorous changed Hakeem's grade in algebra from an "F" to a "D," declaring that an error was made in calculating Hakeem's original grade.

The second teacher the athletic director approached was Mr. Firm, Hakeem's English teacher. Mr. Firm has been at Migraine for eight years and is not at all involved in the school's athletic program. When he was asked to change Hakeem's English grade, Mr. Firm was offended and became angry at the athletic director. Acting on his anger, Mr. Firm decided to speak with the vice principal about the athletic director's suggestion. The vice principal was furious with what he considered to be an attempt to pressure Mr. Firm into acting unethically.

While the processing of Ms. Timorous's change-of-grade form was taking place, the athletic director simply ignored the academic eligibility rule and allowed Hakeem to play in the next game. Ms. Timorous's grade change was approved the following day, and a copy was sent to the vice principal, who immediately went to see Ms. Timorous. After asking Ms. Timorous if the athletic director had influenced her grade change, he told her to prepare for a meeting in which she would be required to defend changing Hakeem's "F" in algebra to a "D."

Despite this grade change controversy, Hakeem's season has continued uninterrupted, and he has continued to perform and represent Migraine High School superbly on the basketball court. The controversy, however, has resulted in a division between the Migraine staff and administration. As word spread about the athletic director pressuring the two teachers, many questions arose. The whole situation has turned into a headache that just will not go away.

Critical Thinking: Finding Common-Sense Solutions

1. If you were Ms. Timorous, would you have provided Hakeem with an opportunity to complete extra credit assignments after being approached by the athletic director? Why or why not?

2. If you were the athletic director, would you have attempted to persuade Ms. Timorous and Mr. Firm to change Hakeem's failing grades given the circumstances? Why or why not?

3. If you were the principal of Migraine High School, would you support 'linking' athletic eligibility rules to academic performance? Why or why not?

4. If you were the commissioner of a national association of interscholastic athletics, would you support legislation that allows athletes to miss class to participate in athletic contests and/or practices? Explain your response.

Critical Thinking: Moral Theory-Based Decision Making

5. If you were Ms. Timorous, how and to what extent, if any, would you have used *strategic reasoning* to decide whether or not you would change Hakeem's grade?

6. If you were Mr. Firm and you were using *teleological moral theory* to guide your reasoning, what moral values would you have emphasized in determining whether or not to change Hakeem's grade? Why?

7. If you were the athletic director and were using *consequentialist moral theory* as the basis for your actions, how would you have responded after finding out that Hakeem had failed two classes, making him ineligible for the playoffs?

Blood On the Ice

Violence in sport can be ugly, especially in professional hockey. Violence from players comes in many forms, ranging from abusive language to full out 'gloves off' fights. This past Monday night in the semi-professional American Hockey Association, an act of violence that seemed to be quite unnecessary took place in a "C" level game ("A" is the category of the highest level of talent and "D" the least).

This incident involved two players on opposing teams. One of the players was Joe Schmoe, a man in his mid-40s who is not a very good skater. The other player was Johnny Superstar, a former first-round draft pick of the best league in the world, the Elite Professional Hockey League. Recently, Superstar has played for the semi-professional hockey league's hometown Hotshots. Superstar is not on the official Hotshots roster, but sometimes plays for them when his friends on the team invite him, which was the case Monday night.

Approximately 10 minutes was left to play in the game when Schmoe accidentally hooked Superstar with his stick. The referees did not signal for a penalty. Superstar was not too happy about this 'no-call' and started skating after Schmoe, yelling threatening comments at him. Superstar then took his stick and tapped Schmoe on the back of his helmet as a slight 'reminder' that hooking will not be tolerated even if the referees do not call it. When the referees saw Superstar's stick against Schmoe's helmet, they signaled for a penalty.

Since Schmoe's team was on offense the penalty would be delayed, meaning that play would not be stopped to enforce the penalty until Superstar's team took possession of the puck. In the meantime, both Schmoe and Superstar continued to yell threats at one another. A few seconds later, Superstar gained possession of the puck and immediately, from a distance of only 12 feet, turned 180 degrees and shot the puck directly at Schmoe's face. Schmoe instantly fell to the ground. Lying motionless and bleeding on the ice, Schmoe's nose was broken and his lip was split in half beginning at the bottom of his nose. The damage to Schmoe's face was severe and would later require cosmetic surgery.

Meanwhile, as Schmoe was being attended to, a melee broke out as both teams emptied their benches and were fighting against one another. Finally, after 15 minutes, the referees were able to stop all the fighting and begin assessing penalties. Superstar was penalized most heavily by being immediately ejected from the game, assessed with a five-minute high sticking penalty for tapping Schmoe on the back of his helmet and also with a match penalty. The rest of the game finished peacefully.

While the fighting was taking place, Schmoe was placed on a stretcher, carried to a waiting ambulance, and transported to the hospital. Immediately upon regaining consciousness, while lying on his hospital bed, Schmoe made it clear that he intended to press criminal charges against Superstar and sue both the American Hockey Association and the Elite Professional Hockey League. Not wasting any time, Tuesday morning the Justice Police Department began an investigation by calling eyewitnesses, which included both referees, Schmoe, Superstar, and the scorekeeper, Ms. Balance. It has been 11 weeks and a judgment has yet to be made regarding the criminal charges against Superstar. If guilty, Superstar could face jail time.

Critical Thinking: Finding Common-Sense Solutions

1. If you were the director of the semi-professional hockey league (recreational "C" hockey league), would you have allowed Superstar to play since he was not officially on the roster? Why or why not?

2. If you were the director of the league, what effect, if any, do you believe Superstar's actions would have on the sport of hockey? The league?

3. If you were Superstar, would you argue that it was your responsibility to enforce Schmoe's hooking infraction since the referees did not? Explain your answer.

4. If you were Superstar, would you regret having shot the puck into Schmoe's face, since the youth of America might be apt to emulate this same behavior? Explain your answer.

Critical Thinking: Moral Theory-Based Decision Making

5. If you were Ms. Balance (the scorekeeper) and, as part of an effort to gain perspective relative to this case, the presiding judge asked you to apply parts

of the *teleology theory* by prioritizing, based on rationale, the moral values of respect and honesty along with the social values of teamwork and leadership, what would be your response to the judge?

6. Do you believe Schmoe's action of hooking Superstar betrayed the integrity of the game? Why or why not? Do you believe Superstar's action of shooting the puck into Schmoe's face betrayed the integrity of the game? Why or why not?

7. If you were the director of the American Hockey Association, would the fact that Superstar intended to injure Schmoe, along with the fact that Superstar has a documented history of violence in hockey games, influence how you would address the situation? Explain your answer. Do you have a premise from which you will base your decision? What supportive rationale would you use in support of your decision?

Re-entering the Game After a Concussion

Joel, the Highview Cougars best offensive and defensive tackle, was having a fantastic game. He was controlling the line on both sides of the ball during the first half of play, had already accumulated 10 tackles and a sack on defense, and made several key blocks on offense. Early in the third quarter, Joel was hit in the head while making a tackle. As he left the field with the emergency medical technicians, he appeared injured and a bit dazed. Coach Davis decided it was best to let him rest a bit and see how the game progressed before considering whether Joel should continue playing.

The game was tied at 14 at the end of the third quarter and while the teams were changing sides for the start of the fourth, Joel walked up and stood next to Coach Davis. The coach asked him how he was feeling. Joel said he was fine and was ready to go back into the game. Coach Davis, however, had yet to hear anything from the EMTs regarding Joel's condition. He looked behind him and saw the EMTs sitting on the bench, seemingly unconcerned that Joel had left the bench and was standing next to Coach Davis with his helmet, looking as if he was going to re-enter the game. Since the EMTs had never approached Coach Davis or any of the members of his staff about Joel's condition, the coach was somewhat unsure as to what to do.

As an amateur coach with minimal medical training, Coach Davis was no expert on diagnosing head injuries. Injuries such as compound fractures or serious joint injuries typically have obvious symptoms that accompany them.

Minor concussions, on the other hand, are more difficult to diagnose. Coach Davis was from the 'old school'; he taught his players to play through all kinds of pain without complaint. Given the tight game and the lack of concern the EMTs were showing, Coach Davis decided to check with Joel once again. "Are you sure you're ready to go back in?" Joel smiled and put his helmet on. Without further consideration, Coach Davis smacked him on the shoulder pads and Joel ran out onto the field. He played a spectacular fourth quarter, finishing with 17 tackles and 2 sacks, as the Cougars emerged victorious, 20–14.

On Monday morning, many players, students, and faculty members approached Coach Davis and praised Joel's toughness and his play on Saturday. The coach was quite proud of Joel and also talked him up to who-ever was interested in listening. After teaching his last morning class, Coach Davis returned to his office to find his principal and athletic director waiting for him. They escorted him to the principal's office where Joel and his parents were waiting. The six of them sat down and a bewildered Coach Davis was surprised to hear that Joel had received a concussion on Saturday and did not remember going back into the game or playing the fourth quarter at all. Joel's parents informed the administrators and Coach Davis that he would be out of school for a couple of days and would not be playing in the final two football games of the season. Mortified at his decision after the fact, Coach Davis now had to explain to everyone in the room why he decided to let Joel go back into the game.

Critical Thinking: Finding Common-Sense Solutions

1. As a coach, develop a plan of action that will help you decide whether a player with a head injury should continue to play. What elements should/must be considered when arriving at a decision relative to playing such a player?

2. Who should have a say in whether an injured high school player returns to action? Justify your answer.

3. What should athletic directors do to help coaches handle a situation such as the one above?

4. What should the EMTs have done in this case?

5. As a parent, if your child has a head injury in a game, what should you do?

Critical Thinking: Moral Theory-Based Decision Making

6. Using *deontological moral theory*, explain why Coach Davis should not have let Joel back into the game.

7. Using *teleological moral theory*, explain how the EMTs should have handled Joel's situation and why.

Key Terms

altruistic—looking beyond one's own good in determining the right action to take in a certain situation; living for the good of others; doing good and not expecting anything in return.

argument—a form of reasoning; a set of statements explaining what a person believes is true and why he or she believes it is true; the content of an argument (its premises and conclusion) must be true if the argument is to be strong.

beneficence—being kind to others; doing good; not harming others.

best interests—bringing about the most good for everyone.

bracketed morality—a morality that grants sport participants additional moral freedom when involved in a sporting contest than what is expected outside of sporting contests; allows sport participants to emphasize self-interest, related to the goals of sport, more than everyday morality; may be used as a justification by players and coaches to support behaviors within sport that may be perceived as questionable by those not operating within its realm.

categorical imperatives—universalizable principles that are good, and under which one would want anyone to act.

compassion (moral value)—merciful; suffering with another; being able to understand another's position, ideas, problems, etc.; being able to understand the injustices or moral problems other persons are facing; a compassionate person is one who sees how cheating hurts and feels badly for those who have had illegal tactics used against them.

conclusions—statements asserting what someone believes; conclusions are only as strong as the premises upon which they are grounded.

consequences of actions—that which naturally follows an action; a result; moral theories contending that the consequences of actions are the primary element in determining the right action to take in a given situation are consequentialist moral theories; actions taken within the consequentialist moral theory are based on the consequences that will follow.

consequentialism—contending that the consequences of actions are the primary element in determining the right action to take in a given situation.

decision maker—person who settles an issue; person who arrives at a judgment or makes a choice, that is, athletes, coaches, and sport managers who are confronted with difficult decisions that call for adherence to a reasoning process or decision-making model to make the right choice.

deontological moral theory—a form of ethics that believes actions that are considered "good for me are good for all"; determines what is right by considering whether an action would be generally accepted if applied to all people; the Golden Rule is representative of deontological moral theory.

diligence (social value)—hard working; industriousness.

discipline (social value)—a systematic self-control directed toward accomplishment.

egoistic—self-interested; devoted to own interests and advancements.

equal opportunity—the same chance; participants who compete under the same conditions have equal opportunity to succeed.

ethics—the area of philosophy that deals with questions about morality and assesses the rightness or wrongness of actions and decisions.

fair play—playing by the rules.

fairness (moral value)—just; impartial; straightforward justice; being objective.

greatest happiness principle—actions are right based on their creation and promotion of the greatest amount of happiness.

happiness—as described by John Stuart Mill, the intended pleasure and the absence of pain.

hedonism—the doctrine that pleasure is the most important pursuit in life.

honesty (moral value)—telling the truth; not lying; upright; faithful.

hypothetical imperative—principles calling for the action that leads to achievement of a desired state, consequence, or desire.

integrity (moral value)—uprightness of character; being honest.

justice (moral value)—fairness; equity; founded on fact.

leadership (social value)—being able to guide; to persuade; having traits that make others want to follow you.

moral dilemma(s)—a situation that calls for actions to determine which option is morally best.

moral egocentrism—in sport, the tendency to interpret the sporting world in terms of self. Putting one's own interests or the team's interest ahead of others, often times to a non-moral end.

moral goodness—condition of virtuousness; relates to persons and their character traits.

moral obligation—moral obligations include moral judgments that people make that affect people's relationships and dealings with one another and that bring the moral value of their motives, intentions, and character traits under scrutiny.

moral principles—statements prescribing or proscribing particular types of action.

moral reasoning—a decision-making process that requires persons to use criteria such as moral values, moral principles, and/or the anticipated moral consequences of actions to determine whether a particular action is right or wrong, or whether we have a moral obligation to act in a particular manner toward others.

moral value(s)—particular traits or characteristics that help people act well toward others, including honesty, justice, kindness, respect, beneficence, and compassion; moral values consist of dispositions that influence one to do what is morally right and carry out one's moral responsibilities to others.

morality—a system of norms, values, and rules that regulate the manner in which human beings treat one another.

non-moral reasoning—does not require that you decide between actions that are morally good or bad, or ethically right or wrong.

premises—statements explaining why someone believes something; part of the content of an argument; if the premises of an argument do not firmly support its conclusion, the argument will be a weak one; premises make up a set of claims from which a conclusion is drawn.

psychological egoism—the view that the ultimate aim of each person is his or her own self-interest.

psychological hedonism—the theory claiming that human beings will seek out actions bringing them the most pleasure and absence of pain.

respect—regarding others with honor; to appreciate others; recognizing and treating others in sport as fellow human beings.

safety—protection from harm.

social values—values such as teamwork, discipline, diligence, and leadership; the cultivation of social values alone is not enough to guarantee the fostering of moral reasoning or action.

sportsmanship—fairness in following the rules of the game; a component of morality in sport that is befitting to sport participants.

strategic obligation—the type of judgment that is arrived at through a process of strategic reasoning that requires people to examine the possible consequences of actions to determine which action will bring the greatest advantage to them personally or to the group they represent (e.g., their team, school, or organization).

strategic reasoning—a decision-making process in which the decision made/action taken is based on that which will bring the greatest advantage or reward to an individual or that individual's 'in-group' (e.g., team, school, organization).

teamwork (social value)—working together; cooperation among members of a group.

teleological moral theory—driven by moral values such as justice or fairness, honesty, compassion, beneficence, and respect; rooted in the work of Aristotle; requires that you consider your purpose as a human being by determining the moral values that make up a morally good person.

utilitarianism—a universal form of hedonism developed by philosopher John Stuart Mill and his predecessor, Jeremy Bentham; emphasizes the good of others instead of the good of the individual decision maker; a consequentialist theory that states that when you are faced with a moral decision, you should choose the act that will bring the greatest amount of happiness to the greatest number of people.

virtues—values; good qualities; characteristics, attitudes, and habits of action that help people do good things.

welfare—the best interests or well-being of a group or individual.

winning at all costs—placing winning ahead of all else; compromising moral values and sportsmanship in the interest of winning.

2 Ethical and Unethical Behavior in Sport

Learning Outcomes

After reading Chapter 2, the student will be able to:

1. State reasons why obstacles are purposefully implemented in sport.

2. Identify the variations of sport in different human cultures.

3. Describe how the various teachings of sport affect strategies, values, and overall types of play.

4. Explain the relationship between achieving excellence and winning or losing.

5. Describe the relationship between a strong emphasis on winning and morally right actions.

6. Contrast the view that cheating is "just another way to gain an advantage" with the view that cheating is wrong in and of itself.

7. Explain the importance of the enforcement of rules in sport.

8. Provide examples of how coaches can influence player behaviors that are reflective of achieving excellence.

Sport is an activity governed by specific rules or customs and usually includes competition that results in winning or losing. It is an activity intensely scrutinized by the public, and public opinion about sport differs widely. These different views about sport are shaped by our upbringings and overall human cultures. The widespread popularity and visibility of sport accounts for its intense public scrutiny. Even for those who do not regularly attend sporting events, the opportunity to be informed and to form opinions is readily available thanks to daily print and broadcast media reports. But we don't all interpret rules the same, which leads to opposing views as to what actions are and are not honorable or moral. And there are many opinions regarding what outcomes should result from sport. Some people believe winning should be emphasized, while others believe that the achievement of a team and personal excellence should be a priority.

This mixture of opinions causes people to act differently under similar conditions. The decisions made and the actions taken by sports persons are influenced by many factors, including the intense public pressure that surrounds sport, the immediacy of decisions made in the heat of a competitive moment, and the fact that many professional athletes are seen as role models. Society often views elite athletes as being worthy of emulation, but many professional athletes and others involved in sport do not always behave in a morally unquestionable manner, on or off the field. In the competitive world of sport it can be difficult to maintain a focus on moral integrity when the emphasis is so often on winning, especially winning at all costs.

Reaching common ground on what acting morally means is important to the function of sport. Rightly or wrongly, people attribute to sport the ability to help people develop character through the learning of moral and social values. The dynamic nature of sport is conducive to such development, as those involved in sporting tests are placed in constantly changing situations that often call for decision making that relates to moral and social values. This chapter will provide you with a better understanding of how to act morally as you navigate the numerous perspectives related to sport. We will examine the role of excellence in sport and learn why the values of fairness and good sportsmanship in the achievement of excellence are important. The influence of such values and how they can help keep winning in perspective and protect the best interests of those involved in sport will also be discussed.

Obstacles, Rules, and Conventions In Sport

The Purposeful Implementation of Obstacles Within Sport

According to Suits, sport philosophers frequently hold that sports is a category of games.[1] Suits goes on to define a game as "a voluntary attempt to overcome unnecessary obstacles."[2(p41)] People use what is known as **conventional logic** in the performance of most everyday activities; that is, they use the most direct and efficient means to eliminate obstacles. In games,

conventional logic: the normal tendency of making the necessary arrangements to bring tasks to closure in the most efficient way.

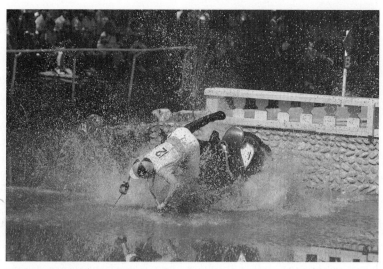

2-1 *In games, the obstacles that are placed in the way to present different types of challenges exemplify alternative logic and require players to use particular kinds of physical skills to overcome these artificially placed obstacles.*

alternative logic: in sport, the purposeful establishment of an inefficient environment, including the placement of obstacles to overcome, in the way of its participants (alternative to arranging the environment in a way to make achieving the task and/or reaching the goal more efficient).

however, players use what is known as **alternative logic,** wherein inefficient environments are created using unnecessary obstacles that must be overcome. Players must use their own unique skills against a competitor to overcome these obstacles.

In track and field, for example, an obstacle in the form of a bar is placed in front of the high jumper and pole vaulter for the purpose of separating the achievement levels of the athletes. The athletes achieving at the highest levels will overcome the obstacle (the bar) at its highest point, and the others will be considered less able and hence ranked at a lower level in terms of talent evaluation since they are only able to clear the obstacle at its lower heights. Thus, as a category of games, sports require a different type of thinking than we engage in normally in our everyday activities.

Morgan refers to this different type of thinking as "gratuitous logic."[3] According to Suits, this gratuitous logic requires us to voluntarily accept rules that establish particular challenges by making us use less efficient means rather than more efficient means in pursuit of a particular goal.[2] The most efficient means to score a goal in field or ice hockey would be to shoot it straight into the net without the challenge of having to overcome the obstacle of a defender or a goalie. Defenders and goalies, however, make scoring more challenging and difficult and provide a way to identify the players and teams that are more talented in scoring and those that are not. The defenders and goalie require the offensive player to alter shots and create various different types of shots other than a straightforward approach in order to score. Since not all players can alter shots equally effectively, those that succeed in scoring are considered more skilled than others. In other words, those players who overcome obstacles more effectively are viewed as achieving higher rates of excellence.

As mentioned, only games include intentionally placed obstacles to be overcome. In everyday life, we generally set about attempting to achieve objectives by using those methods and materials that will help us get the job done as quickly and efficiently as possible. When driving to work, we look for the path of least resistance, trying to avoid highly traveled routes and routes under construction. Businesses do not place obstacles in front of their employees, but instead attempt to remove any obstacles that restrict productivity and prevent progress. When a professor provides a course syllabus to a student, the student usually looks for the most efficient way to complete assignments and achieve the desired grade.

Competitions such as the steeplechase, hurdles, and equestrian events serve as examples of contests that illustrate, literally, the concept of sports' inclusion of the placement and overcoming of obstacles. The winner is declared as the competitor who best demonstrates the ability to most efficiently overcome these obstacles.

"The Unintended Obstacle in Hockey"

As the seconds ticked away ending period number two of the conference championship ice hockey game between Digital College and Bell College, the game was tied 3–3. Before the period ended, Digital College's goalie, Dick, dumped half of the water from his water bottle on the crease in front of his net. When the goalies switched goals at the end of the period, unbeknownst to Ralph (Bell's goalie) he would be defending the goal at which Dick had dumped the water. The first shot of the third, and final, period taken by Digital was a 45-foot slap shot. Ralph anticipated making a routine stick save, but unfortunately when the puck hit the puddle of water in the crease it slowed nearly to a stop, at which time another Digital player stepped in and knocked the puck past Ralph for the score. Digital ended up winning the game 4–3.

Questions
1. Although Digital won the game, do you consider them to be the best team and/or the team that exhibited the highest skill level? Explain your answer.
2. Were both teams presented with the same obstacles?
3. Explain the difference between purposeful obstacles of the game, such as defenders, and the obstacle presented to Bell College by Dick dumping water on the crease.
4. Explain the relationship between fairness and (a) purposeful (intended) obstacles put in place by the creators of the game and (b) unintended obstacles, such as the obstacle Dick created when he dumped water on the crease.

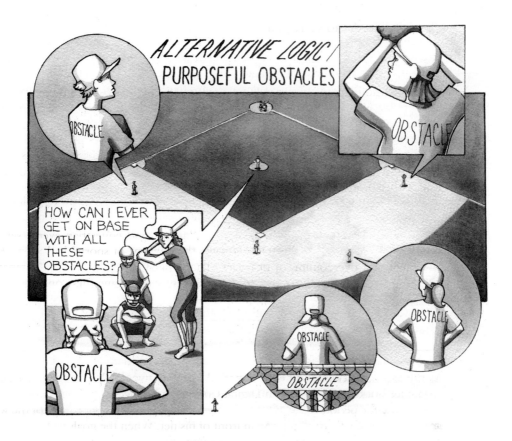

The rules of golf serve as another example of a sport that requires its participants to overcome intentionally placed obstacles. Golf rules require participants to use particular implements (i.e., golf clubs) to achieve the goal of putting a ball into a hole. In golf, obstacles are presented in the form of the fairway, undulations on a putting green, lakes, and the ultimate artificially created obstacle—the bunker or sand trap. The clubs must be used to hit the ball from its location on the ground to the green and, finally, into the hole, no matter which obstacle may present itself on any given shot. Golfers who overcome obstacles most efficiently not only rise above **mediocrity** but also approach a level of excellence and are considered more talented than those who frequently have difficulty doing so.

mediocrity: neither good nor bad; second rate; a mediocre sport performance is an average performance.

Games of sport do not operate solely by placement of inefficient, artificial obstacles to be overcome. To ensure a consistent, level playing field and to be able to determine the outcome of contests, games of sport must be governed by rules, discussed below.

Constitutive Rules

According to Suits, rules that establish the skills and strategies that may be used in the attainment of a game's goal are its **constitutive rules.**[2] Torres noted that constitutive rules are rules that "impose strict restrictions on specific actions and procedures that participants of the game may engage in while trying to attain the prelusory goal."[4(p82)] Accounting for the formalist claim that games must be constituted before they can be regulated, according to Kretchmar,[5] constitutive rules indicate game objectives and the means by which they may (and may not) be pursued.

constitutive rules: regulations that establish the skills and strategies of the game, impose strict restrictions on specific actions and procedures of the game, and indicate the game objectives and the means by which they may and may not be pursued.

To equalize competition, constitutive rules are necessary. Constitutive rules standardize such things as age in Little League organizations; weight classifications in boxing and wrestling; and scholarships, practice times, and eligibility in Division I National Collegiate Athletic Association (NCAA) sports. The standardization of constitutive rules for each sport allows for meaningful comparisons of player accomplishments to be made within the same sport. For example, the length of the game in soccer is the same no matter where the game is played. The number of outs in baseball per nine-inning game is always 27. When a pitcher strikes out 15 batters, that number can be meaningfully compared with the number of strikeouts in another baseball game, since in each nine-inning game, the maximum number of outs possible is standardized as 27.

Constitutive rules also ensure that physical playing environments are standardized. The distance of the rim from the floor in basketball must always be 10 feet; the length of a football field must always be 100 yards; and the movement of air during table tennis tournaments must always be kept to a minimum. In a sense, constitutive rules control for home team advantages. When constitutive rules effectively standardize the environment, home court/field advantages are minimized.

If home team officials do not clearly outline a cross country course for the visiting team, this obviously could cause visiting team runners to be confused and run in the wrong direction, thus losing the race. If, in this case, the visiting team does lose the race, it is not necessarily because they are not the best and fastest team. Excellence may have been achieved by the visiting team, but a win was not recorded because the home team officials did not clearly mark and accurately describe the path of the course. If, however, both teams were aware of the correct path of the course—and all other factors such as the physical talent level of both teams was equal—both teams would have an equal and fair chance to achieve both excellence and victory.

"Bobby Bruiser's Boxing Gloves"

Bobby Bruiser was scheduled to box against Hank Hitter in a summer league amateur boxing competition. Both boxers' gloves were checked prior to the match to make sure they met the correct specifications of weight and size. While in his corner

"Bobby Bruiser's Boxing Gloves" (*Continued*)

immediately prior to the beginning of the fight, however, Bobby's trainer and others in his corner huddled around him while he changed into a pair of gloves that were not as soft and would inflict more pain to his opponent upon contact. Going into round three, both boxers had landed exactly the same number of punches. Then with a minute to go, Bobby landed the punch that knocked out Hank.

Questions
1. Did Bobby break a constitutive rule? Explain your answer.
2. What is the purpose of requiring both boxers to adhere to the standards/constitutive rules that outline standards for gloves?
3. When considering Bobby and Hank, who do you believe is the best boxer? Will Bobby really ever know if he was the better boxer?

Even though golf can be a rather frustrating game, it is one in which millions of people choose to participate. Golfers accept the rules of golf so that they may experience the challenges resulting from those rules. Some of those rules call on golfers to learn to hit different types of shots, and to hit them with enough consistency to get the ball into the hole in fewer strokes than their opponents do. Thus, the rules of golf include the placement of obstacles in the way of participants so that they may use particular skills and strategies to achieve the sport's objective. Participant acceptance of the rules of the sport makes the sport itself possible; unless participants accept and play by the rules with a strong measure of consistency, the game cannot be played.[2]

rule-governed tests: competitive sport; the fact that competitive sport is governed by standardized rules for all participants allows for meaningful outcomes and comparisons to take place.

Sports are also **rule-governed tests** of skill that require athletes and teams to be involved in the same activity so that meaningful and accurate comparisons can be made between them. Not only from day to day but also from generation to generation, meaningful and accurate comparisons of statistics from player to player and team to team are made in sport through rule-governed tests.

Different Human Cultures and the Teaching of Sport

Sports are not simply defined by their rules. Coakley states that:

> "Although definitions of sports vary, those who offer definitions tend to emphasize that sports are institutionalized competitive activities that involve rigorous physical exertion or the use of relatively complex physical skills by participants motivated by internal and external rewards."[6(p21)]

Sports are part of human culture; they are distinctly human activities. The following question serves to establish this fact: Did you learn to play your sport by reading its book of rules? Typically, people answer "no" to this question because they have been socialized into their sport by parents, siblings, or peers. A mother brings her daughter to the NCAA national championship softball tournament and her daughter wants to learn how to play softball. A boy who plays ice hockey teaches his younger sister how to skate and she wants to learn how to become a competitive figure skater. A next-door neighbor introduces his young friend to the game of soccer. Thus, most people learn a sport's rules, skills, and strategies within the social context of that sport.

As Coakley reminds us, "As part of **cultures,** sports have forms and meanings, which vary from one group and society to the next and vary over time as groups and societies change."[6(p5)] In terms of variance over time, even the sport of baseball—a sport that has been a target of criticism for not progressing with the times—has experienced changes in such forms as the designated hitter, modification of the strike zone, and alteration of the height of the pitcher's mound.

> **cultures:** environments that are distinguished from one another based on the differences between various groups and societies; sports and acceptable actions within sport vary from culture to culture; that is, some cultures might quietly accept certain rule breaking in the interest of winning whereas others might not.

Regarding variations of the same sport in different cultures, the sport of football in the United States serves as an example. The southern part of the country includes teams like Florida, Georgia, Louisiana, and Mississippi, and is more known for speed than for brute strength, as has been the case with teams in the midwestern part of the country like Wisconsin, Iowa, and Indiana. When comparing football to other locations throughout the country, football in the South has been described as being different. In the South, football is life.[7(p14)] The entire cities of the local southern teams wear the school colors, university organizations spearhead the fun with tailgate events, parties, and decorations. Classes are often canceled, businesses close, fraternity and sorority members dress up, and eager fans flood into the stadium when the gates open.[7] Here one can see that sporting cultures within the United States itself exhibit differences in strategies and styles.

How one is socialized into sport and the way one is taught to participate in sport is affected by the variance of sport within societies and groups. A sport might gain such a level of importance in some countries or areas within a country that coaches at the high school or even youth levels will teach players **illegal tactics,** some of which might be very difficult to detect, to give their team an edge. In the interest of winning, some sporting cultures might be quietly accepting of such illegal behaviors. In other places, teaching such tactics might get a coach suspended or fired.

> **illegal tactics:** strategies employed or practiced that are against the rules.

Athletes are also taught different styles of play in different places or times. Continuing with examples that demonstrate variations of strategies and style of play in the United States, basketball offers different variations based on its location. For example, high school basketball players in different geographical regions of the country play different styles of basketball. Teams in the midwestern part of the country are generally known for a somewhat methodical, deliberate offensive style that often utilizes several seconds of the shot clock before attempting a shot. But high school teams in the eastern part of the country are generally known for a more fast-paced, offensive style that includes shooting quickly without using many seconds of the shot clock during each offensive possession.

No matter the differences, the ways in which young athletes are taught to play sports affect the skills, techniques, and strategies they learn; the values they cultivate and portray within sports; the views they have of opponents, officials, and fans; and the level of respect they demonstrate toward these individuals and toward their sports. D'Agostino points out that because sports are socially constructed, each one has its own **ethos**—a set of conventions and customs that, to an extent, determine how a game is to be played.[8] Some conventions come into being because the rules of sport require some interpretation by officials, whose job it is to determine when specific skills are being performed illegally.

> **ethos:** unique character of a group or social context (i.e., sport), usually expressed in attitudes, habits, and beliefs.

Differences in the Interpretation of Rules

Good officials strive for a consistent interpretation of rules so they are interpreting rules in the same manner for all parties involved throughout the game. Oftentimes, however, officials interpret rules differently, or a single official is inconsistent in his or her interpretation of the rules. This can lead to misunderstandings about what exactly is considered traveling in a game of basketball, or what is considered interference in a game of hockey, and can make it difficult for athletes and coaches to be sure whether a particular move is acceptable.

> **fairness (moral value):** just; impartial; straightforward justice; being objective.

To maintain **fairness,** it is important that officials be knowledgeable about how skills are to be performed and be consistent in their interpretation of the rules that are set forth for these skills. For example, a home plate umpire in baseball must be consistent in his or her calling of balls and strikes. If an umpire's strike zone is inconsistent from pitch to pitch, it is not fair to the batter or the pitcher. Batters and pitchers both must have a clear understanding of the strike zone so that they can pursue excellence in the skills of hitting and pitching. If umpires are inconsistent in their calling of balls and strikes, they are the ones who determine the performance outcomes instead of the pitcher and batter. For excellence to be achieved there must be a balanced, consistent set of rules that are accurately enforced.

Unwritten Agreements to Overlook Rules Violations

As social constructions, sports also develop many idiosyncrasies over time. According to D'Agostino, some people believe that the rules of a sport may be ignored or suspended by officials during play.[8] Violations of such rules are sometimes intentionally overlooked, allowing players to use tactics that are illegal because they make the game more exciting or allow play to flow better. For example, basketball players at the professional level often times appear to travel or carry the ball while advancing it or moving it to the basket. According to D'Agostino, officials and players at this level have come to a silent agreement that the rules against these two practices will be relaxed somewhat to allow players to be more creative in their play making, which, in turn, will make the game more exciting for fans.[8] In the third period of National Hockey League (NHL) playoff games (and overtime periods should games be tied at the end of regulation play), officials often allow players to get away with minor violations such as slight holds, trips, and interference. These minor violations are ignored late in contests so that the flow of play is maintained.

Finally, baseball umpires in Major League Baseball frequently allow infielders to 'phantom tag' a base or player to avoid possible collisions. The phantom tag most generally takes place when an infielder is attempting to execute a double play. Instead of stepping on second base to force the runner out, the infielder executing the force-out does not actually step on the base but beside it. If the infielder beats the runner to the general area of second base, the umpire recognizes this and calls the runner out, not requiring the infielder to actually step on the base.

The acceptance of such rules violations within sport often goes unquestioned. Players, coaches, officials, and fans patently state that there are unwritten rules that allow such behavior and that the behaviors themselves are simply part of the game. Others, however, disagree with this assessment. Those who disagree claim that since the rules of sport indicate that such tactics are illegal, those illegal tactics should be avoided and should not be tolerated or ignored by officials, administrators, or fans. According to people who believe in absolute enforcement of rules, even when the outcome of a contest may already be known because of a lopsided score, the officials should continue to call each and every infraction, enforcing rules to the letter of the rule since rules guide the actions of players in present as well as future games. These individuals staunchly believe that 'rules are rules' and that rules make a sport the unique activity that it is and should be upheld in all cases.

How can the above dispute be settled? As noted earlier, sports have a dual nature; they are partially defined by their rules but are also human social constructions with customs, conventions, and histories that play an important role in rule interpretation and the defining of moral action within them. This dual nature requires one to seek out a mediating value to help gain an understanding of right action in sport. That mediating value is excellence.

Excellence in Sport

excellence: of the highest quality; fineness; performing in sport in a superior fashion.

Excellence in sport goes beyond winning and effective skill execution. Achieving excellence in sport calls for not only winning and effective skill execution, but also practicing moral values such as fairness, respect, sportsmanship, altruism, honesty, and kindness. In some cases, the emphasis or overemphasis on winning takes place early in a player's career. For example, it is not unusual for Olympic snow skiing hopefuls, with the support of their parents, to begin practicing on skis immediately after they learn to walk. Over the next several years, thousands of dollars are spent on training and education that is often provided at a ski academy. As the parents encourage and cajole with phrases such as "never give up on your goal," the youngster perseveres and makes serious sacrifices. School work, training, competition, and teenage parties with friends all are contending for the youngster's time, but the skiing-related activities always win out. As the young athlete grows into adulthood, he looks back and discovers he missed a part of life that others experienced: childhood. When the overemphasis on winning consumes a child's life to the point where he or she only trains and does not experience a normal childhood, the question as to whether the overall gain is worth sacrificing his or her childhood in the pursuit of athletic excellence is open for debate.

It can be argued that as more and more emphasis has been placed on the external rewards of winning, less and less importance has been placed on the

> **process of competition:** course of actions taken when striving against others to win contests.

process of competition. For example, Olympic athletes work endless hours in the pursuit of the best performance, in hopes of winning a gold medal. In doing so, they are quite aware that tremendous financial opportunities will follow in the form of endorsements, professional contracts, and maybe even motion picture contracts. Outstanding performances by American Olympic medal winners such as sprinter Michael Johnson, figure skater Michelle Kwan, and swimmer Michael Phelps have resulted in lucrative financial opportunities for all three. The desire for such financially related by-products that result from winning can have an effect on players' actions, since these desires may cause them to pursue winning in any way possible, instead of simply pursuing the goal of athletic excellence. "It is not whether you win or lose, but how you play the game" is a phrase that is not reinforced in a win-at-all-costs sport environment. Such phrases do not always relate directly to a product-oriented, produce now sporting world.

Although winning is an important indicator of success and a primary goal of those committed to their sport, it should be recognized that winning is neither the

> **respect for the opposition:** treating opponents with honor; being reverent toward opponents.

only objective nor the only valuable element of sport participation. **Respect for the opposition,** winning and losing with dignity, playing the game fairly, performing to the best of your ability, and demonstrating good sportsmanship before, during, and after the contest are all valuable elements of sport that are not related to winning.

Notre Dame's head football coach, Charlie Weis, demonstrated a valuable element of respect for the opposition after suffering a defeat at the hands of the #1 ranked University of Southern California (USC) during the 2005 season. Weis, with his son, walked into USC's locker room following the defeat and congratulated the winning Trojan football team.[9] Despite losing the game, Weis recognized it as a well-played game by both teams and, although disappointed in losing, demonstrated respect for the opposition and the game as a whole through his actions. Just as importantly, as a highly visible national figure in sports, Weis's actions of respect for the game and opponent can be modeled by sport and non-sport persons alike. If Weis's congratulatory words to the Southern California players extend beyond the locker room and into the mainstream population, this example of good sportsmanship could have a widespread positive effect on mainstream society.

The Importance of Winning

At this point, it might be helpful to point out that the author is in no way claiming that winning is unimportant. Winning in sport *is* important. When people agree to take part in a particular sport, they not only accept its rules and challenges but also implicitly agree to play to win, to do everything they can within the rules they have agreed to play by. In other words, as Delattre points out, competitors implicitly agree to present each other with the best possible challenge as they strive to win the game through the execution of the legal skills and strategies of the sport.[10]

Players have an obligation to pursue victory through practicing and playing hard, while doing so through a strict adherence to the rules. The pursuit of excellence should be the primary goal. If excellence is achieved in the form of execution and performance, winning will frequently follow. Of course, there will be times when another player or team is simply physically superior, but if games are scheduled between similarly talented opponents, the team that achieves or most nearly achieves excellence will usually win. It is not only important to try to win, it is assumed that if you are involved in a sporting contest, you are expected to do your best to win.

The Overemphasis on Winning

Problems arise within sport when winning's importance becomes overstated to the point that athletes, coaches, and administrators adopt a win-at-all-cost attitude. Schools, parents, and society are placing more emphasis on winning in school sports than ever before, at times pressuring athletic personnel to deviate from athlete-centered educational and personal development missions.[11] Furthermore, those involved in the

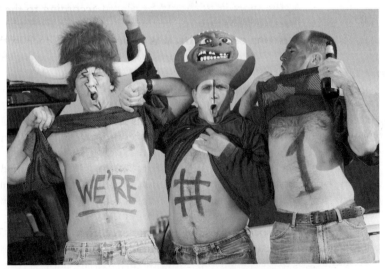

2-2 *The overemphasis on winning can intrude on good moral behavior.*

<table>
<tr><td>circumvention of rules: not blatantly breaking rules but strategically going around them.</td></tr>
</table>

circumvention of rules forget that sports are not simply about winning; sports are about a process of competition through which particular kinds of excellence are what players strive for and hopefully attain.

This overemphasis on winning has trickled down to the Little League baseball level. Birth certificate documents have been falsified in order to make talented players, who in reality are too old to be eligible to play. In the 2001 Little League World Series, Danny Almonte, a star pitcher for the Bronx, was found to be playing under a falsified birth certificate indicating that he was 12 instead of his actual age of 14. Almonte struck out the first 15 batters in the first perfect game pitched in the Little League World Series. Almonte followed up his perfect game with a one-hitter in the semi-finals.[12]

When Danny Almonte broke the constitutive rule of the maximum age limit for Little League competition, he did not achieve individual excellence and his team did not achieve excellence, even though wins were officially posted on their record. True excellence was not achieved because Almonte did not adhere to the rules of the game. Until it was factually discovered that Almonte was too old to play, wins were posted but excellence was not achieved because the wins took place under cheating circumstances. In reality, Almonte's Bronx team was not victorious because they did not abide by the rules to which all agreed at the outset of the game. Winning is only meaningful if those involved in the game have abided by the rules that define that game.

Athletes, coaches, and administrators who focus on the mastery of skills and strategies and the cultivation of discipline in sport performance recognize the importance of excellence, but, as previously stated, many tend to forget that their sport is a unique type of activity. Its rules define its challenges, and those challenges are manifested through the actions of the athletes and the interpretation of the rules. Thus, the sport itself should be played according to the best interpretation of those rules. Within this interpretation, it can be seen what a sport can be at its best; that is, one can see what it is to achieve excellence in the performance of that sport.

The Pursuit of Excellence and Winning

Excellence in sport is attained by individuals and teams to varying degrees at different points in a contest. One myth that has become stronger as winning has received greater emphasis is the belief that only winners achieve excellence in sport. We also live in a 'no-place-for-second-place' society.[13] A no-place-for-second-place society is the type of society in which one forgets that those who lose a particular sport contest can still demonstrate some degree of excellence, and that those who win but play poorly do not display such excellence.

Unfortunately, society does not associate excellence with losing. Teams and players can suffer lopsided defeats yet still exhibit excellence in performing to the best of their abilities. A mature sport eye can easily differentiate between excellence, mediocrity, and poor play, regardless of the score or who is winning or losing.

"Should Excellence Be Fired?"

Coach Good was hired three years ago as the head soccer coach for needy Deprived University. Prior to being hired at Deprived University, Coach Good established himself as a proven winner at three previous colleges. Coach Good's experience at Deprived University, however, has become quite painful. His team has won only nine games in three years, and the community is insisting that he be fired. Feeling the pressure, the athletic director is considering giving in to the community's demands that he fire Coach Good. Although the community at large is outraged, those who understand the game of soccer unanimously attest to the fact that Coach Good has achieved excellence with his team throughout his three years of coaching at Deprived University. Deprived University has the worst facilities in the conference, the least number of scholarships, and is limited primarily to a liberal arts curriculum that is not highly attractive to students. As a result of these adverse conditions, Coach Good, who refuses to cheat, is at a major recruiting disadvantage. Interestingly, despite these disadvantages, Coach Good's teams consistently execute and perform to their highest potential. His players put forth 100% effort at all times, but unfortunately are simply not physically talented enough to win on a consistent basis.

Questions

1. In this case, what is the relationship between winning and excellence regarding Coach Good? The relationship between winning and excellence regarding the Deprived University soccer team?
2. In this case, do the fans associate excellence with winning? Or are the fans okay with the fact that the team performs excellently but does not win?
3. Under the same or similar circumstances, is this community/fan reaction typical of the society in which we live? Is it typical of other societies? Explain your answers.
4. As an athletic director, could you morally justify firing Coach Good? Explain your answer.
5. In your opinion, is there an overemphasis on winning by the community/fans in this case? Is the emphasis on winning appropriate given all of the circumstances? Explain your answers.

Gymnast Mary Lou Retton's perfect score of 10 in the 1984 Los Angeles Olympic Games is an example of achieving excellence.[14] Under an evaluation in which 10 is the absolute top of the evaluation scale, Retton achieved the highest score possible. Achieving excellence in her performance earned her the gold medal in the all-around competition. As mentioned previously, victory and winning are often a by-product of the achievement of excellence. Interesting to note, however, is that even though Retton achieved a perfect 10 by the judges' standards, Retton may have underperformed based on her own personal standards. The same holds true for an athlete who performs poorly in the eyes of others. If the athlete has performed to the best of his or her abilities but does not receive a high score or does not win, he or she still may have achieved excellence based on his or her own abilities and standards.

Bar-Eli et al. point out that individuals with an **ego** (ability) **orientation** define success and failure in terms of winning and losing.[15] Outperforming opponents is a measure of success by ego-oriented individuals as opposed to successfully performing a skill or task. Ego-oriented individuals, may approach competition to seek normative success, or may avoid competition to avoid embarrassment and preserve their self-worth.[16] The ego-oriented athlete wants to outperform his or her opponents and be recognized by fellow athletes as a good athlete. Given the ego-oriented athlete's desire to be perceived as a worthy competitor in athletics, **morally upright** actions may be compromised in the interest to outperform opponents.

> **ego orientation:** competition that is driven by winning and defeating others.

> **morally upright:** ethically respectable and/or honorable.

Achieving Excellence Yet Not Winning

If a major college tennis player is matched against a minor college player, in all likelihood the major college player will have a higher skill level and will win. This is not to say, however, that simply because of losing the minor college player cannot achieve excellence. A freshman cross country runner may run a personal best time but finish last in a race when running against senior elite runners. Despite finishing last and running the risk of being labeled 'the loser' of the race, the freshman has performed to the best of his or her abilities and has achieved a personal level of excellence.

"The Slippery Spot at the Steeplechase"

The women had just finished the steeplechase event and now it was the men's turn. For the men's competition, an upward adjustment of the hurdle in front of the water barrier was required. The coach from the host school and his coaching friend from another school were fixing the water barrier so that it was at the appropriate height for the men. As the two men were adjusting the height, the host coach told his coaching friend to instruct his runner stay to the outside when going over the barrier. Next, without anyone noticing except his coaching friend, the host coach then proceeded to place a slippery substance on the surface to the inside of the barrier. Finishing first and second were the runners of the host coach and his coaching friend, who were the only two runners to pass the barrier on the outside. The others, including the leader, took the inside route, which caused them to slip and fall after stepping on the slippery substance. Suffering the most serious injury was the leader, who tore ligaments in his knee and required complete reconstructive surgery.

"The Slippery Spot at the Steeplechase" (*Continued*)

Questions

1. Describe why placing the slippery substance on the surface would be considered cheating.
2. Is this an example of winning at all costs? If so, what were the costs?
3. Should the two coaches who placed the slippery substance on the surface and instructed their runners to avoid it be punished? If so, what should be the punishment and how should it be carried out?
4. Was this a case in which winning was pursued without compromising excellence? Was this a case in which athletic excellence was abandoned completely to attain victory? Explain your answers.

The myth that only winners achieve excellence is clearly untrue, and watching a single well-played, close contest between evenly matched opponents demonstrates this fact. Losing teams *can* display excellence within a contest. They can mount successful scoring drives with strong execution of offensive skills, make skilled defensive stands, and present their opponents with strong overall challenges. Although losing teams may not come out on top, they *do* display elements of excellence in their play. A poorly played contest by a winner who barely manages to defeat a weak opponent shows that the display of excellence is mutually exclusive from winning. Despite winning, a team might play so poorly that their performance is far from achieving excellence or reaching their highest potential. In some cases, winning teams might be embarrassed or even disgraced by their performance if it is far below their performance capabilities. When teams execute skills poorly or fail to capitalize on scoring opportunities, they do not demonstrate excellence in meeting the challenges set forth by the rules of the sport.

Good coaches and good athletes expect excellent performances from their teams and themselves regardless of their opponent's talent level. If the opponent is physically superior, excellence can still be achieved by the team with inferior talent. Playing to the best of one's abilities can take place under all competitive conditions.

As stated previously, achieving excellence is not directly related to winning. Winning is a simple measure of a team's ability to reach previously established criteria. In many sports, the criteria is as simple as scoring the most runs, running the fastest time, or jumping the highest. Other sports such as gymnastics, boxing, and figure skating require judges to determine which participants most effectively meet the performance criteria that will earn them the title of winner.

Excellence can be achieved even when not winning the contest. The margin of loss could be large or small, and excellence can be maintained in defeat. Unfortunately, communities and fans sometimes fail to recognize excellent performances unless they are combined with winning. And when teams lose by large margins, people often assume that a poor performance caused the loss, when in fact the team that lost by a large margin could still have played excellently. For instance, if a major college Division I power in women's basketball plays against a mediocre Division III team, the major power may be able to win by 30 or more points, but in doing so does not achieve excellence. In fact, if a team can win by more than 30 points and decides to 'take it easy' on the less-talented team by not playing hard or by not attempting to execute with complete efficiency, from a teleological perspective the team should be embarrassed since they are not respecting the game in that they are not attempting to play hard or execute skills to a maximum capacity.

As described in Chapter 1, the focus of teleology is values oriented. In the case of 'letting up' during a sporting contest, the value of respect is being dismissed since part of respecting the game means to play hard and attempt to achieve excellence throughout the contest, from beginning to end. Sports persons must take it upon themselves to recognize excellence without winning, since myriad forces are in place that reinforce winning regardless of the achievement of excellence. In terms of reinforcing excellence, sport might be better served if wins and losses were tallied based on the achievement of excellence instead of outscoring opponents.

Competitions involving youth, such as the youth football league referred to as Pop Warner, are often able to place a higher emphasis on excellence over scoring and winning. In other words, a Pop Warner football team may suffer a four-touchdown defeat as displayed by the scoreboard, but may achieve victory on an evaluation that measures the level of excellence achieved. Conversely, the team that was victorious based on outscoring their opponent by four touchdowns may not have performed to the best of their abilities and, therefore, not achieved excellence. Even though the scoreboard indicated victory, they would not be considered victorious when success is measured based on whether or not excellence/playing to the best of their abilities was achieved.

Excellence might also be measured by exhibiting good sporting behavior and demonstrating proper skill development. Former National Basketball Association (NBA) player and analyst, Bill Walton, believes winning is emphasized to the extent that good sportsmanship is losing out to it. Walton indicated that for young people, the emphasis should be on fundamentals of the game, safety tips, and the importance of qualities such as confidence, hustle, and dedication. Furthermore, concerning young athletes, he believes that attitude, sportsmanship, teamwork, and respect should supersede an emphasis on winning.[17]

Instead of measuring success strictly by wins and losses, achievement of excellence should at least be *a* measure if not *the* measure of success. Although realistic at lower levels of competition, this notion of reinforcing excellence based on achievement has real practical limitations in the world of elite sport given the huge rewards and financial incentives tied to sport at the major college, Olympic, and professional levels.

"Serious Trash Talking"

A football player tackles another player and gets in the tackled player's face and talks trash saying, "You better stay down cause if you get up, I'm gonna break both your legs next time."

"Serious Trash Talking" (*Continued*)

Questions

1. Do you believe that the decline of morally upright behavior (demeaning trash talking) took place because more emphasis was placed on winning than on excellence? Explain your answer.
2. Do you believe it was ego orientation that caused the athlete to try and intimidate through trash talking? Explain your answer.
3. Would you consider this action cheating, gamesmanship, or blatant rule breaking? Explain your answer.

Gaining Advantages to Win

When more emphasis is placed on winning than on excellence, morally right actions may decline. Those involved in sport may look for any way possible to gain an advantage, even if doing so involves the art or practice of winning games by questionable means without actually violating the rules (commonly referred to as gamesmanship, discussed later in the chapter) or engaging in blatant rule breaking. For example, if parents of players in a youth hockey league place a frantic emphasis on winning, the young athletes in the league may be inclined to engage in inappropriate behavior in the pursuit of winning. Under this ego orientation held by some parents, the youth participants may be more inclined to try and intimidate through trash talking or **cheating** in hopes of giving themselves a better opportunity to win. Achieving excellence in this case is overshadowed, if not completely forgotten, and all efforts are focused on winning in any way possible.

> **cheating:** intentionally breaking rules; to deceive.

A real challenge for the sporting world today is to pursue winning without compromising excellence. The pursuit of winning through excellence can include, but is not limited to, the performance of skills, executing plays, and putting forth your best effort. Excellence is compromised if you cheat or circumvent the rules of the game or do not put forth your best effort. Winning cannot be presumed to be a direct result of excellence; those who cheat or circumvent rules may win but they are not achieving excellence while winning.

In more extreme cases, the pursuit of athletic excellence is abandoned completely in favor of cheating to attain victory. Everything from academic fraud to point shaving to sport-specific types of cheating, such as corking bats in baseball, have taken place since the beginning of sport and continue today. The Professional Golfer's Association (PGA), dominated by Tiger Woods over the past several years, serves as a professional sport example in which the top golfers win an assortment of material prizes. The four major tournaments that consist of the United States Open, the British Open, the Masters, and the PGA Championship all provide the top performers with hundreds of thousands of dollars in prize money. Although golf has maintained a reputation for not circumventing rules, areas do exist in which bending the rules may be tempting. And to place themselves in a better position to win and be awarded prize money, some golfers may look for ways to gain unfair advantages. For example, using a club that does not adhere to equipment specifications can result in a longer drive off of the tee box, providing the golfer with an unfair advantage. Unfair advantages jeopardize the sanctity of the sport and provide participants who use illegal equipment with an unfair advantage over rule-following opponents. Performances that result from unfair advantages are less meaningful and less able to be compared with performances resulting from rule-following opponents.

More serious acts have occurred when athletes attempt to remove fellow competitors from competition. In 1994 at a practice rink in Detroit, before the U.S. Olympic trials, a man clubbed U.S. Olympic figure skater Nancy Kerrigan above the right knee with a retractable baton. According to fellow U.S. Olympic figure skater Tonya Harding's husband, Harding approved the assault on Kerrigan.[18] In the 1980 Boston Marathon, Rosie Ruiz allegedly cheated, according to one eye witness, by jumping in the race one-half mile before the end to be the first woman runner to cross the finish line. Extensive raw footage of the race did not show Ruiz passing by several cameras before the finish, nor was there a single photograph that showed Ruiz in the race prior to the finish line.[19]

Pride in the Product

Pride in the product is achieved when an athlete attains excellence with or without victory through the effective execution of skills and strategies. Some sports people will recognize these facts but declare, "Who cares? A win is a win no matter how it is achieved. Why should you care about how the game is played?" Athletes, coaches, and administrators who value their sport and its interests will not adopt such a view. Good coaches and players are not satisfied with just winning. They take pride in creating a good product that reflects positively on them. Coaches and players personally invest themselves in their sport and understand that the performance of their team is a reflection on them. Certainly a level of satisfaction comes with winning, but complete satisfaction only comes with winning and at the same time performing excellently.

> **pride in the product:** being satisfied with a specific outcome, result, or achievement.

The football team that is favored by five touchdowns but, because of several turnovers and overall poor play, needs a field goal to win with no time remaining on the clock does not feel good about the win. No satisfaction should be taken by the league-leading baseball team that requires extra innings to defeat the least-talented team in the league because of committing fielding error after fielding error. Aware of their sub par performance, they can only take pleasure in winning when it is accompanied by personal and team excellence.

Because the talent levels of competitors can differ considerably, winning is not an indicator of personal or team excellence. The goal of athletes is to execute skills and strategies and meet the challenges provided by the best available opponent. Excellence is achieved under such conditions, which is when sports people truly take **pride in winning.** Winning is truly meaningful when it happens to those who effectively execute skills and strategies against a strong opponent. For people who participate or work in sport

> **pride in winning:** having feelings of self-respect when having obtained victory through excellence (pride in winning does not exist when victory takes place by cheating).

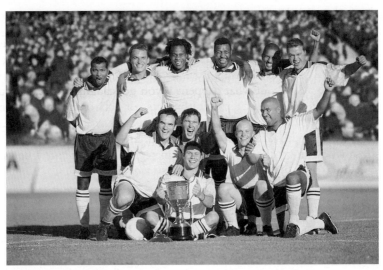

2-3 *Pride in the product is obtained when a sports person achieves excellence with or without victory through the effective execution of skills and strategies.*

for reasons other than achieving excellence within it, excellence is either of secondary importance or is simply identified with winning. In fact, at some levels, millions of dollars are spent on player and coach salaries, prize monies, tickets, promotions, and advertising. When the primary goal of sports is to generate revenue, the pride associated with achieving excellence may be diluted.

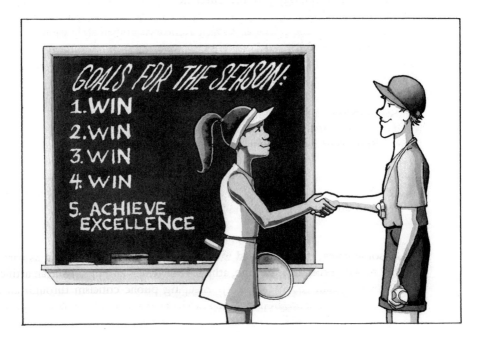

Cheating To Win

What happens to excellence when cheating becomes part of sport? Those who adopt a win-at-all-cost attitude might believe that cheating is okay as long as the perpetrators are not caught. Cheating is simply another tool through which winning may be achieved in sport. But what happens if you get caught cheating? Usually the rules of the game outline particular punishments for acts of cheating. In extreme cases of cheating, or unsportsmanlike behavior, society may also discourage cheating by voicing their disapproval against the inappropriate action. Conversely, if society applauds those who win by cheating, cheating may gain acceptance and be viewed by those in sport as acceptable behavior in the pursuit of victory.

"The Strategic Artificial Apology"

Coach Rehearsal is the head gymnastics coach at Greenleaf High School and is aware that he is breaking a high school athletic association rule that only allows teams to practice a certain number of hours per week. Not worried, Coach Rehearsal is prepared to offer a pre-planned apology to escape any punishments that might result from his actions. Coach Rehearsal has explained this strategy to his assistant coach, who seems confused by the strategy. Some other coaches at the school notified the principal of Coach Rehearsal's extended practices and the principal 'called in' the coach. As planned, Coach Rehearsal put on his best acting face and offered up his imitation of the most genuine apology possible. After hearing the apology, the principal immediately told Coach Rehearsal to be a bit more careful but not to worry about it. After shaking hands with the principal, Coach Rehearsal immediately went to his assistant coach and said, "Okay, since I was able to apologize my way out of that conflict, we have to create an alternative way to get in more practice time." The assistant coach was not quite sure what to think.

Questions
1. Is the principal reinforcing a negative behavior by not punishing Coach Rehearsal? Explain your answer.
2. Is Coach Rehearsal's artificial apology destructive to sport? Explain your answer.
3. When Coach Rehearsal's teams win, are they achieving excellence? Explain your answer.

In some cases, those involved in sport may incorporate cheating as part of their strategy to win. From time to time, athletes may cheat and then issue an artificial public apology to gain societal amnesty. Escaping public criticism through an apology places the athlete in a position in which he or she can cheat repeatedly. Acting contrite and apologetic with the full intention of cheating again once public amnesty is

artificial apology: insincere
repentance; disingenuous
remorse; dishonest regret.

achieved can be described as an **artificial apology,** and is a calculated effort on the part of some to continually gain an advantage through cheating. At some point, society or those issuing the forgiveness for cheating must recognize that individuals who create a repeated pattern of cheating are destructive to the game.

Those who value excellence in sport as a product of a fairly played contest disagree with the claim that cheating is just another way to gain advantage. They recognize what represents excellence in a particular sport and understand that it is partially determined by the rules of that sport. These individuals recognize that if someone is intentionally breaking the rules to meet the challenges presented by an opponent, excellence cannot be truly achieved within the sporting contest.

During the 2005 Major League Baseball season, the Texas Rangers were accused of cheating. Rangers personnel, when playing at home, were allegedly signaling their batters through the use of a high-technology light system in center field. Chicago White Sox pitcher Mark Buehrle complained that Rangers batters were being tipped off as to what type of pitch was coming based on the types of lights or the number of times the lights were being flashed in center field by Rangers personnel. Flashes of light were based on signals from the catcher and the positioning of the catcher's mitt. It is possible, for example, that a flash code could be used for a fastball that would be located inside and a different code could be used for a curve ball with an outside location. Although stealing signs is somewhat common in baseball, to have someone out in center field flashing light signals to batters is cheating, according to Buehrle. [20]

If the Rangers were doing this, it would have to be considered intentionally breaking the rules in order to make the challenges presented by the opponent easier, which would also be unfair. In baseball, batters must rely on their hitting skills to hit all types of pitches without knowing for sure which type of pitch will be thrown to them until the pitch actually leaves the pitcher's hand. The batters with the best hitting skills are the most successful hitters. If, however, a lighting system is being used to tip off the home team hitters as to the type of pitch that will be thrown, those batters are gaining an unfair advantage that, based on the rules of the game, is not allowed.

An offensive lineman who, in order to prevent his quarterback from being sacked, breaks the rule that disallows holding defensive players has not achieved excellence even though the quarterback is protected. The offensive lineman knows that unless he holds he cannot stop the defensive lineman from getting to the quarterback. If the referee does not see the holding violation, excellence is not achieved by the offensive lineman even though it appears that he reached his objective of protecting the quarterback.

Circumventing and Breaking the Rules

Not uncommon in the world of major college coaching is the mindset that it is acceptable and maybe even necessary to circumvent or break recruiting rules since so many other coaches are doing it. Major League Baseball players may have adopted a similar attitude regarding steroid use: "Everyone's doing it so it's okay." If sport is not protected by the enforcement of its own rules, it runs the risk of changing into something other than what its originators and participants intended. The NCAA's Office of Enforcement and Congress have taken on the responsibility of saving their games from disruption or even ruin by punishing those who break rules.

Even if the overemphasis on winning has taken on a life of its own that may be nearly impossible to reverse, small steps can be taken to manage its growth. The players are at the center of the win-at-all-cost issue, and through their actions display what others central to this issue are reinforcing through the rewards spoken of previously. Coaches have a tremendous influence on players and can have a serious local influence on emphasizing the achievement of excellence over winning at all costs. Coaches should reinforce player behaviors that are reflective of achieving excellence. Such behaviors include dedicating oneself to team goals, a willingness to work to improve one's weaknesses, and practicing and playing hard. In fact, when coaches emphasize the achievement of excellence over winning, they might even find that winning will follow.

A basic tenant necessary to the achievement of excellence is performing within the framework of the rules. Again, excellence is not directly related to performance outcomes. In the case of the offensive lineman holding to reach his performance outcome of protecting the quarterback, even though the quarterback is protected, the outcome was not reached while abiding by the rules of the game agreed upon by all persons prior to participation. Thus, excellence is not achieved. Excellence is achieved only if the performance outcome is achieved while abiding by the parameters/rules that are agreed to by those affiliated with the game. When those rules are no longer followed or are broken, meaningful and accurate comparisons can no longer be made.

If a player takes illegal performance-enhancing substances, that player has broken a rule put in place to help ensure that when a home run is hit, it is meaningful and can be compared on an equal basis with another home run hit by a player who has not taken performance-enhancing substances. To place this in a modern context, if Barry Bonds and others are found to have reached record-breaking statistics by taking steroids or other performance-enhancing substances to increase their home run productivity, can those home run statistics be meaningfully compared with others like long-time home run leader Hank Aaron and previous home run leader Babe Ruth?

Challenges defined by rules play an important role in determining excellence within a sport. Challenges that result from such rules in sport that prevent a basketball player from traveling, a baseball outfielder from trapping a ball when fielding it, a football player from crossing the line of scrimmage before the snap, and a hockey goalie from wearing oversized shoulder pads all serve as rules that, if enforced and followed, allow for excellence to take place within the game. A true winner can only be determined when each team or player has an equal opportunity to achieve excellence within the parameters of the rules, which must be enforced consistently. When players and coaches try to circumvent or break these rules, excellence cannot be achieved because the challenges are not equal for all competitors. You may achieve a goal or even victory, but not excellence, since excellence can only be attained if the challenges are met through the rules that define the challenges.

Not abiding by established rules reduces the meaningfulness of the victory and the pride that the winner or winners may take from it. What is worse morally, however, is that the individual or team is using opponents as a means to winning, something that, from the Kantian deontological perspective discussed in Chapter 1, is unethical. To use opponents in this manner is to disrespect them as fellow human beings who are striving for excellence in the game and sport.

Winning by cheating is also morally wrong from a teleological perspective, since if you cheat, you fail to show respect to your sport as the test of skills for which it was intended. Winning by circumventing the rules or not adhering to the spirit of the rules is also morally wrong. Many instances exist in which you can, by definition, be adhering to the letter of the law/rule. However, it is morally wrong when coaches and players are not actually breaking a rule, but 'getting around' the rule to gain a strategic advantage. For example, coaches may look for ways to counter offensive styles of play in basketball. When playing against a fast-breaking basketball team, a team that has a slower approach is interested in keeping the pace of the game slow. One way to do that is to attach tight nets to the rim, causing a made shot to not fall quickly through the net, or in some cases causing the ball to get stuck in the net. Acting in this way does not show respect for the game. Respecting the game means participating in the game under the established rules. It is understood and accepted that a net in basketball should allow the ball, after a made shot, to drop through the net with limited resistance. If a coach intentionally installs a tighter net, he or she is not respecting the intended purpose of the net, but instead manipulating it to gain an unfair advantage. The purpose of the net is to manage the direction of the ball as it falls to the ground so that play can continue with limited interruption after a made shot. Tightening the nets favors the team that does not fast break, since the ball will not drop out of the net quickly after a score, preventing the fast-breaking team from beginning their fast break.

"Blocking in the Back"

As Burnville College's Andy Agile received the opening kick-off, he sprinted up field looking for openings and avoiding tacklers. Heavily reliant on his blockers, Andy especially relied on Bob's blocking skills to create openings. Bob was one of the best blockers on Burnville's team; he had mastered several blocking techniques that 'got around' or circumvented the rules of blocking. One of his most effective techniques was the block to the back. While running down the field, instead of lowering his arms and shoulders, Bob would simply raise both arms completely over his head and push his entire upper body into the back of the potential tackler. In effect, Bob was blocking the player in the back, but in a way that the official would have difficulty in deciding whether or not to make the call since Bob had not made a direct specific hit by lowering his shoulder into the person he was blocking. In this instance, because of Bob's effectiveness in blocking to the back without getting caught, Andy returned the opening kick-off 97 yards for a touchdown.

"Blocking in the Back" (*Continued*)

Questions

1. Is Bob getting around/circumventing a rule to gain a strategic advantage? Explain your answer.
2. As a player, do you believe the meaningfulness of Andy's kick-off return was diminished because of Bob's illegal block to the back that made it able to happen? Explain your answer.
3. Is Bob participating in the game under the established rules of the game? Explain your answer.
4. Is Bob respecting the game? Explain your answer.
5. Regarding Bob's blocking technique, should a coach intervene?

To achieve excellence in sport, certain values must be upheld. For instance, excellence cannot be attained without fair play. An athlete must adhere to the written and morally acceptable unwritten rules of the sport in which he or she has agreed to participate. When you win a contest or score points, you will do so using the prescribed skills of sport, thus showing respect for the sport and the opponent, and also displaying both moral and performance excellence. As stated previously, achieving skill-related objectives such as scoring against an opponent or preventing another player from scoring are meaningful only when completed within the framework of the established rules of the game.

During Michelle Wie's first professional golf match on the Ladies Professional Golf Association (LPGA) tour, she was accused of cheating when it was determined after taking a penalty shot that she dropped the ball closer to the hole than allowed by rule. After *Sports Illustrated* reporter Michael Bamberger told golf officials that he was concerned about the legitimacy of the drop, officials questioned Wie, made some measurements, and then disqualified her for not adding two shots to her scorecard before signing it.[21] Golfers, to a large degree, assume the responsibility of monitoring themselves and their peers to ensure that all are playing within the framework of the

> **punitive action:** inflicting a penalty; in sport, when a person breaks a rule, an authoritative person or body can penalize them.

rules. If a golfer intentionally or mistakenly breaks a rule, their peers may point it out to the officials who may then make a determination as to the **punitive action,** if any, to be taken. In Wie's case it was decided that she would be disqualified from the tournament.

Sportsmanship

Sportsmanship is another important value one must have to demonstrate excellence in

> **sportsmanship:** putting moral standards ahead of strategic achievement in sport; adhering to the spirit of the rules even when doing so may result in strategic loss; respect for the rules, people, and conventions related to sport.

sport. Drewe defines sportsmanship from a practical orientation by stating "the minimum condition for someone to be considered a good sportsperson would have to be someone who played fairly; that is, someone who followed the rules of the game."[22(p128)] NBA guard Dwayne Wade gained an early reputation in his NBA career of being a good sportsman. Playing the game the 'right way'—which is a practical way of making reference to

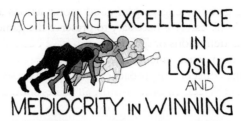

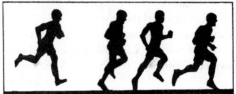

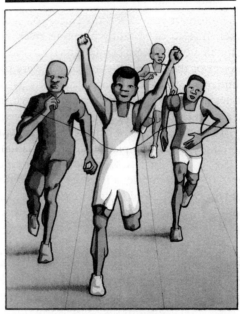

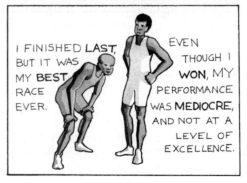

respecting the game or engaging in good moral actions as a participant—as Wade has done thus far in his career is necessary to preserve the game in its intended form.

Additional definitions of sportsmanship have been offered over the years, many of which have taken what Shields and Bredemeier referred to as a "bag of virtues" approach to the concept.[23] Approaches of this kind present sportsmanship as an aggregate of different values. In other words, all values should be taken into consideration. Although some values, such as honesty and fairness, on occasion may be emphasized more than others, a bag of virtues approach to good sportsmanship calls for a collective emphasis of all values and the dismissal of none. When it comes down to it, however, the care and conscientiousness displayed in acts that are considered sportsmanlike are demonstrations of respect. Clifford and Feezell present sportsmanship in terms of respect for opponents, officials, coaches, and teammates, as well as the game and its rules.[24] In this age of overzealous fans, one might add respect for fans to this list as well.

Most unsuitable actions are accounted for and prevented through the structure of the rules; therefore, if you follow the rules, you usually are behaving in a sportsmanlike manner. Instead of blatantly breaking rules, competitive people often look for ways to gain an advantage by bending or circumventing the rules in a way favorable to themselves or their team. If competitors were to naturally take it upon themselves to act under the guidance of the teleological theory, it would not be necessary to establish rules for the purpose of creating an environment of morally upstanding behavior. After all, rules that foster good moral behavior include a strong teleological base. To practice the moral value of beneficence, you would act kindly, which includes not fighting. Hence, a rule is in place that prohibits fighting. To adhere to the value of respect, you would not act disrespectfully, including humiliating opponents through taunting. Hence, a rule is in place that prohibits taunting. To practice the moral value of fairness, you would not act unfairly, including cheating. Hence, several rules are in place to prevent cheating. However, sports persons should take it upon themselves to practice good moral values with or without an established set of rules.

"Creating a Sportsmanship Environment"

The principal of a local middle school has charged the athletic director with creating sports teams in the athletic department that adhere to sportsmanship ideals. Never having formally studied sportsmanship, the young athletic director felt a bit lost and confused with the new task at hand and shouted out, "I am a good sport, and I know good sportsmanship when I see it, but how in the world am I supposed to create it in my athletic department?"

Questions
1. What general advice would you give to the athletic director?
2. If you were the athletic director, how might you utilize the teleological theory to create a sportsmanship environment?

Gamesmanship

Framing sportsmanship in terms of respect also fits well with an emphasis on excellence in sport. If excellence is to be achieved, it will not be by individuals using **gamesmanship** to throw opponents off of their game. The use of gamesmanship tactics are indicative of an athlete who is afraid to face a mentally focused opponent. The athlete who practices gamesmanship attempts to add another aspect to the game, or to develop a competition within the agreed-upon competition, all for the sake of improving his or her odds of winning. Examples of gamesmanship include faking an injury to get a timeout, and faking fouls to disqualify an opponent. You might attempt to determine whether or not an action is appropriate by asking yourself if it is an intended part of the game. In other words, would the founders of the game approve of such an action as a test of someone's skills or abilities? The answer would clearly be "no" in the above two examples.

> **gamesmanship:** looking for any way to possibly gain an advantage, even if doing so involves the art or practice of winning games by questionable means without actually violating or breaking the rules, yet violating the spirit of the rules.

"Obstructing the Passing Runner"

During a 1500-meter indoor track race, two runners, Jan and Shakira, had separated from the pack and were the only ones in contention for victory. As the gun sounded, signifying to the runners that there was just one lap to go, Jan was completely exhausted yet found a way to take a one-step lead in front of Shakira, who had plenty of energy remaining. Knowing that Shakira could easily pass her, Jan blocked Shakira from passing on every attempt. Try as she might, Shakira was unable to pass as Jan continually moved her body in front of Shakira during the final lap. Jan was officially declared the winner of the race as she crossed the finish line one-half step in front of Shakira. Following the race, Shakira told family members that she is a faster runner than Jan even though Jan crossed the finish line first.

Questions
1. Did the fastest runner win the race?
2. Would you consider Jan's behavior gamesmanship? Why or why not?
3. Did Jan achieve excellence in victory? Why or why not?

A somewhat humorous example of gamesmanship has, on occasion, been practiced in basketball. As an offensive team prepares to inbound the basketball from underneath their own basket, one of their players crouches down near the baseline on his or her hands and knees and barks like a dog. The bark distracts the defense for a split second as they look in the direction of the bark. As the defense is distracted, the player in-bounding the ball passes the ball to the offensive player who is standing nearest to the basket and scores just as the defense realizes what has happened to them. Inevitably when this act of gamesmanship takes place, fans of both teams get a chuckle out of it.

This example, however, demonstrates the need for one team to create a non–game-related distraction to gain an advantage. Defeating an opponent who has been mentally distracted through non-game-related factors does not demonstrate the level of excellence that defeating a focused opponent would display. Therefore, if you are devoted to the attainment of excellence within your sport, you would not use such tactics.

Winning by fooling the referees is another way of gaining an advantage through means other than direct game-related skills. When those involved in the game attempt to trick the referees into making or missing a call, they are relying on the officials to help gain an advantage instead of gaining it themselves based on such things as their talent, skill execution, and game preparations.

During the 1999 women's World Cup soccer competition, Briana Scurry blocked a penalty kick by deliberately jumping off the line, toward the kicker, to reduce the angle needed by the kicker to have the best chance of scoring. Afterward Scurry admitted that she stepped forward over the line on purpose, hoping that the official would not make the call against her even though she knew her action was against the rules.[25] In this case, Scurry gained an advantage by breaking a rule. She did so thinking that the official would probably not call this particular infraction—oftentimes officials ignore this rule—and hence would not be able to correct the unfair advantage gained by Scurry. As a result, the perception is that Scurry effectively succeeded in blocking a kick, when in fact the perceived success took place artificially. The game of soccer was intended to measure talent levels and abilities of players based on the established rules. When a player does not follow those rules or, in this case, deceives the official in a way that prevents him from maintaining a fair balance through the enforcement of the rules, the winner may not be the team or person that is the most skilled.

Wanting Excellence From One's Opponent

Competitors wanting to display excellence will sometimes do things that might actually help their opponents, to provide them with a stronger challenge rather than a weaker one. Examples of this are seen even at elite levels of competition.

At the 1936 Olympics Games in Berlin, Germany, the United States' Jesse Owens fouled on his first two attempts in the long jump. If Owens fouled once more he would be out of the competition. To assist him, German long jumper Lutz Long suggested that Owens remeasure his steps so he would begin his jump from 6 inches behind the take-off board. This tactical advice helped Owens to qualify with a clean jump. Owens then went on to win the long jump event on his way to winning four gold medals at the Berlin Games.[26] Examples of sportsmanship such as this one show how it is possible to respect one's opponents while pursuing excellence in sport.

"Forgotten Tennis Racket: To Give or Not to Give"

It is the finals of the high school national singles tennis tournament and Fiona Fling is pitted against the defending champion, Stephanie Stroke. In the midst of the excitement that comes with defending one's title, Stephanie has forgotten all three of her rackets that she always brings for tournament play. Although Stephanie could use one of the several rackets available in the clubhouse, ironically, Fiona has in her possession a practice racket identical to the type Stephanie uses. Fiona is aware of Stephanie's dilemma but is not sure whether or not to offer the racket to her.

Questions
1. If you were Fiona would you provide your identical racket to Stephanie? Explain your answer.
2. Would you want Stephanie to perform at her very best against you, and how might this affect your decision to provide her with your identical racket?
3. How important is it to you that your opponent—in this case Stephanie—achieves excellence during competition against you? Explain your answer.

Keeping Winning In Perspective

As demonstrated above, the strong emphasis on winning in sport only becomes problematic when winning's importance becomes overstated to the point that athletes, coaches, and administrators take on a win-at-all-cost attitude. Such an attitude leads to sayings like, "It doesn't matter *how* you win, just *that* you win." When this view is adopted, the goal of winning is no longer a goal of sport but a desire to which sports people become attached.

On occasion, this absolute desire to win has even turned ugly. Participants in the world of sport who are not satisfied in achieving excellence without winning have turned violent in their pursuit of winning at all costs. Tactics such as humiliating trash talking and mental and physical intimidation have also been used. Winning is an attractive thing. As stated earlier, we live in what Gough referred to as a "no-place-for-second-place" society, in which winners receive an unwarranted amount of credit and too great a share of the accolades, rewards, prize moneys, status, publicity, and endorsement opportunities.[13]

Examples abound of sports persons who receive unusually high amounts of credit for success and winning. The winning Super Bowl team receives monetary bonuses; Olympic champions win gold medals and often times lucrative financial endorsements follow. New York Yankees third baseman Alex Rodriguez's $1 million bonus that he received for winning the 2005 American League Major League Baseball's Most Valuable

Player (MVP) Award symbolizes the exorbitant awards that accompany winning.[27] The $1 million bonus in addition to Rodriguez's $252 million contract exemplifies the amount of money that organizations are willing to spend to win games.

Coaches periodically make adjustments and changes, but generally they coach in a very similar fashion from year to year. Interestingly though, when coaches have better players or their opponents are weaker, they receive tremendous accolades and are recognized as great coaches even though they are doing the same things as when they were losing. This is not to say that champions—players as well as coaches—do not

> **extrinsic rewards:** materialistic prizes or awards; that is, money, medals, and trophies, that are given in sport, usually for winning or outstanding performances.

deserve much of the accolades, but it is to say that when winning comes with so many **extrinsic rewards** it often becomes something that is desired over excellence. Extrinsic rewards that usually come in materialistic form, such as money and medals, can reinforce winning over excellence. Hence, sports people no longer care if they give up their ideals and values to win. Fairness and sportsmanship lose their importance in victory's shadow.

A problem exists with winning when you lose perspective of what it really is and how it is rightfully attained. Winning can only be rightfully attained when participants of the sport play fairly and by the rules. When the goal is to win no matter how it is achieved, winning becomes artificial and without genuine meaning.

So how can sports persons avoid this fate? As stated previously, sport is part of an environment that often encourages and reinforces winning and far too often winning at all costs. In addition, materialistic rewards are all too often incentives for those involved to win. Attempts by those interested in featuring excellent performances over winning certainly would be met with strong resistance by those who gain materially by winning. And the list of those gaining from such benefits is long: players, coaches, athletic administrators, parents, owners, corporations, and others. It is unlikely that NCAA officials, athletic directors, and corporate sponsors would support removing winning as the central focus of sport. That doesn't mean, however, that good moral behavior should not be practiced.

Good Moral Behavior In Sport

There are abundant examples of good moral behavior in sport, but those examples do not often get the high public exposure that immoral actions do. Examples of good moral actions that have taken place in sport include the swimmer who, after finishing second, swims across lane lines to congratulate the winner; the second place runners stating that they ran their best race and were defeated by a better athlete and were proud to finish second; or members of a team expected to win telling the media that they did their best and simply were defeated by a better team.

Additional examples of good moral behavior practiced by athletes and coaches include genuinely congratulating opponents with a handshake after the game, accepting officials' decisions without question, and acknowledging concern for an injured player by offering applause as they make their way from the field to the sideline. Even though these and more acts of good moral behavior generally are not feature stories in the media, it is important that those close to the game understand the necessity of reinforcing such good moral behavior. Hopefully, the reason that bad behavior is reported more often than good behavior is because bad behavior has not yet become the norm, which thus makes it more 'newsworthy.'

Moral Values and the Achievement of Excellence

Values such as fairness and sportsmanship should be cultivated to achieve moral excellence in addition to physical excellence in sport. This can be accomplished by focusing athletes' attention on the process of competition. If coaches explain the importance of values and their relationship to excellence, young athletes may be better able to understand the importance of values for themselves and their sports. The same understanding can be achieved in elite athletes through the reinforcement of moral values. Coaches and players must go further than explaining and understanding; they must *practice* moral values. A coach must exercise every opportunity to not only teach moral values, but also compliment and reward athletes for practicing good moral values.

For example, a basketball official may inadvertently call a foul but on a wrong, more talented player. Even though it might hurt her chances to win the game, an opposing player might point out the error to the official. In pointing out the error, the player is respecting the game in that she wants it to be played as fairly as possible and wants the achievement of excellence to determine the winner instead of an error that may provide an unearned advantage to her team.

Many athletes are at an age when fun and skill acquisition and development are important. Youths who participate in sport are especially impressionable to the words and actions of their coach. Coaches who overemphasize winning and underemphasize fair play and sportsmanship could be compromising young athletes' development as human beings. These coaches often play only their best or key players, rather than playing everyone on their roster and giving all players game experience. In more extreme cases, coaches break rules that specifically address the provision of equal playing time for youth. Coaches may be influenced by players, parents, fans, or become overcome by their own emotions and personal desires to win. All of these reasons may cause coaches to break rules that call for the equal participation from all their players.

According to Weinberg and Gould, coaches forget that their yelling, screaming, and use of sarcasm (behaviors that may be symptomatic of an overemphasis on winning) have negative psychological and emotional effects on athletes and may contribute to athletes losing self-esteem.[28] Even simply ignoring or giving only passing attention to 'benchwarmers' during practices sends a message that these players are not appreciated and that the coach has little confidence in them. Players—especially those at the youth level—are deserving of the opportunity to develop as human beings through sport experiences realized through participation. Equal participation can assist in this quest. In some cases, youth league administrators have assumed the responsibility of structuring their league rules in a way that requires coaches to provide all participants with playing time, regardless of talent levels.

There are additional ways in which coaches can cultivate and reinforce the importance of moral values in their players. Coaches should praise players who perform special roles in practice, such as emulating the strengths and tendencies of the opposition through the scout team; designating specific roles for non-starters or benchwarmers when they enter a game; continuing to coach when the outcome of the game has already been determined; and praising players who do not frequently receive playing time.

"Talent, But No Work Ethic"

Katrina is a benchwarmer, yet comes to practice on time every day, treats her teammates with respect, is willing to do the dirty work in practice, and patiently waits, without complaining, for an opportunity to play in a game. Britney, on the other hand, is a starter with an abundance of talent, frequently arrives late to practice, trash talks to her teammates, only wants to participate in scrimmage-related drills, and takes the fact that she is a starter for granted.

Questions
1. In the interest of achieving excellence, how would you manage this situation?
2. If you were the head coach, what specifically, if anything, would you do to encourage good moral behavior in Britney?
3. If you were the head coach, what specifically, if anything, would you do to discourage Britney's immoral behavior and foster her moral growth?

As youth increase in age and advance to higher participation levels, rules governing equal participation may no longer exist, but it does not mean that behaviors that foster the development of the participants as human beings should cease. Nor does it mean that the emphasis on achieving excellence and the adherence to strong values should cease. Coaches at all levels can influence and foster the growth of all of their athletes as human beings, starters as well as non-starters. Coaches should be aware of this fact and try to regularly provide substantive feedback to all of their athletes. Focusing on the improvement and character growth of their athletes can help coaches keep winning in perspective and even may be advantageous in the long run. Remember, not all athletes learn and can display strong skills immediately. If coaches help each athlete, a benchwarmer might develop into a starter or key reserve and could play an important role when a starter is injured. This frequently takes place at the youth level, but examples also exist at elite levels.

Ben Roethlisberger, a relatively unknown quarterback in college, completed an uncelebrated career at Miami of Ohio. Although Roethlisberger may not have been a household name, he was drafted by the National Football League (NFL) Pittsburgh Steelers. Roethlisberger's coaches worked with him and spent time helping him make the difficult transition from a low-profile college to the ultimate competitive football challenge, the NFL. In the end, the coaches' and Roethlisberger's efforts turned out to be valuable investments when Roethlisberger was called on to enter a game, replacing quarterback Tommy Maddux, who at the time sustained an injury. Spending the time with this 'no name' quarterback paid off, as Roethlisberger won his first game and continued to win, establishing the NFL record of 14 consecutive wins including a Super Bowl victory by a rookie quarterback in his first NFL season.[29]

In youth sport, where players often experience growth spurts and physical maturation at different stages, the potential for significant improvement over a short period of time is even greater than at the elite level. If taught the proper fundamentals and skills at a young age instead of being ignored, the benchwarmer who at a young age is at a lower physical maturation level than others could very well end up surpassing those who reached their level of maturity at younger ages. These successes, however, will be made more difficult if coaches spend all of their time teaching skills and providing performance-related feedback only to those youth who at the present time are the ones most athletically gifted. If coaches, in the moment, ignore participants that do not yet have the physical prowess, those participants will not be prepared to take advantage of their physical maturation if and when it does take place. They will lack the individual and game skills, as well as the confidence necessary to compliment their newly developed physical abilities, to achieve higher levels of success. Thus, by assisting all athletes' development, coaches are fulfilling their responsibilities to their athletes by helping them achieve the short- and long-term goals they set for themselves in their sport.

By emphasizing skill development, fun, and moral values like fairness and sportsmanship, coaches can help to put winning in its proper place and help athletes to focus on committing themselves to excellence in competition. For example, coaches can teach the skill of spiking in volleyball, and players can practice and perfect it to the point where spiking results in scoring in practices and games, which brings about an enjoyable sense of accomplishment. Organizations, teams, and players are well served if the practice of physical skill is balanced with the practice of moral values. When this is done, athletes will strive to win, but will not do so at the expense of their own moral integrity or the integrity of their sport.

Of concern, however, is that sport may not help develop character. When it comes to reasoning morally in sport, people often see only the goal of winning and fail to understand that sport is an activity that is dependent on values such as fairness, honesty, and respect for their moral status. Sports interests can be disrupted and overshadowed by the external environment. For example, it is in the interest of college football to foster clean competition, build individual character, and help provide healthy physical fitness levels for players. The external environment that surrounds major college football, however, can make these interests more difficult to achieve. The NCAA has created a post-season environment in college football that has an intense focus on winning. Millions of dollars are provided to teams that receive post-season bowl invitations, with the largest amount of money going to those teams that play in the elitist of the bowl games, the Bowl Championship Series (BCS). This money-driven external environment often helps create a situation that is at odds with building individual character.

The Good of the Game

Finally, it must be remembered that as evolving social constructions, sports cannot merely be defined in terms of their initial or traditional rule structures. The constitutive rules do frame the challenges that make particular sports what they are, but certain elements of them may be changed to improve sports. Unfortunately, many changes at the professional and major college level are made primarily to help attract fans and make greater profits. For example, in 1986 the three-point line was added in men's basketball largely to increase scoring and to provide an exciting offensive facet to the game of basketball. The excitement of the three-point shot continues today as college basketball enjoys large television audiences and in-person attendance. Sentiment has been expressed, however, that the line be moved back farther, as the three-point shot has gone from being used sparingly during its early years to monopolizing offenses during its later years. In other words, the three-point shot is now favored disproportionately over inside play.

Similarly, in hockey a series of rules changes were implemented to make the game more exciting and bring back fans after the NHL missed the entire 2004–2005 season due to a labor impasse. Those overseeing sports at this level tend to view 'the good of the game' as what is economically best for particular sports, without recognizing that sports have other interests that require maintenance and protection. These **internal goods** (the skills and strategies that make a sport a unique type of activity) are, to some extent, defined by the rules. However, internal goods are not just so many words in a rule book, but are real-world actions. There is some flexibility in how the skills and strategies of a sport may be manipulated, but there is also a point at which those who know the sport would say that a rule change is compromising a particular skill or strategy.

> **internal goods:** the skills and strategies, to some extent defined by rules, that make a sport a unique type of activity; that is, ensuring, through rules, a balance between offense and defense allowing for player talent and skill execution to determine the superior offense or defense.

Furthermore, those involved in changing rules must be aware of disrupting the balance between offense and defense. If a rule change is put in place to make the game more offensively exciting, making it nearly impossible for the defense to have a fair and equal chance in stopping the offense from scoring, the offensive play might be more exciting, but the excitement may soon diminish since scoring comes too easily. The fans may no longer respect scoring as an accomplishment resulting from excellent skill execution, but instead see it as a result of an advantage provided from a rule.

When the pitcher's mound is lowered in baseball, the skill of pitching or hitting might be compromised if it sways the balance between the two skills toward one or the other. The change should only be made to create a fair balance between hitting and pitching. In other words, hitters and pitchers of equal talent in their respective skill areas should have an equal chance of succeeding. If a rule change provides one with an advantage, the change is not made for the good of the game. Rule changes for the good of the game will create competitively equal environments and situations for offenses and defenses, and more broadly, will result in the game being played as its founders intended. Thus, it is necessary for rules committees and governing bodies to protect the elements that make a sport unique from changes that threaten its integrity.

It is sometimes necessary for those who are part of a sporting community to protect the internal goods of their sports. All those involved in sport have a responsibility to behave as caretakers of the game, including administrators, coaches, players, fans, and community members. They should all take it upon themselves to make sure the game does not deteriorate into an artificial replication of what was once a respected and solid product.

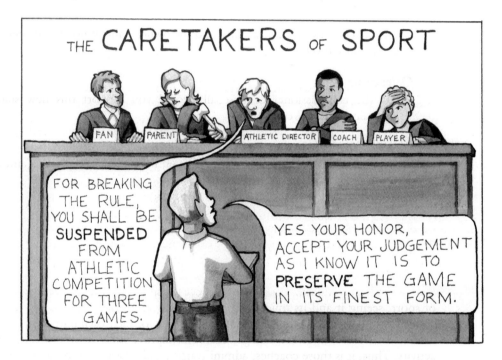

At the professional level, some of these individuals may make rule changes based on whether the changes increase interest in the sport and profits, not on whether they improve the sport as a test of skills. If rules committees are too focused on profits, this scenario becomes more likely. However, if the focus of the rules committee is to protect the sport and its primary challenges, then its members will avoid compromising them for money and recognition. In their attempt to change rules to draw more fans, rule makers/changers have to be careful not to disrupt the balance, in team sports, between offense and defense. If fences of baseball are moved in, making it easier to hit more home runs, fans may ultimately lose interest if the batter has an unfair advantage over the pitcher. Fans enjoy home runs, but they want a home run to be a meaningful accomplishment that results from a batter executing his skill more effectively than a pitcher executing his. Home runs are supposed to be reserved for those who execute perfectly. If you can hit a home run without executing the skill of hitting perfectly, the home run becomes less meaningful and fans could ultimately lose interest.

"The Short Baseball Fence"

Professional baseball's Butane Silver Birds are proposing a new stadium that will feature a home run fence that is on average 70 feet shorter than the typical professional field in the league. Silver Birds players want the fence because it will be a way for them to pad their home run statistics; fans also want this short fence because they enjoy the excitement that comes with home runs; and the owner wants it because he believes it will result in more revenue.

Questions
1. As the commissioner of baseball, would you support this new stadium? Explain your answer.
2. Are you concerned that the good of the game might be compromised by a much shorter fence? On what might such a concern be based?
3. As commissioner, what obligation do you have to meet the wants and needs of the players, fans, and owners?

The value of respect is important. If the governing body is one that holds respect for the sport and its unique history and excellence, its members will reason with the best interests of the sport in mind. Maintaining respect clearly plays an important role in protecting sport from those only interested in using it for their own gains or as a means to their own ends. Those with respect for sport view themselves as caretakers of sport, seeing it and its uniqueness as being invaluable as an end in and of itself. Caretakers of the game do not set out to use sport for their own purposes; they protect it and allow only those changes that will improve it as its own unique kind of activity. Thus, it is those coaches, administrators, and players who place winning and its accompanying extrinsic rewards in perspective who are best able to focus on the good of the game and be strong caretakers of the sports they represent.

Conclusion

As demonstrated in this chapter, sports are unique activities in which rules, conventions, and moral values and actions all play a role in determining what is morally acceptable and unacceptable behavior. By emphasizing values such as fair play, sportsmanship, and respect, as well as defining excellence in sport and the good of the game, athletes, coaches, and administrators can improve the moral environment of their sports. When improving the moral environment, these individuals not only help to keep winning in perspective, but also establish themselves as members of sporting communities and caretakers of their sports. Thus, we see that moral reasoning can help individuals recognize their responsibilities to their sport and to others who participate in it and enjoy it, and help motivate them to act on these responsibilities to morally strengthen their sport.

References

1. Suits B. The elements of sport. In: Osterhoudt RG, ed. *The Philosophy of Sport: A Collection of Original Essays.* Springfield, IL: Charles C. Thomas Publisher; 1973:48–64.
2. Suits B. *The Grasshopper: Games, Life and Utopia.* Toronto: University of Toronto Press; 1978.
3. Morgan WJ. *Leftist Theories of Sport: A Critique and Reconstruction.* Chicago, IL: University of Illinois Press; 1994.
4. Torres CR. What counts as part of a game? A look at skills. *Journal of the Philosophy of Sport.* 2000;27(1):81–92.
5. Kretchmar RS. A functionalist analysis of game acts: Revisiting Searle. *The International Association for the Philosophy of Sport.* 2001;28(2):160–172.
6. Coakley J. *Sport In Society: Issues and Controversies.* 8th ed. New York: McGraw-Hill; 2004.
7. Whiteley J. College football in the South: Don't forget to deck out the dog. *Christian Science Monitor.* 2000;93(18):14.
8. D'Agostino F. The ethos of games. *Journal of the Philosophy of Sport.* 1981;8:7–18.
9. Roberts A. WHO, ME? Notre Dame has great coach, great man. December 12, 2005. *The Ball State Daily News* website. Available at http://media.www.bsudailynews.com/media/storage/paper849/news/2005/12/12/Opinion/Who-Menotre.Dame.Has.Great.Coach.Great.Man-1308247.shtml. Accessed March 13, 2007.
10. Delattre EJ. Some reflections on success and failure in competitive athletics. *Journal of the Philosophy of Sport.* 1975;2:133–139.
11. Gould D. Are high school sports good for kids? College of Education, Michigan State University Department of Kinesiology. *Institute for the Study of Youth Sport* website. Available at: http://ed-web3.educ.msu.edu/ysi/coaches/FAQ/askexperts2.htm. Accessed March 19, 2007.
12. ESPN. Almonte, Bronx team records wiped away; August 31, 2001. *ESPN* website. Available at http://espn.go.com/moresports/llws01/s/2001/0831/1246234.html. Accessed March 13, 2007.
13. Gough RW. *Character Is Everything: Promoting Ethical Excellence In Sports.* Fort Worth, TX: Harcourt Brace College Publishers; 1997.
14. USA Gymnastics. Favorite Olympic memories: Mary Lou Retton. *USA Gymnastics* website. Available at http://www.usa-gymnasticsolympics.com/2004/history/rettonmemory.html. Accessed March 14, 2007.
15. Bar-Eli M, Tenenbaum G, Pie JS, et al. Aerobic performance under different goal orientations and different goal conditions. *Journal of Sport Behavior.* 1997;20(1):3–15.

16. Yun Dai D. To be or not to be (challenged), that is the question: Task and ego orientations among high-ability, high-achieving adolescents. *Journal of Experimental Education*. 2000;68:311–331.

17. Walton B. Good sportsmanship is losing out to winning. *USA Today* website. Available at: http://www.usatoday.com/news/opinion/editorials/2005-12-20-walton-edit_x.htm. Accessed February 20, 2008.

18. Buckley S. Gillooly pleads guilty, says Harding approved plot; February 2, 1994. *Washington Post* website. Available at: http://www.washingtonpost.com/wp-srv/sports/longterm/olympics1998/history/timeline/articles/time_020294.htm. Accessed March 11, 2007.

19. Globe Staff. Rosie Ruiz pulls the ultimate prank; April 21, 1980. *Boston.Com Sports* website. Available at: http://graphics.boston.com/marathon/history/1980.shtml. Accessed February 18, 2008.

20. Associated Press. Buehrle accuses Rangers hitters of cheating. *ESPN* website. Available at http://sports.espn.go.com/mlb/news/story?id=2147225. Accessed: March 11, 2007.

21. Associated Press. Wie's disqualification put in motion by reporter. *ESPN* website. Available at http://sports.espn.go.com/golf/news/story?id=2193534. Accessed: March 11, 2007.

22. Drew SB. *Why Sport? An Introduction to the Philosophy of Sport*. Toronto: Thompson Educational Publishing, Inc.; 2003.

23. Shields DLL, Bredemeier BJL. *Character Development and Physical Activity*. Champaign, IL: Human Kinetics; 1995.

24. Clifford C, Feezell RM. *Coaching For Character*. Champaign, IL: Human Kinetics; 1997.

25. CNNSI. Scurry admits she stepped forward; July 14, 1999. *CSN/SI* website. Available at http://sportsillustrated.cnn.com/soccer/world/1999/womens_worldcup/news/1999/07/13/scurry_penalty_ap/. Accessed March 14, 2007.

26. Owens J, Neimark P. *Jesse: A Spiritual Autobiography*. Plainfield, NJ: Logos International; 1978.

27. CBC Sports. Alex Rodriguez wins AL MVP; November 15, 2005. *Canadian Broadcaster Centre* website. Available at: http://www.cbc.ca/sports/story/2005/11/14/al_mvp051114.html. Accessed March 14, 2007.

28. Weinberg RS, Gould D. *Foundations of Sport and Exercise Psychology*. 3rd ed. Champaign, IL: Human Kinetics; 2003.

29. Bell J. Roethlisberger, defending Super Bowl champs Steelers stumble to 1–3 start; October 12, 2006. *USA Today* website. Available at: http://www.usatoday.com/sports/football/nfl/steelers/2006-10-12-steelers-cover-x.htm?POE=SPOISVA. Accessed March 14, 2007.

The Mission of High School Athletics

Coach Moore arrived at school early one spring morning to prepare to teach her mathematics classes. Her Morris County High School Spartans had just completed a lackluster 3–12 basketball season in which they failed to live up to expectations. Coach Moore took over the traditionally weak women's program two years ago, and her players loved her. While she was strict with them, she always gave them motivating constructive criticism that would help them improve their skills and their teamwork. While the team was a cohesive unit and showed marked improvement in practice over the two-year period, it had yet to find success in competition. Although somewhat disappointed, Coach Moore remained optimistic and believed in a few years her program would grow to be a successful one.

As Coach Moore was organizing her lessons for the day, Pam, her athletic director, stopped by her office. Looking very serious, she asked if Coach Moore had a few minutes to talk. The two sat down and Pam started talking about the season that had just passed. She conveyed her dissatisfaction regarding the team's performance, and said that Coach Moore's job could be in jeopardy if she did not improve the team's record, significantly, by the next year.

Coach Moore was stunned and asked Pam to evaluate her performance as a coach. She wanted to know how she could improve what she was doing and what adjustments to make for the following year. Pam proceeded to praise her hard work and dedication to the kids and to the program. She had noted the improvements in individual and team skill level and the strong cohesion the team displayed. Pam also had no major complaints about the behavior of the athletes or the work that Coach Moore had done. But the record was still not good enough.

Since it was nearing time for class, Coach Moore had to excuse herself from the conversation to go teach. The two agreed to meet later that afternoon to continue the discussion. On the way to class, Coach Moore could not stop thinking about her dilemma. "How am I supposed to improve on what I am doing if I do not receive constructive feedback concerning my performance as a coach?" she thought.

As she returned to her office, Pam was thinking the very same thing. She really had no issues with Coach Moore's work, just her basketball team's record. "Maybe I shouldn't be so worried about the record," Pam thought. "Coach Moore is an excellent teacher of skills and the girls really appreciate her. But the administration of the school says we need to win to receive more media coverage. What should our focus be as an athletics program?"

Critical Thinking: Finding Common-Sense Solutions

1. What should be the mission of high school interscholastic athletics programs?

2. As an athletic director, what advice can you give to coaches who are doing their job well but are not winning? How can you help them become more successful?

> **Critical Thinking: Moral Theory-Based Decision Making**
> **3.** Using teleological ethical theory, describe an ideal mission of high school sports.
>
> **4.** Should high school coaches be fired if their programs are unsuccessful? Justify your answer through principles of moral reasoning.

Key Terms

alternative logic—in sport, the purposeful establishment of an inefficient environment, including the placement of obstacles to overcome, in the way of its participants (alternative to arranging the environment in a way to make achieving the task and/or reaching the goal more efficient).

artificial apology—insincere repentance; disingenuous remorse; dishonest regret.

cheating—intentionally breaking rules; to deceive.

circumvention of rules—not blatantly breaking rules but strategically going around them.

constitutive rules—regulations that establish the skills and strategies of the game, impose strict restrictions on specific actions and procedures of the game, and indicate the game objectives and the means by which they may and may not be pursued.

conventional logic—the normal tendency of making the necessary arrangements to bring tasks to closure in the most efficient way.

cultures—environments that are distinguished from one another based on the differences between various groups and societies; sports and acceptable actions within sport vary from culture to culture; that is, some cultures might quietly accept certain rule breaking in the interest of winning whereas others might not.

ego orientation—competition that is driven by winning and defeating others.

ethos—unique character of a group or social context (i.e., sport), usually expressed in attitudes, habits, and beliefs.

excellence—of the highest quality; fineness; performing in sport in a superior fashion.

extrinsic rewards—materialistic prizes or awards; that is, money, medals, and trophies, that are given in sport, usually for winning or outstanding performances.

fairness (moral value)—just; impartial; straightforward justice; being objective.

gamesmanship—looking for any way to possibly gain an advantage, even if doing so involves the art or practice of winning games by questionable means without actually violating or breaking the rules, yet violating the spirit of the rules.

illegal tactics—strategies employed or practiced that are against the rules.

internal goods—the skills and strategies, to some extent defined by rules, that make a sport a unique type of activity; that is, ensuring, through rules, a balance between offense and defense allowing for player talent and skill execution to determine the superior offense or defense.

mediocrity—neither good nor bad; second rate; a mediocre sport performance is an average performance.

morally upright—ethically respectable and/or honorable.

pride in the product—being satisfied with a specific outcome, result, or achievement.

pride in winning—having feelings of self-respect when having obtained victory through excellence (pride in winning does not exist when victory takes place by cheating).

process of competition—course of actions taken when striving against others to win contests.

punitive action—inflicting a penalty; in sport, when a person breaks a rule, an authoritative person or body can penalize them.

respect for the opposition—treating opponents with honor; being reverent toward opponents.

rule-governed tests—competitive sport; the fact that competitive sport is governed by standardized rules for all participants allows for meaningful outcomes and comparisons to take place.

sportsmanship—putting moral standards ahead of strategic achievement in sport; adhering to the spirit of the rules even when doing so may result in strategic loss; respect for the rules, people, and conventions related to sport.

3 Moral Education and Development Through Sport

Learning Outcomes

After reading Chapter 3, the student will be able to:

1. Create arguments for and against sport as a positive character builder.

2. Describe both positive and negative aspects of sport and its impact on academic achievement and self-identity.

3. Identify and explain how particular outside influences have a deteriorating effect on the good moral standing of sport.

4. Name and describe differences between positive and negative role models in sport.

5. Identify and explain the similarities between an American capitalistic society and sports competition.

6. Identify and explain the moral potential of sport.

"Sport builds character!" This old saying is one that still strongly influences people today, as evidenced by the increasing number of children who participate in youth sport leagues across the United States. There is still a belief that sport is an educationally important and developmentally valuable activity for children. According to Rudd, generally when an athlete or team is believed to have displayed character, the word "character" is associated loyalty (social value): being faithful/devoted to a person, ideal, or custom.

perseverance (social value): persisting; not giving in.

work ethic (social value): a disciplined effort of labor; for example, in sport, working on a skill daily, without exception.

moral character: the evaluation of the moral quality of a person based on his or her practice and demonstration of moral values, or lack thereof, such as honesty, fairness, and responsibility.

social character: the evaluation of the social quality of a person based on his or her practice and demonstration of social values, or lack thereof, such as teamwork, loyalty, self-sacrifice, work ethic, and perseverance.

moral responsibility: an obligation to do the right thing; a duty to behave in an ethically good manner; for example, the notion that elite athletes have a moral responsibility to be positive role models.

role model: someone who serves as an example; in sport, athletes who are looked up to.

with a host of moral and social values such as teamwork, **loyalty,** self-sacrifice, **perseverance, work ethic,** and mental toughness.[1]

There is a distinction to be made between **moral character** and **social character,** however. Rudd and Stoll point out that character development literature, newspapers, media, and personal communication with coaches, parents, and the general populace defines character from a social rather than a moral perspective.[2] Social character is denoted by such social values as team work, loyalty, self-sacrifice, work ethic, and perseverance, as opposed to moral character, which is denoted by such moral values as honesty, fairness, and responsibility.[2] An argument can be made that experiencing these values in the form of memorable sport lessons may help children develop into morally and socially responsible individuals.

In this chapter we will examine the ways in which sport can help build and influence character development, and whether or not a focus on competition is detrimental to good character building. Whether or not the elite athlete has a **moral responsibility** to be a **role model** for young athletes, and whether young athletes should view elite athletes as heroes or role models also will be discussed. The pros and cons of competition will be examined, along with a discussion on how those in sport can help to actualize the moral and social value of competitive sports and athletics.

Sport and Character Building

Character Building and Positive Outcomes of Sport

In *Character Development and Physical Activity*, Shields and Bredemeier noted that sport's reputation as a strong builder of positive character and teacher of positive values is not clearly evidenced in the literature.[3] Sport does, however, have some positive qualities. According to Seefeldt and Ewing, sport participation has been shown to decrease the likelihood of delinquency in young adults.[4] And in a study conducted by Kirkcaldy et al., a strong association was found between participation in sports and the type of personality that tends to be resistant to drug and alcohol addiction.[5] Evidence that indicates sport's capacity to build character is important, since so many young people are drawn to particular sports.

Anecdotal examples exist as to how values learned through sport might be carried over to the workplace. For example, the discipline required to attend practice can be applied to arriving to work on time. Leadership required to 'go the extra mile' in preseason conditioning can be applied to the need to motivate others at work to achieve a company sales goal. Sportsmanship fostered from shaking hands with the opposing player or team can be carried over to the workplace when an employee gracefully accepts not being promoted. And fair play practiced in sport by not cheating can be implemented at work when completing employee performance appraisals fairly and without personal bias.

Although the transfer of sporting behavior to off-field life has not been empirically substantiated to date, through their observations of sport and their direct dealings with athletes, coaches commonly make the claim that sport does build character. Legendary UCLA men's basketball coach John Wooden addressed the importance of character and what character does for an individual with the following statement: "Ability may get you to the top, but it takes character to keep you there."[6(p199)] Wooden further elaborated, "Be more concerned with your character than your reputation, because your reputation is what people may think of you, while your character is who you really are."[6(p199)]

From an educational perspective, a compelling argument sometimes made to justify and attract funding for sport programs is the one claiming that sport builds character.

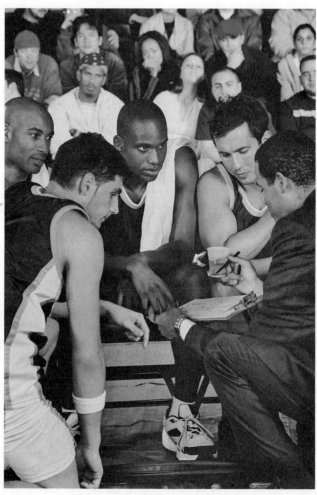

3-1 *Coaches commonly make the claim that sport builds character in participants.*

It is not unusual for educational institutions to have a mission statement that includes character development in students. If sport participation is perceived to enhance character development in students, sport will then be recognized as an entity that fits with the educational mission. When coaches, athletic directors, and other athletic personnel convince—empirically or anecdotally—board members, boosters, and other decision-making administrators that sport does in fact build character, sport programs likely will be looked upon more favorably and supported.

Negative Outcomes of Sport

There are those who would argue that sport participation is not an educationally valuable experience for children that cultivates moral values. Situations in which athletes, coaches, and administrators behave badly often support that belief. For example, instances of **trash talking** and verbally disrespecting opponents have always existed, but seem to be on the increase. Veteran National Football League (NFL) football player and 2006 Super Bowl participant Chris Gray of the Seattle Seahawks has first-hand experience with the propensity for trash talking in the NFL. Earlier in Gray's career when he played for Miami, he was the recipient of trash talking from defensive lineman John Randle. Knowing that Gray was from the South, throughout the game Randle referred to him as David Duke, the former Ku Klux Klan leader. Gray then informed Randle that he was a Christian, at which time Randle started to call him the "Christian Boy."

> **trash talking:** verbal chatter; trash talking is usually delivered during a game or practice, usually directed at an opponent for the purpose of gaining an advantage by attempting to make an opponent mentally weak or by mentally strengthening/motivating oneself.

Players are not the only ones who at times display a lack of good moral behavior. Coaches occasionally teach athletes illegal tactics and break recruiting rules designed to maintain fairness in competition. For example, during the 2003 season, the University of Washington men's basketball program was placed on probation for both gambling and recruiting violations. The gambling violations included auctions involving the men's basketball championships in which groups of individuals, including the former head coach, bid on several teams in the tournament, a violation of National Collegiate Athletic Association (NCAA) rules. The recruiting violations included the continued use of a yacht to transport recruits even after the NCAA informed the university that such behavior could be a violation of NCAA rules.[7]

Administrators display poor moral values when they tolerate and utilize discriminatory hiring practices. An NFL hiring policy was created that requires interviewing at least one minority for head coaching positions, but accusations of discriminatory hiring are still made. To help prevent such discrimination at the collegiate level, offices of affirmative action throughout American colleges and universities are required to implement fair hiring practices. Despite affirmative action hiring procedures, administrators sometimes circumvent them to hire friends.

Fans also display a lack of moral values at times, such as during the 2003 French Open when the crowd behaved inappropriately toward Serena Williams. After a linesman did not call a ball out and Serena stopped play to point to the spot where the ball landed, the crowd reacted negatively, an inappropriate behavior by tennis spectators.[8]

Appropriate behavior does not allow for verbally displaying biases for or against those participating in the sport.

Effect of Sport on Academic Achievement

Sports are meaningful to young people; they are activities in which young people can excel when, perhaps, they are not excelling or enjoying academic subjects. In some cases, sports can spur individuals to work harder on academics and stay in school when they might otherwise have quit. Eccles et al. found team sports to be a promotive factor for academic outcomes.[9] Athletic departments have instituted athletic eligibility policies that require students who participate in athletics to perform at predetermined levels of academic acceptability. If they do not perform to these levels, students are not allowed to participate in sports. These sport eligibility requirements often motivate students who participate in school sports to do well academically and, in some cases, to stay in school. The enhancement of academic achievement makes for a more educated individual, which is good for society.

According to Eccles et al., participation in sports can facilitate connections in the school context that satisfy adolescents' developmental needs for social relatedness and competence.[9] They also suggested that sport participation often leads to not only better academic achievement and reduced likelihood of dropping out, but also higher education aspirations.[9] Yin and Moore also found that drop-out rates were significantly lower for athletes.[10] Note, however, that sport may not have a positive effect on academic achievement. Results of a study by Din[11] indicated that no significant differences were found between rural high school students' grades during the pre-sport season and the post-sport season, which suggests that participation in school-sponsored sports activities does not necessarily have a positive academic effect. Plausible additional reasons exist to support this view. Probably the most obvious reason is that the amount of time required for school athletics takes away time spent on academics; that is, practices and games require several hours per week that could instead be spent on studying.

Sport as a Means of Enhancing Self-Identity

Yin and Moore also found that participation in interscholastic sports is positively related to self-concept during early adolescence.[10] Young people look to sport as a means to create an identity for themselves; making a team and belonging to a team are ways to prove they are part of something good. Students who play on a sports team are viewed as having athletic talent by mere virtue of the fact that they 'made the team.' This positive outside perception enhances self-identity.

Bluechardt et al. also studied how sport affects self-image and found that participation in school athletics programs can have a positive, immediate effect on self-image during the adolescent years, particularly if the activity is a team sport.[12] Kirkcaldy et al. showed that 9th and 10th grade students who "frequently" participated in sports displayed significantly higher self-images than those who "never or seldom" participated in sport and physical activity.[5] Thus, as adolescents go through a period of trying to determine who they are and how they fit in with society, their participation in sport can provide them with a sense of self.

Sport can also provide participants with a general sense of security. Being part of a team that has scheduled practices, games, and training sessions throughout the year provides participants with a sense of stability that is often difficult to come by during adolescence. In a study examining the effects of sport participation on adolescent self-image, Kirkcaldy et al. found the association between sport participation and self-image to be substantial and highly significant statistically.[5]

Steiner et al. suggest that athletic participation has distress buffering properties.[13] In a stress-filled society in which short-term relief often is found in the form of prescribed or over-the-counter medication, athletic participation is a healthy alternative. Certainly a stress-free, healthy individual would be more likely to make better overall and ethical decisions than would a stressed, unhealthy individual. Oftentimes bad decisions are made when a person is under high levels of stress. If participation in sport can relieve such pressures, those who participate may be more likely to make overall good decisions.

In a broadly generalizable study conducted by Marsh and Kleitman from the National Education Longitudinal Study (NELS) data set, athletic participation was shown to benefit most of the diverse grade 12 and postsecondary outcomes that were used to represent the effects of schooling.[14] These outcomes were school grades, coursework selection, homework, educational and parental aspirations, self-esteem, number of university applications, subsequent college enrollment, educational and occupational aspirations, and highest educational level. If the benefits are as numerous as Marsh and Kleitman claim, then sport truly is a worthy enterprise. One can, without hesitation, profess sport to be a valuable undertaking if it truly has a positive effect on its participants' academic and professional success.

"Running Track is Good for Me"

Sitting in homeroom waiting for the bell to ring, Teri told a classmate seated beside her, "You know, if I were not a fast runner for the track team, I would not be good at anything and I would not have any friends. To tell you the truth, I probably would not even come to school. The only reason I did my stupid homework last night was because Coach Proper told me if I didn't do it, she wouldn't let me play. Coach Proper also told me that I am fast enough without taking drugs and that she'd kick me off the team for cheating if she learned that I was taking them."

Questions
1. Is this scenario realistic in the real world? Why or why not? If it is, recount a similar real-world scenario.
2. Do you think the positive effects resulting from Teri's sport experiences are commonplace in the world of sport? Explain your answer.
3. Do you believe Coach Proper positively influenced Teri's academic achievement, self-esteem, and value system? If so, how?

Sport Participation and Development of Character

As Coakley points out, research on sport and character development shows that not all sport experiences help every participant build positive character.[15] Moral values such as fairness, **responsibility,** and honesty enhance moral character development. Social values, on the other hand, enhance social character development and include teamwork, loyalty, self-sacrifice, work ethic, and perseverance. But a child who participates in sport does not simply absorb moral and social values often attributed to competitive athletics. Put another way, sport does not necessarily instill positive moral and social values in its participants. And before a legitimate conversation can take place supporting the view that sport builds character, the evidence must show this. Coaches, athletic directors, and even parents commonly speak to the positive character building that takes place, but the evidence supporting these claims is far from conclusive and cannot be generalized to all sport participants.

> **responsibility (moral value):** duty, obligation. ✔

For example, a study by Eccles et al. found that sport participation was linked to increased alcohol use.[9] Alcohol consumption is negatively associated with sport participation, but it's not the only negative association. At some point, those who participate likely are exposed to negative sport-related experiences such as **hazing,** verbal abuse, circumventing rules to gain an advantage, cheating, and humiliating trash talking. The question to ask is, are these negative experiences a direct result of sport participation or do particular individuals involved in sport have negative behaviors that are revealed through sport? It could be argued that certain negatives behaviors are specific to individuals and will always be exhibited through various mediums, including sport, school, home life, or work.

> **hazing:** any activity expected of someone joining a group (or to maintain full status in a group) that humiliates, degrades, or risks emotional and/or physical harm, regardless of the person's willingness to participate.

Research cited by Shields and Bredemeier[3] found no strong relationship between sport participation and prosocial behavior. In fact, you do not have to look beyond a newspaper's sports page or ESPN's Sports Center to learn about athletes behaving badly. It is true that you cannot link an individual's inappropriate behavior to athletics simply because they participate in sport; but if athletes are found to consistently behave inappropriately, it does become difficult to establish a strong argument that sport participation influences good social behavior.

Does this mean sport has no educational value for those who take part? Does it mean that sport does not teach unique values or teach values more effectively than other activities in which children become involved? Involvement in sport does not automatically infuse good moral habits in its participants, although participants may learn moral habits more effectively through sport than through other activities. Those who oversee and participate in sport must commit themselves to creating a sporting environment conducive to moral values. Players, coaches, athletic directors, league commissioners, and even fans must dedicate themselves to the goal of utilizing sport as a vehicle to foster moral values.

Despite the element of competition that sometimes impedes progress in the area of ethics, an emphasis on moral values must be a high priority for sports-related people. More specifically, players can treat opposing players with respect by competing hard and not engaging in trash talking as a way to humiliate an opponent. Coaches can positively reinforce good moral behavior in athletes. Athletic directors can reward players and coaches alike with end-of-the-year sportsmanship awards. League commissioners can take a serious, no-nonsense approach to enforcing rules that prevent poor ethical behavior such as fighting and dirty play. Fans can behave respectfully to officials, opposing fans, coaches, and players when attending games.

Potential Moral Value Loss Through Sport Participation

According to research by Lumpkin et al., the longer a person is in sport, the more **morally callused** they become, that is, the less respect they show for opponents, officials, coaches, and teammates.[16] If this assertion is true, it would seem that youth sport participants are probably behaving in line with the highest of ethical standards, and, arguably, professional athletes are the least in tune with ethical standards. Even though youth athletics on many occasions is overly competitive, there does seem to be a refreshing element of respect involved. In some cases, prior to competition, players read a sportsmanship creed and then during competition adhere to the creed. There is often an emphasis on social aspects of the game, such as complimentary food for all participants afterward, not keeping score, and equal playing time for all participants.

> **morally callused:** having become hardened to doing the right thing; the consideration that the longer a person is in sport, the less regard he or she has for the adherence to moral values in the sporting environment.

Respect and general sportsmanship often seem to diminish as age and talent level increase, however. For example, at the most elite levels such as professional and Olympic sport, the respect for fellow competitors might be emphasized to a lesser extent than at lower levels since winning is so important. Super Bowl, Final Four, Stanley Cup, World Series, and Olympic competitors, for the most part, are interested mostly in winning. As discussed in Chapter 1, Shields and Bredemeier put forth that the context of sport has a "bracketed morality," which allows athletes more latitude for **egoistic reasoning** and self-interested action.[3] However, this does not give athletes, coaches, and administrators the right to ignore the interests of others or the interests of the sport.

> **egoistic reasoning:** using logical thought for the purpose of one's own interests.

The context of sport can play a role in fostering unsportsmanlike thinking and behavior. According to Jones and McNamee, it has been argued that sport participation contributes to, detracts from, or is neutral when it comes to fostering certain valued traits and dispositions in its participants.[17] They concluded that participation in sport is often accompanied by less mature moral reasoning, which reflects the self-interested nature of the activity.[17] When discussing dangerous sport, Russell indicated that criminal-like behavior, plain and utter recklessness, or poor judgment are not judged or constrained by the normal conventions or inhibitions of ordinary life.[18] For example, punching someone in a hockey game results in a penalty, but punching someone in the workplace (i.e., outside of sport) may result in assault charges.

There is a near dearth of cases in which criminal charges have been filed for acts of violence that have taken place during sporting contests. In essence, sport participants are allowed to behave in violent ways that would be considered inappropriate, unacceptable, and illegal in mainstream society. Fighting serves as a common example of illegal behavior that is acceptable in hockey and commonly takes place in the other three major sports—football, basketball, and baseball. At this level of play, you would likely have a difficult time making the argument that allowing and/or encouraging fighting is conducive to moral character development.

Possibly the most famous case of a criminal act in sport that did not result in criminal punishment was the Latrell Sprewell and P.J. Carlesimo choking incident in the National Basketball Association (NBA) in 1997. After a practice session, Sprewell, a player for the NBA's Golden State Warriors, physically grabbed his coach, P.J. Carlesimo, around the neck and chocked him until players restrained Sprewell. Had this same incident taken place in a non-sport environment, such as the corporate world, Sprewell would have been fired and maybe even sentenced to jail time if convicted of assault. In 2007, Chris Simon of the New York Islanders was suspended for a league-record 25 games for a vicious on-ice, two-handed stick attack to the face of Ryan Hollweg of the rival New York Rangers. Factoring into the decision not to criminally prosecute Simon was the fact that Hollweg did not express an interest in doing so.[19]

"Never Back Down From a Fight"

As usual, after arriving home from his eighth grade basketball practice, Josh immediately went to the computer to check his e-mail. Josh's mother, who was in the kitchen preparing dinner, leaned over the counter and asked Josh, "What did you learn in practice today?" Still concentrating on his e-mail, Josh replied, "Coach told us never to back down from a fight." Josh's mom, unsure if she heard Josh correctly, asked, "Did you say that your coach told you never to back down from a fight?" Josh, slightly annoyed, replied, "Yes, Mom, Coach told us that if we were ever challenged in a game or practice, we should 'punch the person out' before they 'punched us out.'" Disturbed by what she was hearing, Josh's mother replied, "I will have none of this; I am calling the principal immediately to stop this teaching of bad character." Upset at his mother's reaction, Josh pleaded, "Please Mom, don't call the principal. When it gets back to Coach that I'm the reason, Coach will no longer start me and he might even lose his job. Besides, it's important that we learn to stick up for ourselves through fighting."

Questions
1. Do you think Josh's mother was correct in intervening by calling the principal? Explain your answer.
2. In this case, do you believe teaching Josh to never back down from a fight is a positive character trait or a negative character trait? Explain your answer.
3. As a result of Josh's coach teaching him to never back down from a fight, will Josh be better prepared for life after sport? Explain your answer.

Sport as a Different Type of Venue for Demonstrating Moral Behavior

Sport is a unique environment in that the behavior of its participants and spectators is out in the open for the public to see and comment on. If a participant breaks a rule, the infraction may be seen by parents, friends, and members of the community. Because sporting events take place on a public stage, and very often are televised, the public openly scrutinizes those involved. Fans voice their opinions throughout their communities in response to print and broadcast media reports and coverage, including the subplots that often include on- and off-court behaviors of players. If players or coaches act unethically, their actions will be observed and reported both informally and formally.

You would think that being on a public stage would be a deterrent to unethical behavior, but in a win-driven society that is not always the case. During the 1980s, Bill Laimbeer of the Detroit Pistons may have been the roughest team member of the physically aggressive Pistons. Public perception of Laimbeer was conflicting, in that some people saw him as a tough, hard-nosed player, while others saw him as a dirty, unethical player. This example is indicative of society's conflicting perspective on acceptable ethical behavior in sport that plays out in the limelight. Public opinion of Bill Laimbeer could be formed because as an NBA player he was on display during games.

Being on public display does not mean that sport is a teacher of good or bad values, however; it simply indicates that the values and character of athletes, both good and bad, are on constant display. In other areas of life, such as in corporate America, most employees are unknown outside of the workplace and therefore escape public criticism and scrutiny. Employees at a brokerage firm, construction company, or automobile manufacturing plant do not open themselves up for criticism by exposing themselves to the general public during their workday. This is not to say that there aren't unethical employees in non-sport entities. More often than not, however, non-sport entities are free from large-scale public criticism because their day-to-day work and behavior is largely private. Criticisms of individuals in most non–sport-related enterprises are limited to their direct supervisors, who have a vested interest in quality performances.

Moral Issues in Sport

Unfair Advantage Seeking

Previous discussion addressed the importance of keeping winning in perspective and not allowing the desire to win to assume such importance that it overshadows other moral values. When the goal of winning becomes all-consuming, sport runs the risk of de-emphasizing the importance of other moral values. For instance, athletes, coaches, and administrators might dismiss sportsmanship in the interest of winning. Winning can be overemphasized to the point that the inherent spirit of sport itself is imperiled.

In the past few years, several NCAA rules in college athletics have been broken. A coach paid tuition for players and tried to conceal it. Coaches provided meals, transportation, lodging, and clothes to athletes. A football coach took part in impermissible pools, gambling on the NCAA men's basketball tournament. An athletic department booster provided recruits with and undercharged them for boat rides, which is against NCAA rules. A basketball coach was photographed partying and drinking with college students from the opposing team the night after a game. Another basketball team was banned from a conference tournament for using an ineligible player. Allegations of academic fraud led to one former statistician admitting to delivering and being paid for 17 pieces of coursework for three players in 2000.[20]

Most of these actions are infractions of NCAA rules, but they are not uncommon in intercollegiate sports. Other violations include providing money to a prospect in an effort to persuade them to play for a university; making arrangements for a prospect to meet with an NBA coach; giving tickets to sports agents who have illegally cultivated business relationships with players; and coaches making impermissible recruiting contacts both inperson and with phone calls.

Condoning Violence and Overly Aggressive Play

Intimidating violence during play is accepted by some football and hockey coaches, who pass the behavior along to players. Pain-inflicting hits are praised by fans, coaches, and even sport administrators. To reinforce hard hits, coaches verbally praise those who hit the hardest and 'reward' them with such things as decals for helmets and cash payments. In football and hockey, hitting as a way to perform a game-related task is generally understood to be not enough; players are expected to deliver a pain-inflicting blow in a physically punishing way to make opponents lose their concentration, execute poorly, or sustain serious injury.

Allowing overly aggressive acts in sport can have a deteriorating effect on good moral behavior. The common acceptance of aggressive techniques that are not directly related to the goals and objectives of the game creates an environment of violence that has a destructive effect. The baseball pitcher who throws at a batter's head, the boxer who punches below the belt, and the football player who chop-blocks an opponent below the knees are all engaging in acts injurious to not just opponents but to sport itself.

According to Cluff,[21] the Denver Broncos of the NFL have long been accused of using unethical blocking techniques. Cut blocks—hits below the waist—are legal as long as they are done on the front side of the defender. When a player blocks another low and on the back side, it is against the rules. In 2004, Broncos offensive lineman George Foster cut-blocked Cincinnati defensive tackle Tony Williams and broke his ankle. Foster's block was considered unethical and a 'cheap shot' because Foster initiated the block just as Williams was turning around.

Playing for Profit

For administrators such as athletic directors in Division I intercollegiate athletic programs and officers in professional sport organizations, profits can be as influential a force on their actions as winning. The firing of coaches at major college and professional levels can be the result of a lack of revenue generation. Winning can be an important and influential factor driving decisions to replace coaches, but revenue is often a bigger factor. Not surprisingly, winning is a strong, if not the strongest, driving force behind revenue generation. Money from gate receipts and television contracts increases as teams win more. Coaches understand the absolute necessity of revenue generation and its direct relationship to winning and to keeping their jobs, and might be tempted to do almost anything it takes to win. Rule breaking, dirty physical play, and intimidation are examples of unethical practices that coaches might resort to if they succumb to the pressures related to revenue generation and winning.

Furthermore, as profits tend to be greater for winning programs and franchises, administrators may be willing to overlook or cover up violations of rules and regulations such as those related to eligibility and recruiting in college athletics. For example, it would be unethical for a general manager of a professional sports team to trade a player who was known to be injured to another team. Yet many of these kinds of unethical behaviors take place in sport, all in the name of winning and revenue generation.

Major college coaches who are fired for rules infractions often are rehired by another school within one or two years. Those responsible for the hiring (athletic directors) and those who endorse it (presidents and board members) usually are aware of a coach's past history of ethical and unethical practices. An organization that hires such coaches anyway is, for all intents and purposes, endorsing these unethical practices, most likely for the purpose of revenue generation and winning. For example, in 2003 Mike Price was hired as the head coach of the University of Alabama, but was quickly fired after it was learned that he was drinking heavily and involved with dancers at a strip club.[22] Price, who has a history of winning college football games, was hired eight months later as the head football coach of the University of Texas at El Paso.

Athlete Behavior

The behavior of professional and elite amateur athletes may also contribute to the questionable moral climate of sport today. The antics and idiosyncrasies of today's elite athletes make entertaining sound bites and video clips for the media. And whether done for the sake of the truth, the public's right to know, or simply as a way to increase ratings, media personnel rarely miss an opportunity to report any outrageous, unusual, or controversial behavior by athletes. As Barry Bonds learned during his efforts to surpass Babe Ruth and Henry Aaron to become Major League Baseball's all-time home run leader, the close scrutiny of the media is ever-present. Bonds' athletic and personal life were put under a microscope. The press reported on accusations and, ultimately, court testimonies, proving that Bonds took steroids, as well as a domestic controversy with a woman, and the longer-than-expected recovery from a knee injury during the 2005 season that included somewhat secretively performed medical procedures.[23]

Those aspects of Bonds' life that were reported could all be considered morally questionable, but, to be fair, if the average person's life was as carefully scrutinized as Bonds', in most cases some unusual and probably even frowned-upon behaviors would be discovered. It's too easy, and unfair, to blame athletes as the sole contributors to the

PREMIUM HIGH SCHOOL FOOTBALL TALENT FOR SALE

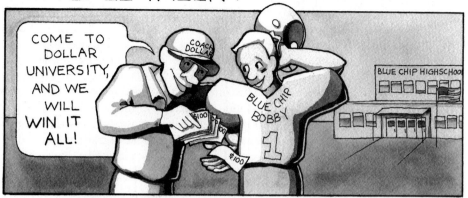

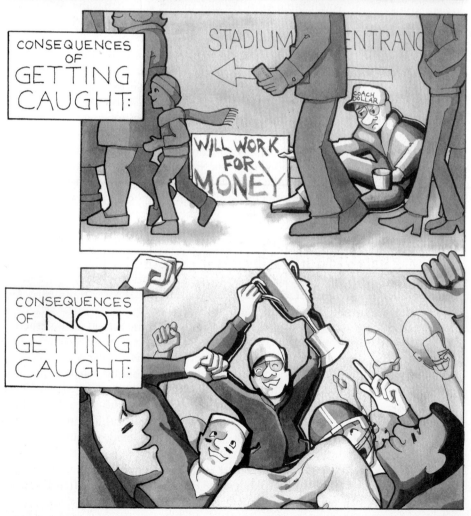

morally questionable environment of sport today. Some television executives make decisions to place violence, trash talking, and other crude or unsportsmanlike behavior on the air. And viewers tune in. The American Broadcasting Corporation (ABC) was criticized for airing a commercial during the 2004–2005 season that featured then-Philadelphia Eagle Terrell Owens and actress Nicollette Sheridan from the television show Desperate Housewives. The commercial included a sexual overtone that was perceived by some people as distasteful and lacking in morality. The challenge for those serious about eliminating unsportsmanlike behavior associated with professional sports is human nature itself. The viewing audience arguably is drawn to the crude and outrageous, whether it occurs on a talk show or on the playing field.

emulate: imitating; modeling behavior; in sport, athletes who are perceived to be role models may be emulated by youth athletes who aspire to reach an elite athletic status.

Unethical and inappropriate behaviors by elite athletes that are reinforced by the press deserve special attention since, unfortunately, youth often **emulate** and model such behaviors. When elite athletes react to what they perceive as inappropriate fan behaviors by entering the stands and even sometimes confronting fans, those athletes are breaking a rule that strictly prohibits such behavior. Behaving in that way could send the wrong message to youth that it is acceptable to disrespect established rules.

During the 2005–2006 NBA season, Antonio Davis of the New York Knicks did just that when he entered the stands in Chicago after noticing that his wife was being harassed by a Bulls' fan.[24] Although Davis' actions were, in his eyes, well intended, he broke an established rule. By entering the stands, he may have sent an unintended message to impressionable youngsters that it is acceptable to take matters into your own hands, disregarding the rules. Everyone involved in sport must understand the huge influence that elite athletes have on young people. They, and even some adults, often mimic the actions of athletes, whether or not those actions are morally problematic. For better or worse, athletes frequently are looked upon as role models.

"Pressure to Cover Up a Violation"

Prior to Super University's last football game of the season against their arch rival, Super University's head coach learned that his starting quarterback may have accepted cash payments from a booster, which is a clear violation of the rules. After asking around, the head coach felt certain that his starting quarterback had, in fact, accepted money from a booster affiliated with the program. Unsure what action to take, the head coach immediately met with his athletic director and explained the situation. Without batting an eye, the athletic director replied, "We have to cover this up. If we don't, it will taint the image of our program and could even destroy the program if the wrong people find out. One thing is for sure, if we do not cover it up it will take center stage and overshadow the big game this weekend against our arch rival, making it less likely that we will be offered a television contract next year for the same game."

"Pressure to Cover Up a Violation" (*Continued*)

Questions

1. If you were the athletic director, what advice would you have given the head coach? What is the rationale supporting your advice?
2. Do you think there were outside influences that made the athletic director decide to cover up the problem? If so, what were the influences? If not, explain your reasoning.
3. In this situation, what could be done to preserve the good moral standing of sport?

Athletes as Role Models

Almost everyone who loved sports when they were young had athletic role models they wanted to emulate. The same holds true today. Young people want to be like their role models and often copy the on-court and off-court mannerisms and behavior of outstanding athletes. This would not be a problem if all athletes were good sports persons, played fairly, respected others, and manifested the best values that sport has to offer. However, that is not always the case.

In particular, youth frequently look up to gifted athletes who are so successful at their sport that they achieve superstar status. Major League Baseball (MLB) player Cal Ripken Jr., who played shortstop for the Baltimore Orioles, was one of the top sports figures in competitive sport, a baseball superstar. During his playing career, Ripken was a role model to youth throughout the world. Fortunately, Ripken's overall values and character were decent and well serving to those who emulated his on- and off-field behavior. As an athlete, Cal Ripken Jr. held and practiced a respectable set of moral values that could serve as a guide not only for youth but also for adults, including other professional athletes.

Young people frequently demonstrate their idolization of elite athletes by purchasing and wearing replica sport jerseys of their favorite players. They often do so because of an athlete's exceptional field play, not because of displays of good moral character. During the 2005–2006 season, Los Angeles Lakers guard Kobe Bryant performed the extraordinary feat of scoring 81 points in an NBA basketball game, placing him second on the all-time single game scoring list behind Wilt Chamberlin's 100-point performance. The day after Bryant's record-setting performance, apparel companies manufactured and sold Los Angeles Lakers jerseys printed with the number 81 along with Bryant's name. Thousands of young people bought these jerseys. They didn't do so because Bryant displayed good moral values; the phenomenal 81-point performance was reason enough to idolize Bryant.

Young people often do not examine such things as character and values when selecting role models. They frequently are attracted to and try to emulate highly successful athletes regardless of any histories of on-field or off-field unscrupulous and unsportsmanlike behaviors. Because young people are so impressionable, who they choose to emulate is obviously of great concern, especially if that role model displays negative traits.

Athletes as Negative Role Models

Athletes who behave well on and off the field often are overshadowed by those who behave poorly. And many of today's athletes prefer to be viewed as **anti-heroes** rather than as role models. They display attitude or in-your-face behaviors and receive endorsements and media attention because of their outlaw personas. Mike Tyson, one of the most recognizable names in sport, is a perfect example. As a professional boxer, early in his career Tyson performed extraordinarily well, earning him the reputation of being the best boxer in the world. But it was his out-of-the-ring record of breaking the law that earned him a criminal reputation. Clearly, Tyson's values and overall character left a lot to be desired. Throughout his life, Tyson has had numerous brushes with the law, including the serious charge of rape for which he was charged, prosecuted, convicted, and ultimately sentenced to significant jail time.

> **anti-heroes:** in the context of sport, participants who choose to be the antithesis of a role model.

This kind of behavior in role models is of genuine concern to parents and society alike. In attempts to develop their own athletic talents, youth may not only emulate the athletic talents of athletes like Tyson, but also their lifestyles and behaviors outside of sport. Some athletes may disagree with the notion that they have a responsibility to serve as positive role models, but it is an inescapable fact that many young people look up to and aspire to be like their favorite sports figures. And although some athletes do not want to serve as role models, others do make a conscious effort to behave appropriately since they know that many young people look up to and aspire to be like them. Like it or not, because youth so often emulate the behavior of elite athletes, elite athletes should, ideally, set positive examples to follow.

The majority of high-profile athletes fall somewhere between a positive role model like Cal Ripken Jr. and a negative role model like Mike Tyson. It is unrealistic to expect that every elite athlete be of upstanding moral character and demonstrate strong moral values. Being an elite athlete does not equate with being an elite individual. All human beings are fallible and susceptible to error. Perfect behavior by anyone, not just athletes, is an unrealistic expectation, but a certain level of acceptable behavior in sport can and should be expected. And calculated efforts to exploit or hurt others go beyond human fallibility and should not be tolerated. For example, during the 2006 lacrosse season, members of the Duke University men's lacrosse team were accused of raping and assaulting a woman they had hired to dance at a party. Lack of evidence eventually vindicated the Duke team of the most serious charges of rape, but the team was far from removed from grossly inappropriate behavior. It was reported by Wilson and Bernstein[25] that an e-mail from a Duke lacrosse player stated that he was going to

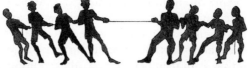

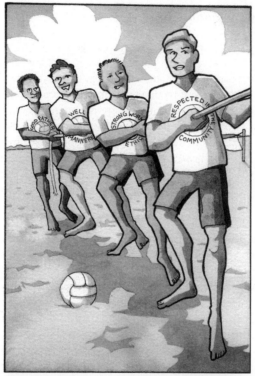

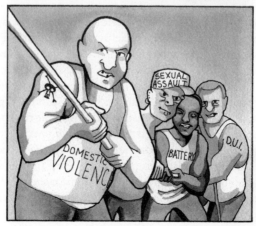

have strippers over and planned on killing the women as soon as they walked in and then proceed to cut their skin off while having sexual gratification.

A similar situation took place during the 2005 NFL season when a member of the Minnesota Vikings football team hired strippers to dance for several Vikings players on a boat that team members rented. Allegations of inappropriate sexual behavior were extensively reported. Given the widespread attention the incident received from the national press, it begs the question whether the inappropriate actions by the Duke lacrosse team were in some way modeled on the Vikings' behavior of the year before.

The Influence of Elite Athletes on Youth

As stated previously, sport in and of itself does not promote moral values. Those involved in sport choose to behave or not behave in a morally good way. When those involved choose to behave morally, sport is perceived as a facilitator of moral values. When those involved in sport do not behave morally, sport is labeled a facilitator of immorality. Individuals with strong moral integrity often make good moral choices, and those with weak moral integrity often make bad moral choices. Thus, to strengthen the **moral fabric of sport,** efforts should be made to recruit players with moral integrity, and leaders should serve as models of morality and expect and encourage sound moral behavior in their players. It is important that those involved in sport display strong moral character and values because, as stated earlier, young people so often model their behavior after the athlete they admire or the team they follow.

> **moral fabric of sport:** underlying standards of right and wrong on which sport must be grounded to maintain its integrity. ✓

When athletes go after fans who have cursed or thrown things at them; when they trash talk in a manner that is threatening or humiliating; when they show disrespect for officials, coaches, or teammates; or when they cheat or break rules to look good or to improve their team's chances of winning, these are actions that young people may mimic and repeat in their own games. Tenenbaum et al. asserted that "modeling is extremely dangerous in that young athletes who choose highly aggressive role models are more likely to become aggressive players themselves."[26(p320)]

One example of aggressive behavior took place during the 2004–2005 NBA season when players from the Indiana Pacers and Detroit Pistons went into the stands and a brawl ensued between players and fans. The brawl began when one of the NBA's top defensive players, the Pacers' Ron Artest, left the court and was involved in a physical altercation with a fan. Artest has gained a reputation of being a negative role model in part from being at the center of and, arguably, initiating the brawl. After receiving a season-ending suspension, Artest returned for the 2005–2006 season only to become embittered with the Pacers management and refusing to play. The Pacers then attempted to trade Artest to the Sacramento Kings, but Artest publicly expressed his disinterest in playing for the Kings and finally both parties agreed to a contract. Such recalcitrant behavior from talented players like Artest could send the message to youth that as long as you possess exceptional talent, it is okay to behave inappropriately.

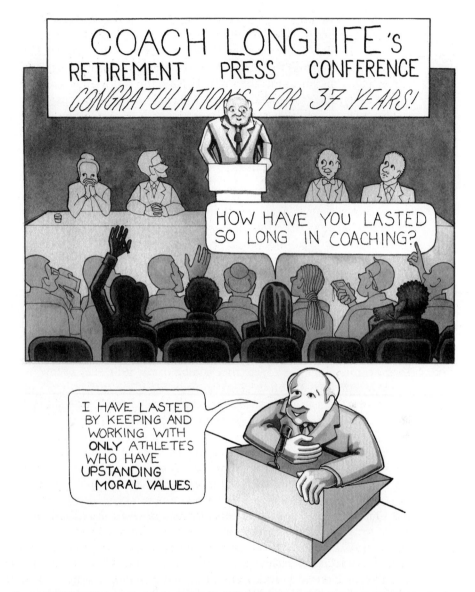

Jones and McNamee caution against quick judgment of the moral character of athletes and suggest that any attempt at assessing the moral characters of those involved in sport must start from a far more complex and less structured account of moral character and the world in which they play.[17] One perspective might be to not to expect or require that athletes adhere to high moral standards simply because they have elite status. Former NBA player and current NBA analyst Charles Barkley's cry of "I am not a role model" represents the side of the debate that does not require a higher standard of moral behavior by athletes or the responsibility of being a positive role model for youth.[27]

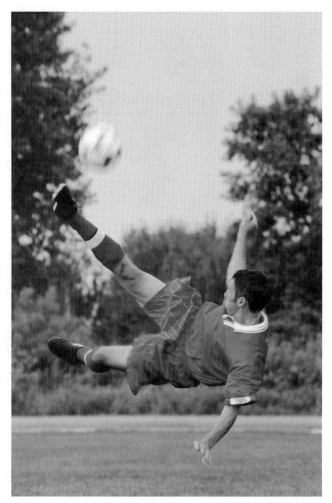

3-2 *Youth may aspire to be like elite athletes and model their behavior.*

As endorsers, entertainers, and celebrities, athletes' actions and images are transmitted to millions of homes around the world, shining a light on not only their athletic talents but also their personal qualities and traits. If youth choose to emulate the athletic and personal qualities of elite athletes, it can be argued that elite athletes have an obligation to present themselves in a morally upstanding manner.

Special Responsibilities of Athletes

In what he terms the "special responsibilities argument," Feezell claimed that celebrated athletes "have special responsibilities to be good role models."[28(p23)] There are athletes who do recognize the importance of personal accountability within and outside of sport. These athletes do see that it is important to help young athletes recognize that there are morally better ways of living and participating in sport, and demonstrate this through the examples they set both on and off the playing surface.

Athletes such as Shaquille O'Neal of the Miami Heat and Cal Ripken, formerly of the Baltimore Orioles, not only show young people how to play the game, but also how to act toward opponents, officials, fans, teammates, and coaches. Many professional athletes also dedicate time and money to their communities, not for good public relations or tax purposes, but because they want to help others. These individuals see themselves as having responsibilities to model morally good behavior and give back to the community.

"The Hiring Committee Punches Back"

After an outstanding two years of professional baseball cut short by an injury to his arm, Patrick Punch is interested in teaching and coaching at his high school alma mater. Given his superb high school, college, and professional playing performances, Patrick is sure that he will have no problem landing the head coaching position. After all, he has the appropriate degree and is so well known throughout the community, what could possibly cause the committee to select a candidate other than Patrick? Unfortunately, however, when the time came for the selection committee to make a choice, the unthinkable happened: he was not hired as the head coach. When Patrick asked why, the committee gave him the politically correct answer that the candidate offered the position had more years of real coaching experience. Interestingly, though, the rumor being passed around informally as to why Patrick was passed over differed considerably from the politically correct response. Rumor had it that Patrick's reputation for fighting in bars was the real reason he was not offered the position.

Questions
1. Had you been on the hiring committee, would you have not hired Patrick because of his history of bar fighting? Explain your answer.
2. Do you think Patrick's history of bar fighting would prevent him from being a positive influence on high school baseball players? Explain your answer.
3. Do you believe Patrick was at a disadvantage because he was so well known and constantly in the public eye that everyone knew of his every action, both good and bad? Explain your answer.

Even with such good examples, it is unlikely that athletes who do not see themselves as role models will change their behavior. It is for this reason that those closest to young people should acknowledge their own responsibility as role models for young people. This means acting appropriately since young people often mimic the actions of their parents, siblings, peers, and coaches. Part of this responsibility is to help young-sters place in proper perspective the behavior of athletes that may not be based on sound moral values.

The Importance of Moral Exemplars Outside of Sport

As Feezell points out, it would be more honest to deny that celebrated athletes are moral exemplars, since all in society share a collective responsibility to shape society and cultures in a way that youth can safely look for moral exemplars in various walks of life outside of sport.[28] Society might be better off if individuals actively discour-aged the notion that elite athletes have a special responsibility to formally serve as role models. Young people need help in understanding what behavior is acceptable on and off the field, and what behavior is unacceptable. There are persons other than athletes who may be better suited to provide such guidance. When parents, relatives, friends, coaches, and teachers serve as good examples, youth can develop their ideas about fair play and sportsmanship from them and thus help sport begin to live up to its character-building potential.

Furthermore, and as importantly, it might be preferable that those who are clos-est to youth are the ones to engage them in communication so as to assist them in choosing good role models from the sporting world. It may be that the most persua-sive role model is one who knows a youngster personally and is interested in his or her positive growth to adulthood. The athlete who truly cares about a youngster may be more inclined to put forth a genuine effort to behave appropriately, much in the same way a father and mother should for their children. In the event that an athlete errs in his or her behavior, if someone close to and trusted by the youngster can point out that no one, including athletes, are perfect, it might help the youngster to differenti-ate between proper and improper behavior.

One way to learn the difference between right and wrong actions is through mis-takes that elite athletes make. In other words, even when athletes do not behave as good role models, if addressed by and discussed with a trusted adult, the athlete's inappropriate behavior can serve as a learning experience for a youngster. Caring and knowledgeable adults can point out that athletes are not perfect and then help youth differentiate, through real-world sport examples, between appropriate and inappro-priate behavior on the part of athletes. In doing so, young people might gain the abil-ity to identify and understand appropriate and inappropriate behavior in order to make good behavior-related choices on their own.

Examples of Good Sportsmanship

The Pac-10 Conference reinforces sportsmanship by offering annual sportsmanship awards to players on teams in the conference. Grayling Love was the recipient of the Pac-10 Sportsmanship Award in 2004. Love was a starter as a sophomore in 2003 for the Arizona State football team and earned 2nd team All-Pac-10 honors. He volunteered to let a senior offensive lineman star in his spot for Senior Day. The game was against in-state rival Arizona.[29] A second example of good sportsmanship took place in 1940 in a game between Dartmouth and Cornell that Dartmouth ended up winning on a fifth down play. Later, after reviewing the films, it was discovered that Dartmouth had been allowed a fifth down on its winning drive. Upon learning the news, the Dartmouth president, Edmund Day, announced that Dartmouth would forfeit the win.[30]

Another example of good sportsmanship took place at the 2006 Winter Olympics in Turin, Italy during a cross country skiing race. In the women's team sprint, Canadian Sara Renner was in the lead and beginning an uphill portion when her left ski pole broke. Renner frantically tried going uphill with just one pole but struggled to make progress. Seconds later, three other skiers passed her. Finally, from one side of the course, a man stepped forward and handed Renner his ski pole. Even though the pole was larger than Renner's other pole, she was able to get up the hill at a faster rate than without a pole and remain competitive. Renner and her teammate finished with the Silver medal. Unbeknownst to Renner at the time, the man who came out of the crowd to hand her his pole was Bjoernar Haakensmoen, the coach of Norway's cross country team.[31]

The Moral and Social Value of Competition

Ethical Problems and Competition

Does competition lead to ethical problems in sport, or is it the attitudes that many sport people have about competition that leads to ethical problems? Simon questioned whether or not there is anything inherently unethical about sport competition or competition in general.[32] The competitive aspect of sport may make it a morally questionable activity. And emphasizing the defeating of an opponent and the seeking of one's own advantage may influence those who play sport to become morally insensitive toward others as they adopt a win-at-all-costs attitude.

Morally insensitive behavior may take place in the form of humiliating trash talking, coaches screaming obscenities at players, and sacrificing time spent with family to perfect one's athletic skills. Having complete disregard for the consideration of others' feelings is a type of moral insensitivity that can take place in sport because of a win-at-all-costs attitude. For instance, players may shout abusive words at opposing players as they attempt to distract their opponent during competition, and coaches may use humiliating language toward athletes and refer to such language as motivational. In professional sport, sports agents may adopt a calloused, morally insensitive approach during contract negotiations to get the best deal for their clients. To acquire the most talented players, general managers might engage in immoral behavior, regardless of who might be negatively affected in the process, such as players and players' families.

When winning is the highest priority, means to achieve it sometimes do not include moral sensitivity if it does not support the larger goal to win. Without respect for moral sensitivity, sports people are more likely to behave immorally. That is, if sports people view sport from a morally insensitive perspective, they might be more likely to cheat or use violence and gamesmanship to gain advantages. Delattre[33] and Simon[32] claim that those with morally insensitive attitudes also tend to view opponents as enemies to be conquered or obstacles to be overcome rather than as fellow human beings questing for the same prize. During a 2005 interview with CBS's 60 Minutes, former Oakland Raider linebacker Bill Romanowski talked about surviving in the NFL with overpowering strength sometimes induced by steroids and hatred. Romanowski described how, after a game, he started the mental process of hating the next week's opponent as well as their family, coaches, and fans.

"Coach Capital Takes Offense at Ms. Includeall"

Coach Capital arrived in his office Monday morning at his seventh grade teaching and coaching job to find a note from the principal. The principal, Ms. Includeall, requested that Coach Capital meet with her regarding sport participation opportunities at the school. She began the meeting by saying, "I think we should create enough sports teams so that everyone has a chance to play. Our students need to feel included and appreciated." Coach Capital's response was, in part, based on his coaching philosophy that had evolved over the past several years: "The last thing I am interested in is a lecture on sensitivity training. I will cut the weakest players and only the best players will survive the cuts and make the team. How in the world do you expect any of these players to survive in the real world if they do not learn now that they must be better than their competition if they want to reap the rewards? Our society is one based on capitalism that rewards those who produce at higher levels than others. You are simply wrong and I do not plan on changing my ways any time soon to reward the weak." Ms. Includeall was speechless, as this was not the response she expected.

Questions
1. Do you side more with Coach Capital or Ms. Includeall, and why?
2. If you were the coach, would you support the creation of more teams so that everyone could participate? Why or why not?
3. Should sport reflect the principles under which its society governs? In other words, should sports in America be a direct reflection of capitalism (as Coach Capital seems to believe)? Explain your answer.

Sports as a Zero or Negative Sum

Problematic is the fact that sports are **zero-sum** or negative-sum contests in which there is one winner and one or many losers. While this undoubtedly does create tension between competitors, it does not itself make sport competition something that is inherently objectionable. As Simon noted, when people agree to take part in sport, they agree, in principle, to accept the rules of a zero-sum or negative-sum game.[32] If they understand the rules of the game and are not coerced into playing, then they freely choose to participate in an activity in which they know there will be a winner and a loser(s).

For example, when Olympic hopefuls train to qualify for the Games, they are fully aware that the odds are stacked against them in that sometimes only as many as three participants in certain events qualify. Participants not only accept but also thrive on the fact that there will be a winner and a loser. The risk of losing is accepted because winning is more meaningful if it is achieved over a challenging opponent. Thus, unless the rules of the sport call for ethically questionable behavior, there is nothing inherently objectionable in taking part in sports as zero-sum or negative-sum contests.

Sport Framed as Militaristic

Sport competition can become morally questionable when it is framed as a battle or war and when opponents are cast as enemies to be conquered. This analogy is one that has been popular in sport over the years and has influenced the thinking of many coaches. These military analogies have not helped to endear sport to those who find its competitive aspect objectionable. Furthermore, the analogies have provided objectors with copious amounts of ammunition for their arguments. It is important to make clear that athletes can never be compared with soldiers because of the stakes under which athletes play and soldiers fight. To serve as an athlete is to play hard and put your athletic reputation on the line. To serve as a soldier is to work hard and put your life on the line. Similarities do exist, however, among leaders of athletes (coaches) and leaders of soldiers (officers). Both coaches and officers have as an objective to unite a collection of individuals together to form a cohesive unit to achieve a common goal. Officers and coaches must gain the respect of their players and soldiers to effectively and efficiently accomplish the goal of victory in sport and in combat. Often, coaches and officers implement similar conditioning, motivation, and discipline as they pursue their respective goals.

Given some of these similarities between coaching athletes and directing soldiers, several military analogies have evolved over the years to describe sport. Militaristic terms and phrases such as "in the trenches," "offensive weapons," "low scoring battle," and "throwing a bomb" are often used to describe sport actions—in this case, more specifically, in football. However, sport does not have to be viewed as a battle or war of sorts. In fact, minimizing or eliminating a battle or war-like attitude in sport might aid in fostering ethical behaviors in competitive play.

Competing in the Spirit of Friendship

Stressing the view that opponents are friends or partners and not enemies can help lessen the animosity between opponents and can help make sport a fairer and more ethical form of activity. Could it be, though, that if athletes view competition as a friendship or partnership, the intensity of their play will decrease and they will not put forth as much effort to win? Might competitive athletics become more like

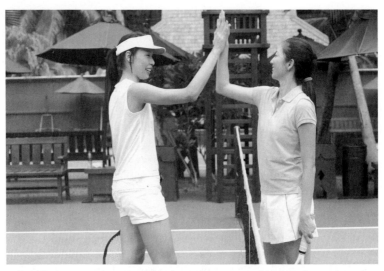

3-3 *Stressing that opponents are friends and not enemies can decrease animosity and make sport a more ethical form of activity.*

recreational games? Several authors have explored this possibility. Delattre,[33] Clifford and Feezell,[34] Shields,[35] Hyland,[36] and Simon[32] have all suggested that it is possible to compete in the spirit of friendship.

We need look no further than some recreational contests between friends to recognize that friends compete fiercely against one another. Friends often play against each other with great effort and intensity and exhibit true competitive spirit. Such examples demonstrate that competitive athletes do not have to lose their edge to preserve fair play and sportsmanship, and that it is possible to play hard and still show respect to an opponent who is also a friend. What is most valuable about viewing competitions as friendships or partnerships is that such an outlook can help to remove the unnecessary animosity that often is created between opponents. This, in turn, could help to decrease instances of cheating, unsportsmanlike behavior, and violence. When players perceive opponents as fellow human beings worthy of their respect, they may be less likely to do things that harm or humiliate them and more likely to play fairly.

A case in point that still arises in conversation today is the friendly, yet extremely intense, rivalry that began during the 1979 NCAA National Championship men's basketball game between Larry Bird of Indiana State and Earvin "Magic" Johnson of Michigan State. Bird and Johnson competed aggressively during the game but established a friendship that remained throughout their professional careers and included world championships for Johnson with the Los Angeles Lakers and Bird with the Boston Celtics. Although Bird's and Johnson's level of competition against one another was of the highest intensity, they maintained a friendship throughout their NBA career that continues in their post-playing careers.

In some ways, athletes today are friendlier with one another than ever before. Players at all levels share a bond in that they all experience the demands that come with participating in competitive athletics. Given the constant strife between management and players' unions in professional sports, through their unions players have united in solidarity for causes like job security, which can be viewed sometimes as even more important than what takes place on game day. And coaches at all levels can take the enemy mentality out of the sport environment by emphasizing very tough play without a focus on hateful and injurious tactics.

Understanding Competition as a Mutual Quest for Excellence

Simon claims that "competition in the context of sports is most defensible ethically when understood as a mutual quest for excellence in the intelligent and directed use of athletic skills in the face of challenge."[32(p38)] This **mutual quest for excellence** might be interpreted as placing a primary emphasis on self-performance instead of on performance against opponents. In other words, after a contest, instead of walking away feeling like you have beaten an opponent, someone who seeks to achieve excellence through the directed use of skills might walk away knowing that their personal performance was one of their best and as a result they ended up winning.

> **mutual quest for excellence:** in sport, when participants place a primary emphasis on self-performance instead of on performance against opponents.

Those who view sport competition as unethical are not focusing on the nature of sport or its necessary elements, but rather on the negative attitudes that some people have toward competition and their opponents. These negative attitudes are not held by everyone, however, and are not a necessary part of sport. For example, coaches who impress upon their athletes the need to humiliate and degrade their opponents in the interest of competing effectively perpetuate the notion that competition causes unethical behavior when, in fact, it may very well be the attitude taught by the coach that results in the unethical behavior. As stated before, sport in and of itself is not bad but can appear so when those involved behave unethically. People involved in sport must make a conscious decision as to how they will act. Those who act unethically often do so when an over-emphasis is placed on winning and an under-emphasis is placed on the process of competition. By changing people's attitudes toward sport competition and helping them to see sport as a mutual quest for excellence, the focus can once again be directed on how the game is played, not on who wins. This emphasis on process helps keep winning in perspective.

"Precious Carrie"

Pausing from reading the local newspaper, Carl Concern said to his wife, "I am not at all sure I want our daughter Carrie to go into sports. Every day I read another article that talks about the trouble that athletes are getting into and much of it seems to take place in practice and games. Here it says that a lacrosse player was thrown out of

"Precious Carrie" (*Continued*)

a game for slashing an opposing player with her stick. As she was leaving for the locker room, she yelled profanities at the opposing coach and several players from the other team. To make matters worse, she continued her tirade by cursing out her own coach and some fans as well. I am afraid that our precious Carrie will be inflicted with this same type of attitude if she gets involved in sports. Or do you think it is just the sport of lacrosse that is the problem?" Mrs. Concerned replied, "I am not sure who is at fault, but I do not want to take a chance. I am going to persuade our Carrie to become involved in the band so that we have nothing to worry about."

Questions
1. Do you believe that Mr. and Mrs. Concern have a legitimate worry that sport will teach their daughter immorality? Explain your answer.
2. In this case, how could Mr. and Mrs. Concern reduce the potential that Carrie might learn immorality through sport participation?
3. Based on what they read in newspaper articles, to what extent should parents make decisions related to their children participating in sport? Explain your answer.

Actualizing the Moral Potential of Sport

As posited at the beginning of the chapter, sport has the potential to be a valuable educational activity that teaches young athletes lessons and moral values that will play important roles in their lives outside of sport. But what can be done to ensure that sport reaches its character-building potential?

Sport is confronted with the tremendously daunting task of morally enhancing those involved in it. To this end, temptations to achieve victory at any cost must be smothered. Behaving immorally to achieve victory can have a contagious effect on the sporting community, but so can behaving morally. If the majority of sport teams in a league are behaving morally, other teams in the league are pressured to respond in kind. When all sports teams are abiding by the rules and behaving morally, victories are more meaningful. If sport can reach the point where moral behavior is the rule instead of the exception, then one can say that sport does in fact create and reinforce moral behavior.

Cultivating Sport's Character-Building Potential

Sport's character-building potential can be realized if those in leadership positions—coaches, athletic directors, principals, and commissioners—recognize and reinforce the acts of good character that take place. In turn, acts of bad character should be ignored and/or punished and under no circumstances rewarded. Unfortunately, society does at times seem to reward those who display bad character. With somewhat of a perverted mindset, a part of American society takes an interest in and even shows a liking for those with a rebel mentality. Outrageous behaviors draw media attention and thus, unintentionally or intentionally, often are reinforced by the public's thirst for more. But good morals should never take a backseat to bad behavior; strength of character should always take precedence over revenue generation and the desire to win.

Although youth leagues have become quite competitive, and the increasing emphasis on and rewards for winning have narrowed the gap between youth and professional levels in sport, youth leagues have not yet been *completely* overcome by the expectation to win. The cultivation of sport's character-building potential probably still occurs most easily at the youth level. But immoralities must be removed before character can be cultivated through sport participation, and the largest and most deeply rooted potential for immoral actions is in the zealous emphasis society places on winning. If an emphasis on winning can be tempered by a strong encouragement to behave morally, sport can succeed in helping build good character.

This encouragement begins at the top, through sound leadership from athletic directors, principals, league commissioners, and university presidents who demand that participants display good moral values, and who strongly believe that the purpose of sport is to build character. Coaches should praise athletes for good moral behavior privately and publicly, at press conferences, banquets, and other social functions. Negative acts in sport should be ignored or even punished. And as difficult as it may be, players who continually display negative character traits should be reprimanded and, if necessary, removed from the sport altogether. Negative character traits should not be allowed to flourish. If leaders of sport are truly committed to ensuring that sport produces positive character outcomes in its participants, they may need to take unpopular stances. Leaders may need to modify or remove environments that tempt sport participants to behave badly. In other words, a change of attitude is required.

Aside from changing attitudes, Clifford and Feezell believe that it is important to begin actively teaching values such as fair play, sportsmanship, honesty, and respect.[34] These values can be taught in a variety of mediums. A committed emphasis can be placed on curriculums at all levels, beginning with elementary and continuing through

> **fair play codes of conduct:** systematically arranged and comprehensive collection of rules to foster honest competition in sport.

college. Leagues and sport programs can also place an emphasis on values by reinforcing good behaviors and punishing bad behaviors. **Fair play codes of conduct** should be at the center of all programs, and administrators, coaches, and adults should lead by example.

How Values Help to Strengthen Sport Morally

Values help to strengthen sport morally when individuals focus on competing with the achievement of excellence in mind. To attain excellence, athletes must consider how they will compete and in what ways, if any, they will practice moral values. If values guide athletes' actions, they are more likely to compete fairly and decently. Sport will be strengthened morally if values are made its central focus. If sport takes on a

> **values-centered approach:** ✓
> primarily focusing on values; in
> sport, strengthening sport morally
> by having a commitment to values;
> for example, include only persons
> of upstanding moral character in
> sport.

values-centered approach, its by-products will be values oriented. The first step in a values-centered approach is to involve in sport only those persons who are values oriented. Athletes, coaches, and administrators must have a strong sense of values and be committed to practicing and expecting good moral behavior on a daily basis. When those involved in sport are committed to practicing strong moral values, sport is perceived as a vehicle that manufactures good morality. Everyone involved in sport must be open to and have a commitment to good moral behavior.

An overall commitment to good morality must be prevalent, and persons affiliated with sport must be proactive in their efforts to influence and reinforce good moral behavior. Others who might be tempted to stray will have a better chance of making good moral choices instead of bad ones if the sporting environment is filled with individuals who have and practice good moral values. From Little League to the Major Leagues to the Olympic level, everyone involved in sport must continually practice and insist on good moral behavior from themselves and everyone around them for sport to succeed as a character-building endeavor.

Conclusion

The debate over sport's moral status and its character-building potential will continue for years to come. Although research indicates that, in many cases, sport is not teaching positive moral values and behavior, a change in reasoning and behavior may help to alter this pattern. Athletes, coaches, and administrators at all levels can assist in this process, but because of their celebrity status and widespread visibility, professional and elite athletes potentially have the greatest influence on whether sport is seen as a positive character builder. If they were to emphasize important moral values such as fair play, sportsmanship, and respect, they would send a message to younger athletes that moral integrity and excellence matters more than winning. In embodying these values, elite athletes would also help to demonstrate how sports can be morally good and valuable activities. Because sports are socially constructed activities, it is athletes, coaches, administrators, and fans who develop and give sport its identity. If these individuals want sports to be morally educational experiences, they must take the initiative and organize them as such. If sports are organized as morally educational experiences, the members of sporting communities will be helping sport actualize a greater degree of its character-building potential while also improving its moral condition.

References

1. Rudd A. Which character should sport develop? *The Physical Educator*. 2005;62(4):205–211.
2. Rudd A, Stoll S. What type of character do athletes possess? An empirical examination of college athletes versus college non-athletes with the RSBH Value Judgment Inventory.

The Sport Journal. 2004;7(2). Available at: http://www.thesportjournal.org/2004Journal/Vol7-No2/RuddStoll.asp. Accessed March 21, 2007.

3. Shields DLL, Bredemeier BJL. *Character Development and Physical Activity.* Champaign, IL: Human Kinetics; 1995.

4. Seefeldt VD, Ewing ME. Youth sports in America. *President's Council on Physical Fitness and Sports Research Digest.* 1997;2(11):1–11.

5. Kirkcaldy BD, Shepard RJ, Siefen RG. The relationship between physical activity and self-image and problem behaviour among adolescents. *Social Psychiatry & Psychiatric Epidemiology.* 2002;37:544–550.

6. Wooden J, Jamison S. *Wooden—A Lifetime of Observations and Reflections On and Off the Court.* Chicago, IL: Contemporary Books; 1997.

7. National Collegiate Athletic Association. Report by the Committee on Infractions. *National Collegiate Athletic Association* website. Available at: http://www2.ncaa.org/portal/media_and_events/press_room/2004/october/20041020_washington_infr.html. Accessed March 21, 2007.

8. Washington M. Crowd behavior affected Serena (evil French alert); July 18, 2003. *ESPN* website. Available at http://www.espn.go.com/tennis/french03/s/2003/0605/1563653.html. Accessed March 21, 2007.

9. Eccles JS, Barber BL, Stone M, Hunt J. Extracurricular activities and adolescent development. *Journal of Sport and Social Issues.* 2003;59:865–889.

10. Yin Z, Moore JB. Re-examining the role of interscholastic sport participation in education. *Psychological Reports.* 2004;94:1447–1454.

11. Din F.S. Sport activities versus academic achievement for rural high school students. *National Forum of Applied Educational Research Journal-Electronic* [serial online]. 2005–2006;19(3E). Available at: http://www.nationalforum.com/Journals/National. Accessed May 24, 2006.

12. Bluechardt MH, Wiener J, Shephard RJ. Exercise programmes in the treatment of children with learning disabilities. *Sports Medicine.* 1995;19:55–72.

13. Steiner H, McQuivey RW, Pavelski R, Pitts T, Kraemer H. Adolescents and sports: Risk or benefit? *Clinical Pediatrics.* 2000;39:161–166.

14. Marsh HW, Kleitman S. School athletic participation: Mostly gain with little pain. *Journal of Sport Exercise & Exercise Psychology.* 2003;25:205–228.

15. Coakley J. *Sport in Society: Issues and Controversies.* 8th ed. New York: McGraw-Hill; 2004.

16. Lumpkin A, Stoll SK, Beller JM. *Sport Ethics: Applications for Fair Play.* 3rd ed. New York: McGraw-Hill; 2003.

17. Jones C, McNamee M. Moral reasoning, moral action, and the moral atmosphere of sport. *Sport, Education and Society.* 2000;5(2):131–146.

18. Russell JS. The value of dangerous sport. *Journal of the Philosophy of Sport.* 2005; 32:1–19.

19. Eltman F. Criminal charges won't be filed vs. Islanders' Simon. *Democrat and Chronicle.* March 20, 2007:4D.

20. Bennett C, Carey J, O'Toole T, Timanus E. Seven college scandals: One year later; June 14, 2004. *USA Today* website. Available at: http://www.usatoday.com/sports/college/2004-06-14-scandals-update_x.htm. Accessed March 23, 2007.

21. Cluff C. Notebook: Chargers' Chatman has people talking; October 31, 2004. *The Seattle Times* website. Available at: http://seattletimes.nwsource.com/html/sports/2002077627_nflnotes31.html. Accessed March 22, 2007.

22. Price calls SI report an 'absolute lie'; May 7, 2003. *ESPN* website. Available at: http://espn.go.com/ncf/news/2003/0507/1550422.html. Accessed March 21, 2007.

23. 'Tired Bonds may miss season'; May 22, 2005. *WSB-TV* website. Available at: http://www.wsbtv.com/sports/4307910/detail.html. Accessed March 22, 2007.

24. Horng E. Knicks player confronts fan bothering his wife; January 19, 2006. *ABC News* website. Available at http://abcnews.go.com/Sports/story?id=1522271. Accessed March 22, 2007.

25. Wilson D, Bernstein V. Duke cancels lacrosse season and announces wide critiques. *The New York Times.* April 6, 2006: C15, C17.

26. Tenenbaum G, Sacks DN, Miller JW, Golden AS, Doolin N. Aggression and violence in sport: A reply to Kerr's rejoinder. *The Sport Psychologist.* 2000;14:315–326.

27. Associated Press. Barkley in Hall, urges young players to plan; September 8, 2006. *NBC Sports* Website. Available at: http://nbcsports.msnbc.com/id/14736771/. Accessed February 22, 2008.

28. Feezell R. Celebrated athletes, moral exemplars, and lusory objects. *Journal of Philosophy of Sport.* 2005;32(1):20–36.

29. Pac-10 Sportsmanship Award. *Pac-10* website. Available at: http://www.pac-10.org/school-bio/saac-sportsmanship.html. Accessed March 22, 2007.

30. Kerkhoff B. Crossing boundaries; October 22, 2006. *Kansas City Star* website. Available at: http://www.kansascity.com/mld/kansascity/sports/15818396.htm. Accessed March 22, 2007.

31. Romano J. 'Cheers' to this reason to cheer; February 27, 2006. *St. Petersburg Times* website. Available at: http://www.sptimes.com/2006/02/27/Columns/_Cheers__to_this_reas.shtml. Accessed March 22, 2007.

32. Simon RL. *Fair Play: The Ethics of Sport.* 2nd ed. Boulder, CO: Westview Press; 2004.

33. Delattre EJ. Some reflections on success and failure in competitive athletics. *Journal of the Philosophy of Sport.* 1975; 2:133–139.

34. Clifford C, Feezell RM. *Coaching for Character.* Champaign, IL: Human Kinetics; 1997.

35. Shields DL. *Opponents or enemies: Rethinking the nature of competition.* Paper presented at the Inaugural Conference of the Mendelson Center for Sport, Character and Culture, South Bend, IN. May 2001.

36. Hyland DA. Competition and friendship. *Journal of the Philosophy of Sport.* 1978;5:27–37.

Losing the Game for a Higher Draft Choice

The snow was blowing and the temperature was below freezing as the opening kick-off soared through the air to begin the last game of the season between the Wilmington Wolves and the Canton Coyotes of the Pro Football League (PFL). Coyote Stadium has 75,000 seats and for this game, less than 10,000 of them were filled. Bad weather was only part of the reason for the poor attendance; the fact that both teams had a combined total of only nine wins was also keeping people away.

The Wolves had absolutely nothing to play for and neither did the Coyotes. But wait a minute. Maybe the Coyotes did have a reason to play this game. If they won the game, would they make the playoffs? No. If they won the game, would they increase their overall standing in the league? No. But what about losing the game? If the Coyotes lost the game, they *would* improve their draft selection. In other words, if they lost, they would have the worst record (instead of the second-worst record) in the league. Having the worst record would allow the Coyotes to select first in the draft. Anyone who knows anything about this year's draft knows that Terry Tosser has the best quarterback statistics of anyone in college and will, without question, lead any team—even the Coyotes—to the playoffs next year.

The coaches are faced with a dilemma. If the Coyotes are victorious they will not gain anything, materially, from the win; but if they lose the game, the top draft choice will be theirs. The coaches are torn as to what strategy they should undertake.

Critical Thinking: Finding Common-Sense Solutions

1. If you were the Coyotes coaches, would you make a 100% attempt to win the game? Explain your reasoning.

2. As the commissioner of the PFL, if you became aware that your coaches were devising a game plan to *not* give the team the best chance for victory, what action(s), if any, would you take?

3. As a paying spectator, regarding making the strongest attempt to win, what would you expect from the Coyotes coaching staff?

Critical Thinking: Moral Theory-Based Decision Making

4. What moral responsibilities, if any, do the Coyotes coaches have to their players, fans, opposing team, and the game to make every attempt to win?

5. Can you create a sound rationale supportive of losing the game to gain a higher draft choice? Explain your answer.

6. Discuss *mutual quest for excellence* and how it would be affected by a strategy by the Coyotes to lose the game.

Fisticuffs Among Parents

Recently, a massive brawl involving adults broke out at a Saturday morning youth (third and fourth grade) recreational basketball league game. The fight started when the father of one of the players went onto the floor and accused an opposing player of playing 'dirty' against his son. The father then got in the 'dirty' player's face and said, "Let's see how you like it," at which time the father assaulted the player by pushing him down to the floor. The assaulted player's father then made his way onto the floor to defend his son as a full-scale brawl erupted.

The brawl lasted more than 20 minutes as parents from both teams began screaming, throwing chairs, and fighting in any manner possible. As the coaches tried, unsuccessfully, to break up the brawl, youngsters from both teams tried to stay out of harm's way. Unfortunately, a few kids were knocked to the floor and injured during the melee. Parents sustained minor injuries too, such as lacerations and broken noses.

After receiving a call, police arrived and gained control of the situation 10 minutes and 17 arrests later. It is important to emphasize that none of the youngsters—players or students—initiated the fighting in any way. The fighting took place exclusively among the adult spectators, including mostly men but also three women. These three women, none of whom were related to any of the kids or the fathers that started the brawl, were directly involved in the fight. In all, approximately 70 people were involved in the fight as either participants or peacemakers.

This is the first time anything like this has ever happened in this youth recreation league. The purpose of this program is to get kids involved in basketball at an early age to foster growth and learning and to improve their talent for advanced levels of competition. Several individuals—including, but not limited to, the league director, parents, players, fans, and law enforcement—now have some difficult decisions to make.

Critical Thinking: Finding Common-Sense Solutions

1. If you were the director of the league, would you disband it? Why or why not? To what extent would you consider the overall benefits gained by the hundreds of kids participating in the league in making your decision?

2. Is it fair to punish all of the players for the negative actions of the adults? Explain your answer.

3. Which parents should be punished and why?

4. Should competition and scoring be taken out of this youth basketball league? Why or why not?

5. What steps need to be taken by the league director to ensure this type of incident does not happen again?

6. As the director, would you set up workshops for parents, coaches, and players to help them understand good sporting behavior? If so, describe how you would design these workshops.

7. As a parent, how would you explain to your children what took place?

Critical Thinking: Moral Theory-Based Decision Making

8. What values should be considered when deciding how to manage the after effects of this situation?

9. How can moral reasoning be used to effectively arrive at a decision that is most beneficial to all parties (youth participants, coaches, parents/fans)? What moral theory or theories might best help you make this decision?

The Exploitation of a Modified Learning Disability

Prospect Middle School boys basketball coach and special education teacher, Coach Owen Overlook, is gaining a reputation for not holding one of his star athletes accountable for inappropriate off-court behavior. The star athlete, Duncan Downs, is an eighth grader who has established a history of behavior problems that commonly include fighting and other acts of disrespect. Many of the inappropriate occurrences have occurred in the classroom.

On one occasion during a physical education class, Duncan was removed from class for verbally abusing the teacher and other classmates. Undeterred by this removal, Duncan arrived for class the next day and was again disruptive when he repeatedly interrupted the teacher's instruction, even after receiving a warning from the teacher. When asked to leave, Duncan refused to do so and increased his verbal abuse toward some students. Duncan was then told to go directly to the in-school suspension room, but he did not comply with this directive either. Since Duncan refused to listen, security finally was called to escort him to the in-school suspension room.

Because of his history of bad behavior and his belligerent attitude when he entered the in-school suspension room, the monitor in charge refused to accept Duncan. Security then escorted Duncan to the office of the assistant principal, Ms. Mindful, where she met with him for several minutes before assigning him to the football coach for the remainder of the day.

The following evening, while attending a varsity basketball game, Duncan's disorderly ways continued when he got into a fistfight with a high school student. After security removed the two students from the gym, because of his troubled past at the school Duncan was kicked off of school grounds for the remainder of the game. The following day, the high school principal, who had attended the game, contacted Ms. Mindful and informed her that Duncan had been kicked out of the varsity basketball game the previous night. Ms. Mindful agreed that Duncan should be restricted from attending any more athletic events for the remainder of the year and phoned Coach Overlook to inform him of this decision.

Coach Overlook responded to Ms. Mindful by explaining that Duncan's unacceptable behavior is caused by an emotional disorder and that a careful review of Duncan's Individual Education Plan (IEP) will indicate this. Annoyed at Coach Overlook's response, Ms. Mindful said that she was more interested in disciplining Duncan than reviewing his IEP. Coach Overlook continued to explain that because of his disability, Duncan is simply unable to control himself and may be in need of more special services.

Ms. Mindful repeated her concerns to Coach Overlook about Duncan's behavior outside the school setting, referring to the varsity basketball game at which Duncan got into a fistfight. The coach said that he understood what happened since he was at the game and witnessed the event first-hand, but he did not feel the need to discipline Duncan. After hearing this, Ms. Mindful became furious that Coach Overlook decided to do nothing about Duncan's violent behavior even though it took place right under his nose. Taking matters into her own hands, Ms. Mindful contacted the athletic director. After Ms. Mindful explained the situation, the athletic director responded by defending Coach Overlook. The athletic director explained to Ms. Mindful that he considered the district fortunate to have a person like Coach Overlook, since he is not only an excellent teacher but also a superb human being. After hearing these comments, Ms. Mindful is sure that the athletic director will not discipline Duncan and unsure what to do next.

Critical Thinking: Finding Common-Sense Solutions

1. If you were Coach Overlook, would you consider using sport-related punishments, such as game suspensions, to discipline Duncan even though his inappropriate behaviors took place outside of his sport? Explain your answer.

2. If you were Ms. Mindful, in what way, if any, would Duncan's high-profile status as a star athlete affect your actions regarding his inappropriate behaviors?

3. If you were Ms. Mindful, to what extent, if any, would you consider Duncan's IEP when deciding what should be done concerning his disrespectful and, in some cases, violent behavior? Explain your answer.

4. If you were the athletic director, after hearing Ms. Mindful's concerns what would you have done?

Critical Thinking: Moral Theory-Based Decision Making

5. Using the *consequentialist theory* as your basis, if you were Ms. Mindful, what action(s) would you take regarding Duncan's inappropriate behaviors?

6. If you were the athletic director and were *morally reasoning* your way to a decision—basing your decision on what is in the best interests of Coach

Overlook, Ms. Mindful, and Duncan—concerning Duncan's disrespectful and violent behavior, what decision would you make? Identify some characteristics of your decision that demonstrate that it is in the best interests of Coach Overlook, Ms. Mindful, and Duncan.

7. Using *strategic reasoning* as your guide, if you were Coach Overlook, what action(s) would you take regarding Duncan's inappropriate behaviors?

Key Terms

anti-heroes—in the context of sport, participants who choose to be the antithesis of a role model.

egoistic reasoning—using logical thought for the purpose of one's own interests.

emulate—imitating; modeling behavior; in sport, athletes who are perceived to be role models may be emulated by youth athletes who aspire to reach an elite athletic status.

fair play codes of conduct—systematically arranged and comprehensive collection of rules to foster honest competition in sport.

hazing—any activity expected of someone joining a group (or to maintain full status in a group) that humiliates, degrades, or risks emotional and/or physical harm, regardless of the person's willingness to participate.

loyalty (social value)—being faithful/devoted to a person, ideal, or custom.

moral character—the evaluation of the moral quality of a person based on his or her practice and demonstration of moral values, or lack thereof, such as honesty, fairness, and responsibility.

moral fabric of sport—underlying standards of right and wrong on which sport must be grounded to maintain its integrity.

moral responsibility—an obligation to do the right thing; a duty to behave in an ethically good manner; for example, the notion that elite athletes have a moral responsibility to be positive role models.

morally callused—having become hardened to doing the right thing; the consideration that the longer a person is in sport, the less regard he or she has for the adherence to moral values in the sporting environment.

mutual quest for excellence—in sport, when participants place a primary emphasis on self-performance instead of on performance against opponents.

perseverance (social value)—persisting; not giving in.

responsibility (moral value)—duty, obligation.

role model—someone who serves as an example; in sport, athletes who are looked up to.

social character—the evaluation of the social quality of a person based on his or her practice and demonstration of social values, or lack thereof, such as teamwork, loyalty, self-sacrifice, work ethic, and perseverance.

trash talking—verbal chatter; trash talking is usually delivered during a game or practice, usually directed at an opponent for the purpose of gaining an advantage by attempting to make an opponent mentally weak or by mentally strengthening/motivating oneself.

values-centered approach—primarily focusing on values; in sport, strengthening sport morally by having a commitment to values; for example, include only persons of upstanding moral character in sport.

work ethic (social value)—a disciplined effort of labor; for example, in sport, working on a skill daily, without exception.

zero-sum—when there is one winner and one loser.

4 Performance Enhancement Issues in Sport

Learning Outcomes

After reading Chapter 4, the student will be able to:

1. Describe ways in which winning and achievement reinforce performance-enhancing substance use.

2. State some perceived problems associated with performance-enhancing substance use.

3. Explain how the potentially dangerous side effects of performance-enhancing substances determine whether harm or coercion is prevalent in a particular environment of performance-enhancing substance use.

4. List some factors that influence the banning of performance-enhancing substances in sport.

5. Differentiate between an earned advantage and an unearned advantage in sport.

6. Summarize arguments for and against drug testing.

This chapter, through the use of moral theory, addresses performance-enhancing substance issues in sport. Praise, rewards, achievement of personal bests, and breaking records all motivate and reinforce athletes to do what it takes to win, which includes taking performance-enhancing substances. The reasons athletes use performance-enhancing substances vary from wanting to gain a competitive advantage, to feeling coerced into taking substances to remain competitive with those who are already taking substances to enhance performance.

The health risks posed by adverse side effects of performance-enhancing substances are of concern with regard to adult athletes, but of even more concern for youth who participate in sport. Unfortunately, scientific evidence that links adverse side effects to performance-enhancing substances is not conclusive, even though anecdotal evidence makes a strong connection between performance-enhancing substances and poor health.

It is helpful to examine from a moral perspective differences in training methods and why some types of training should be against the rules and other types should be allowed. Sport governing bodies and Congress have intervened through legislation to help provide athletes with incentives not to use performance-enhancing substances.

The criteria used to determine whether a performance-enhancing substance should be banned from a sport includes but is not limited to the degree of physical harm a substance causes an athlete, confidentiality rights of athletes, and other legal issues. Again, moral theory is helpful in making decisions with regards to banning substances and testing for banned substances.

Each of the above topics and more will be discussed in this chapter to give the reader insight into the complexities of the issues surrounding performance-enhancing substance use. This chapter will help readers develop their own views concerning performance enhancers and decide for themselves whether these substances have a place in elite athletics.

Performance-Enhancing Substances

Performance-enhancing substances are taken for the strict purpose of providing a competitive advantage—a competitive advantage that is often considered unfair. These substances come in many forms and types and are associated with adverse health effects. Steroids, androstenedione, and human growth hormone are used to enhance strength and speed in sports such as football and sprinting. Beta blockers are used to reduce heart rate and steady the nerves in sports such as rifle shooting, archery, and golf. Erythropoietin and blood doping increases the oxygen-carrying capacity of the blood in distance runners, cyclists, and triathletes. Even pain killers enhance performance by blocking pain that may prevent an athlete from pushing his body to its limit. Those competing in sports such as boxing or wrestling, in which competitors are matched against opponents within the same weight class, may opt to take diuretics to lose or "make" weight.

Muscle enhancers allow athletes to train longer and more intensely and reach higher levels of achievement than athletes of comparable skill and talent level who are participating naturally, without artificial substances. Positive test results aside, anecdotal evidence indicates that these substances help Major League Baseball (MLB) players to hit more home runs and National Football League (NFL) players to increase muscle mass and gain strength.

Examples abound of athletes from all different walks of life who have taken performance-enhancing substances. San Francisco's Barry Bonds of MLB has taken steroids (according to Bonds, unknowingly). After testing positive for erythropoietin (EPO), star Spanish cyclist and Spanish Vuelta winner Roberto Heras had his Spanish Vuelta title stripped by the Spanish Cycling Federation. Softball players from the University of Washington took, based on a team physician's recommendation, narcotics so they could play through injuries. Players from the 2004 number-one nationally ranked high school football team from the state of Texas admitted to using steroids. Finally, 15 years after her participation in the 1972 Olympics, East German swimmer Kornelia Ender admitted that, as a 13-year-old Olympian, East German officials had given her unidentified substances for weight gain.

Natural Training vs. Artificial Substances

Athletes who train naturally, without the aid of artificial substances, must work hard to produce outstanding athletic performances. On the other hand, athletes who inject artificial substances or take pills for performance enhancement do not have to work as hard to achieve the same results.

For example, outstanding performances in endurance events such as track and field's 10,000-meter run and long-distance swimming events require high levels of red blood cells in the participant's body. Because red blood cells carry oxygen and oxygen delays fatigue, athletes participating in endurance events desire to increase their red blood cell count. It is considered natural to increase red blood cells through high-altitude training. On the other hand, the injection of the hormone erythropoietin (EPO), which stimulates red blood cell production, is considered an artificial aid. The difference lies in the fact that high-altitude training is hard work and requires a daily work regimen that is physically and mentally taxing. The injection of EPO, however, can provide the same benefits with limited training and stress on one's body.

Effects of Performance-Enhancing Substance Use Over the Athletic Career

Often, concerns related to performance-enhancing substances pertain to the onfield performance of athletes. The major concerns are how substances affect game-day performance and how the users are affected by negative side effects of the substances. To gain a full understanding of the short- and long-term impact of performance-enhancing substances, however, one must have an understanding beyond game-day performance. For the purposes of discussion in this chapter, the effects of performance-enhancing substances can be placed into three categories: 1. immediate effects, 2. effects during the athletic career, and 3. post–athletic career effects.

Immediate Effects

Immediate effects are the athletic successes experienced as a result of substance use and abuse. Performance-enhancing substances may be used in addition to or as replacement for training to gain a competitive advantage. The effects are immediate when the athlete experiences improved athletic performance.

Effects on Athletes During Their Athletic Career

When athletes use performance-enhancing substances early in their careers, they set a performance standard that is difficult to maintain without the continued use of drugs throughout their entire athletic career. The pressures to continue at established levels of performance come from many areas: coaches, fans, sport administrators, and even family and friends. If an athlete's successful performances are a result of performance-enhancing substances, he or she is faced with the dilemma of continuing to use and continuing to succeed, or stopping use and stopping success.

Post-Career Effects

Following the use of performance-enhancing substances throughout an athlete's career, he or she must deal with long-term side effects. Although all substance side effects are not scientifically known or proven, many are. For example, athletes who use steroids during their athletic careers run the risk of continued physical and psychological damage when their careers are over. In deciding whether to use performance-enhancing substances, athletes should be aware of the potential long-term negative side effects that they will have to deal with after their playing days are over. These side effects are discussed in the next section.

Risks and Side Effects

The use of any substance for the purpose of enhancing sports performance, including over-the-counter supplements—the composition and quality of which are not under federal regulation—may pose significant health risks to young people.[1] Risks may be categorized as, but are not necessarily limited to, physical, psychological, and emotional. Millman and Ross[2] categorized the primary toxic side effects of steroids as follows: reproductive or virilizing and feminizing, hepatic cardiovascular, and psychological. More specifically, Federman[3] reported that the potential adverse effects of anabolic steroids include but are not limited to physical effects such as liver abnormalities, kidney problems, gynecomastia, testicular atrophy, hypertension, myocardial infarction,

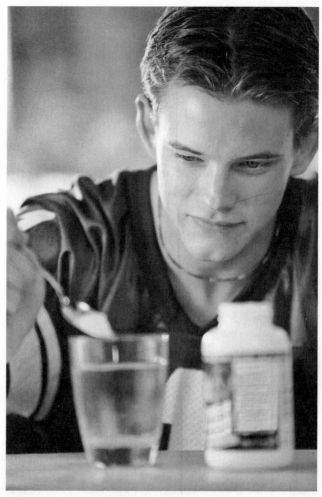

4-1 *Performance-enhancing substances can cause harm to the user and to others.*

stroke, loss of hair, acne, and psychological effects such as aggressive behavior, mood alterations, and psychoses.

Some past, isolated examples suggest that muscle-enhancing substances may even cause birth defects in users' children. Birth defects in children have been linked to East German athletes who were administered substances to enhance their Olympic performances.[4] NFL players and Olympic athletes who took steroids during their careers may suffer from liver damage and depression well after the ending of their careers.

Various Perspectives Regarding Side Effects

Various perspectives exist concerning the seriousness of the **side effects** of performance-enhancing substances. For example, Evans[5] acknowledges the adverse effects of anabolic steroids but also points out that the effects of "serious short-term use . . . are benign and reversible."[p174] Evans further states that the incidence of complications associated with the use of anabolic steroids as performance-enhancing substances is unclear, because drug use in athletes is not well defined.

> **side effects:** the unintended or adverse physical, psychological, and emotional effects that result from taking performance-enhancing substances.

Lack of Scientific Evidence and Risk

In former Major League Baseball player Jose Conseco's book "Juiced," Conseco points out the difficulties in gaining scientific evidence that pertains to the effect of performance-enhancing substances.[6] Because many performance-enhancing substances are against the rules, it is difficult to find users to volunteer for scientific research studies. In essence, athletes are serving as an uncontrolled and informal testing sample for performance-enhancing substances. The lack of formal scientific research makes for an environment in which athletes have to assume the risk of unknown negative side effects if they choose to use performance-enhancing substances.

Anecdotal Evidence Supporting Risk

There is an abundance of anecdotal evidence that links health risks to steroids. For example, Steve Courson and Lyle Alzado, former NFL players during the 1970s and 1980s, openly spoke of the negative effects of steroid use on their own health. Courson, a former Pittsburgh Steeler Super Bowl Champion, stated on many occasions that steroids took a toll on his health. Alzado, who had an outstanding career as a defensive end with the Denver Broncos, Cleveland Browns, and Los Angeles Raiders, died from brain cancer at the age of 43 in 1992.[7] Although Alzado blamed steroid use for his untimely death, it should be noted that medical science did not state or confirm that steroid use was the cause of Alzado's death.

Athletes Choosing to Assume Risk in Sport

Risk takes on many forms in sport. It is inherent in most sport competitions, and athletes willingly assume a level of risk when they choose to participate in a sport. Baseball players assume the risk of getting hit by a pitched ball; football players assume the risk of getting injured from a hard hit; and hockey players assume the risk of being involved in a fight. Should athletes, though, be asked to assume risks not inherent within their sport, such as the short-term and long-term side effects believed to be associated with performance-enhancing substances?

It is problematic that often athletes choose to assume the health risks that come with using performance-enhancing substances. Unlike assumed risks that are a known part of particular sports, the use of performance-enhancing substances provides health risks not completely known. Despite rules in place to prevent the use of performance-enhancing substances in sport, athletes still use them.

Harm Issues Related to Performance-Enhancing Substances

harm issues: in athletics, issues related to the potential for injury resulting from taking performance-enhancing substances; of primary concern is the taking of performance-enhancing substances by athletes who would prefer not to, but feel the need to do so to compete with athletes who are taking them.

Harm issues relating to performance-enhancement in sport are worthy of close examination. Who is placed at risk when athletes choose to use performance-enhancing substances? At first glance it may appear that the only person in harm's way is the athlete who is using the substances. This inquiry, however, should not begin and end with the user, because athletes using substances to enhance performance may not only be putting themselves at risk, but other participants as well. If, for example, steroids are commonly being used in the sport of football, players not using steroids may be physically inferior in terms of strength and speed and be at a higher level of risk for injury.

Coercion

The nature of sport is competition, and if one athlete's performances are enhanced by taking substances, the pressure for other athletes to do so to remain competitive is real.

coercion: compulsion by force; force or the power to use force to secure compliance. In the context of competitive sport, coercion makes reference to athletes who are pressured to take performance-enhancing substances.

Does such pressure amount to **coercion?** If a participant feels coerced into taking performance-enhancing substances to "keep up" with those already using them, it is still important to note that no one has to act on feelings of coercion when deciding whether to use substances to enhance performance. Even though the choice may be a difficult one, athletes still have the option to refuse substances even if that choice means no longer being able to compete effectively in their sport.

Pertaining to steroid use, Simon[8(p75)] points out that "sometimes athletes may clearly be victims of coercion." For example, a teammate may fear losing a starting position and a competitor may fear losing a contest that would have easily been obtained if he or she had used performance-enhancing substances. Furthermore, if use of performance-enhancing substances for a sport become the norm, those who wish to excel in that sport might feel the need to take the same performance enhancers just to keep up.[4] In examining this question with a specific focus on steroid use, Simon contends that there is "at least a presumption in favor of prohibiting steroids in athletic competition" on the grounds that "athletes who use steroids have no right to put other athletes in the position of either damaging their health or competing under a significant disadvantage."[8(pp78-79)] Whether athletes who use illegal performance enhancers are "coercing" other athletes into using them is questionable. But as Simon[8(p78)] notes, "The choice either of using a potentially harmful substance or of being non-competitive may be unethical if imposed on others."

Fost,[9] on the other hand, interprets coercion somewhat differently, believing that there must be an element of threat, force, or depriving someone of something to which they are entitled. Fost[9] explained further by noting that no one is entitled to be a professional athlete and those who do participate in American sports are free to walk away at any time. Based on Fost's explanation, taking performance enhancers to keep up with others may not truly be coercion.

Distinctions might be made between degrees of coercion. A less intense form of coercion, referred to as **soft coercion** is described as the potential for coercion, or at least intense social pressure.[4] The terms "overt" and "subtle" might be used to distinguish between different intensities of the coercion. An example of **overt coercion** took place before the fall of communism, when young East German members of the women's Olympic swim team were forced by their country and coaches to take regular doses of the anabolic steroid known as Oral-Turinabol.[4]

> **soft coercion:** in sport, the self-imposed pressure to take performance-enhancing substances to remain competitive with those who are already taking them.

> **overt coercion:** in sport, an open form of force or pressure applied to players to take performance-enhancing substances by those who have an interest in the enhanced performance of players.

Even though it may be difficult to pinpoint a specific percentage of athletes using performance enhancers, it is clear that some athletes are using them and others are faced with the choice of whether to take them and risk the adverse health effects. If teammates or opponents feel pressured and choose to use performance-enhancing substances to remain competitive, then their choice is one that is not completely free. Strictly enforced rules against the use of performance-enhancing substances might be considered, to keep athletes who do not wish to take the risks associated with performance-enhancing substance use from feeling pressured to do so.

Why Use Performance-Enhancing Substances?

Professional and amateur athletes use performance-enhancing substances for a number of reasons. Performance enhancers are used by less-than-average athletes to make the team, by average athletes to earn a starting spot or gain more playing time, and by elite athletes to achieve record-breaking performances and experience the thrill and celebrity-like status that comes with winning and being the best. And, sadly, although the testing is scant, one would be naïve to believe that youth have not at least dabbled in performance-enhancing substances. In short, all athletes are susceptible to the temptation of taking substances to perform at higher levels.[10]

Achievement and Desire to Win

The thrill of winning and of achievement takes place at every level of competition. When a young girl scores her first soccer goal, she is ecstatic. The little league player who gets a base hit celebrates when arriving at first base. Leading the team in tackles is one of the best achievements a defensive high school football player can experience. A figure skater who skates a perfect "10" cannot perform better.

Athletes who complete performances of a lifetime often enjoy the good feelings that come from achieving such special accomplishments. Good feelings come from the fans, friends, coaches, and omnipresent adulation directed at the athletes as a result of their special athletic achievements.

However, even though the good feeling that comes from winning is a natural one, the process by which the athlete won may have been dubious. More than ever, the public is questioning the authenticity of personal bests and extraordinary player performances due to the presence of performance-enhancing substances in sport. The most serious questioning of substance-enhanced performances takes place at the elite levels of competition. Professional, Olympic, and major college sports have been the primary focus of drug testing for performance-enhancing substances.

At the very top and gaining extensive media attention was Barry Bonds' pursuit of the all-time MLB home run record. The accusations and questions against Bonds go back as far as 1998, when it is thought that he began using performance-enhancing substances, including steroids and human growth hormones, to enhance his home run hitting performance. Concerns related to the legitimacy of Bonds' record-setting performances have been expressed by MLB, sports writers, and fans.[11]

Although the use of performance-enhancing substances in interscholastic sport is gaining more and more attention, its use in youth sport still does not command the attention from its governing bodies as it does in the higher-level sports. As winning and achievement become more emphasized at all levels, including youth sport, the motivation to perform at higher levels increases. Thus, the likelihood of youth using performance-enhancing substances increases. Youth sport organizations should proactively prevent the use of performance-enhancing substances before it becomes as prevalent at that level as it seems to be in many higher-level sports.

"The Shattered Long Jump Record"

As a senior in high school, Mark was feeling a well-deserved sense of satisfaction with his second-place finish in the long jump at the state track meet. This day was particularly special in that Mark achieved a personal lifetime goal of recording a jump beyond 25′ for the first time in his long jumping career. The winner this year was Tyrone, who shattered the record by jumping 27′7″. Following the conclusion of the long jump, it did not take long for the fans, coaches, and athletes to come up with an explanation for Tyrone's extraordinary performance: human growth hormone (HGH). Rumor had it that for nearly the entire past year, Tyrone, under the watchful eye of his personal trainer, had been taking HGH, which is known to increase muscle mass and one's ability to be explosive in sprinting and jumping. Mark was infuriated when he heard the rumor and demanded that the state officials do something about it. He exclaimed to his friends, "This is absolutely not fair! I earned my personal best by lifting weights and running all summer, and all Tyrone did was get his hands on HGH." When Tyrone heard the rumor, he told his friends, "Hey, the

"The Shattered Long Jump Record" (*Continued*)

state High School Athletic Association has not banned HGH, so I did nothing wrong."

Questions

1. Do you agree with the comment Mark made to his friends when he said that he had worked out all summer and thought it was unfair that "all Tyrone did was get his hands on HGH"? Why do you agree or disagree?
2. Do you agree with Tyrone's belief that he did nothing wrong since the state has not banned HGH? Why do you agree or disagree?
3. Following this state track meet, as the president of the state High School Athletic Association, what actions, if any, do you take? Immediately? In the next few weeks? In the next few months?

Praise and Rewards for Winning

Praise and rewards that accompany winning performances, such as compliments from coaches, fans, and family, as well as medals, cash, and prizes, can be addictive to athletes. How addictive are these rewards and to what lengths will athletes go to attain them? For some, doing what it takes to win and to be known as the very best might, in their view, require the use of performance-enhancing substances.

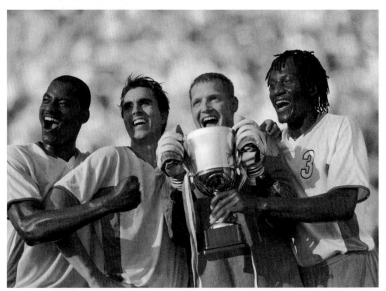

4-2 *To be known as the very best, athletes might be tempted to use performance-enhancing substances.*

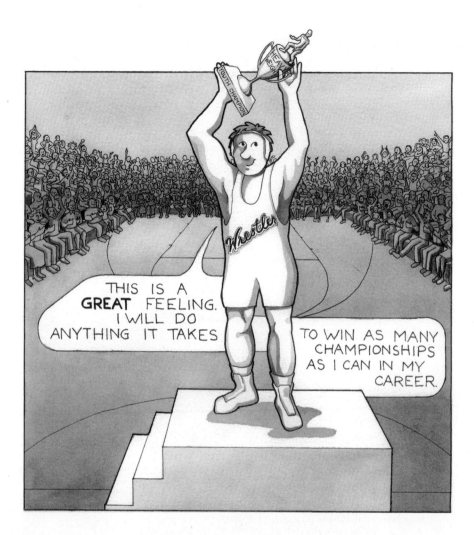

Such was the case with NFL defensive end Lyle Alzado. Alzado, who admitted to using steroids to enhance his professional football career, was the beneficiary of numerous awards and accolades for his achievements as a defensive end in the NFL.[7]

Improved Performances

Besides achievement, winning, praise, and rewards, the desire for improved performance alone may help perpetuate the use of performance-enhancing substances. If athletes improve dramatically or record unusually strong performances after using such substances, they may begin to enjoy and crave the accompanying internal high and positive external reinforcement. As a result, the athlete may choose to engage in the repeated use of performance enhancers in an attempt to experience these feelings over and over again.

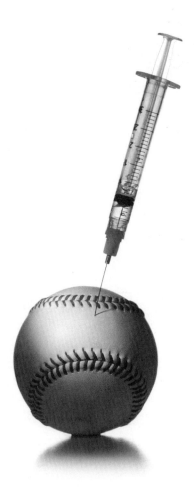

4-3 *Major League Baseball has come under intense scrutiny as a result of allegations of anabolic steroids use by some of its players.*

Moreover, from an organizational perspective, it is quite possible that the same type of "highs" and external reinforcements may take place more broadly across sport organizations. When MLB experiences improved league performances in the form of increased home runs, league officials are well aware of the resultant increase in league revenue through gate receipts and broadcasting contracts. It is quite possible that increases in revenue cause league officials to turn a blind eye to the likelihood that the new and improved performances are a result of performance-enhancing substances.

What about other sports, such as football and track and field? It is possible that organization and league improvements resulting from team successes cause organizations to take a less-than-proactive approach to the prevention of performance-enhancing substances. Because a primary goal of organizations is to improve performance, those at the top might be hesitant to remove anything that reduces performance, including the use of performance-enhancing substances.

Sport Statistics and Performance-Enhancing Substances

Athletes who take steroids and other performance-enhancers frequently perform at higher levels than those who do not take them. This creates a question as to whether statistics should be valid during a time when performance-enhancing substances were thought or known to have increased home runs in baseball, tackles in football, or amount of weight lifted in weight lifting, or to have decreased times in track and field sprinting events.

naturally talented athletes: players whose athletic abilities are not the result of the use of artificial substances; players who are born with above-average physical abilities, such as speed, jumping ability, and strength.

From a fan's and parent's perspective, performance-enhancing substances may be perceived as problematic in that the most skilled and **naturally talented athletes** may not win. In other words, the best player or team may not achieve victory. Part of a team legitimately being the best is winning while training naturally. On the other hand, in the case of sports statistics achieved by athletes known to have taken performance-enhancing substances, one could argue that it is not at all a problem because the goal of sport is to perform at the highest level no matter the methods.

Banning Performance-Enhancing Substances

What criteria should be used to determine whether a performance-enhancing substance should be banned and who influences the decision? The application of moral theory can serve as a basis for such decisions. Several groups and persons can influence the process of determining whether to ban a substance, ranging from sport governing bodies to fans. The best interests of athletes at all levels, including youth, should be considered. If the choice is made to ban performance-enhancing substances, it is important to develop policies effective in carrying out the ban.

The Role of Governing Bodies

To reduce the use of performance-enhancing substances in sport, governing bodies have implemented testing procedures for the purpose of at least deterring substance use. Because these testing procedures are expensive and budgets are limited, not all organizations can afford them. Governing bodies must weigh the benefits included in spending money on testing for performance-enhancing substances against spending money on other benefits for athletes, such as training facilities, participation opportunities, and more qualified coaches.

Major governing bodies such as the National Collegiate Athletic Association (NCAA), International Olympic Committee (IOC), MLB, NFL, National Basketball

Association (NBA), and National Hockey League (NHL) have come to recognize the problematic nature of performance-enhancing substances. The lengthy list of substances banned by these organizations is evidence of their view that performance-enhancing substances are neither good for athletes nor the game. The banning of performance-enhancing substances is, in part, an attempt to help maintain or improve the levels of integrity and fairness within sports and sporting communities.

The attempts by sport governing bodies to reduce or eliminate performance-enhancing substances from their sports have been met with resistance. For years, the commissioner of MLB, Bud Selig, has found it challenging to legislate, implement, and enforce effective procedures to prevent or at least reduce the use of performance-enhancing substances by MLB players. Concerned with the loss of rights, the Player's Union of Major League Baseball has fought against strict, no-nonsense testing procedures of players and punishments of players who test positive. Not until Congress intervened in 2005 were more stringent policies against performance-enhancing substances enacted. The intervention by Congress was a strong influencing factor in getting tough with the testing for steroids in MLB.

Created in 1999, The World Anti-Doping Agency (WADA) was founded by Richard W. Pound, who is also its chair. According to Pound,[12] there was a need to protect the integrity of sport and the health of athletes. To meet this need and to combat doping in sports effectively, there needed to be a harmonized, global strategy that combined and coordinated the resources of both sports and governments. Operating as an independent foundation, the World Anti-Doping Code (Code) was developed by harmonizing the many sets of anti-doping rules. On January 1, 2004, the Code came into effect, and by the time of the opening ceremony of the Athens' Olympic Games, all but one of the Olympic international federations, and all 202 national Olympic committees had accepted the Code and incorporated its provisions into their own rules.

On May 25, 2005, Don Catlin, through testimony to the U.S. Senate Commerce Committee, provided insights regarding the difficulties and effectiveness of drug testing of athletes. Catlin, the former director of the UCLA Olympic Analytical Laboratory (at this writing, UCLA's lab was the only lab in the U.S. accredited for sports doping control by the WADA), indicated that, without adequate funding and independence, anti-doping efforts are doomed to always be thwarted by the cheaters. Testing, according to Catlin, is far from perfect, and athletes determined to cheat have little trouble beating the test. Especially problematic are the legions of doctors telling athletes how to beat the test. Given the cheaters' penchant for staying a step or two ahead of the testers, it is vital to keep the advances in testing secret. If the cheaters learn that the substance they are using can be detected, they will move in the direction of a different drug, for which testing has not been conducted.[13]

In the end, governing bodies must decide how to make decisions regarding which substances to ban and which to allow in athletic training and competition. But on what criteria should they base their decisions? Will governing bodies support legislation against performance-enhancing substance abuse, or will they choose to allow those involved in sport to make choices regarding the use of performance-enhancing substances? It is likely that those making decisions will base their decisions on one or a combination of moral reasoning decision-making models.

To Ban or Not to Ban: Applying Moral Theory

On the surface, the solution for ridding sport of performance-enhancing substances seems simple: provide a strong reason for athletes not to use performance-enhancing substances by banning athletes who do use them. But why is the use of such substances unethical in the first place? For the answer to this question, the consequentialist and teleological moral theories are useful. Consequentialist moral theory requires one to take into account the best interests of those affected by an action in determining whether it is morally sound or flawed. Given the negative moral consequences associated with performance-enhancing substances, one might determine through consequentialist moral theory that it is not in the best interests of athletic communities to permit their use in competitive sports.

Through consequentialist moral theory, the use of performance-enhancing substances might also be believed to be acceptable. In other words, an athlete may believe his best interest lies in being able to perform at his best in an athletic event, because outstanding performances and personal bests might bring about fortune, fame, and professional and personal opportunities leading to a better life beyond sport. Thus, depending on each athlete's situation and perspectives of what is important, the consequentialist theory could be used to justify the use or the non-use of performance-enhancing substances.

Rather than focusing on consequences, a teleological moral theorist would emphasize the importance of the values of respect, beneficence, and compassion regarding this issue. If athletes respect opponents and teammates as human beings, they should not take performance enhancers and put their fellow human beings in a position in which they feel obliged to take potentially harmful substances to remain competitive. As good moral athletes, they should act with beneficence and compassion and not take performance-enhancing substances. Acting upon these same values, and out of a responsibility to protect the athletic communities of their sports, governing bodies should consider outlawing performance-enhancing substances to stop athletes from taking risks that are not essential to participation in their sports.

Given that performance-enhancing substances provide athletes with advantages that are not natural, should these substances be made illegal in sport? The emphasis here is on the moral value of fairness. Is the advantage that performance-enhancing substances give athletes in some way unfair? Moral theorists will approach this question in different ways. Teleological theorists will ask whether the morally good athlete would use substances or techniques that go above and beyond what might be considered natural. Deontological theorists will ask whether it is good and appropriate for *all* athletes to take performance-enhancing substances.

The Importance of Effective Prevention Policies

Because of public and, in turn, congressional pressure placed on organizations such as MLB, league rules and enforcement measures against performance-enhancing substances have become more strict. For example, in 2006, the U.S. Sentencing Commission, on a directive from Congress, made an emergency change to the federal sentencing guidelines to make the penalties for steroid use more severe. The sentencing guideline also provided for stricter sentencing against athletes using masking agents to hide their steroid use, against coaches who pressure athletes into experimenting with the substance, and against individuals who distribute steroids to athletes.[14]

These stricter sentencing guidelines may very well help prevent the use of performance-enhancing substances in sport. In the past, in many sports, athletes did not have to concern themselves with punishments such as suspensions and expulsions from their sport because drug testing was virtually ineffective. If drug testing and punishments against those testing positive are proven to be effective, the pressure placed on athletes to use performance-enhancing substances will diminish.

Governing Bodies' Responsibility to Youth

As elite athletes are a key part of the problems related to the use of performance-enhancing substances, sport governing bodies must step forward and act. In an effort to protect youth, governing bodies must legislate against performance-enhancing substances and diligently enforce their own rules. Otherwise, they risk sending mixed messages to children in telling them not to use performance enhancers, but rewarding athletes who do use them.

Do youth take performance-enhancing substances because they see outstanding substance-enhanced performances by adult athletes? Are these young people placing themselves at risk by taking performance-enhancing substances because they are aware that elite athletes whom they desire to "be like" are taking them? Regarding the use of anabolic steroids, Lydic[15] spoke of the enormous influence that high profile athletes exert on younger, aspiring athletes. Drug use, according to Lydic,[15] encourages drug use by others.

During a 2002 interview of six high school baseball players, the trickle-down effect of performance-enhancing substance use from MLB to high schools was discussed. All six of the players interviewed hoped someday to play in the major leagues. One player, who was 17, mentioned that he would probably take steroids if it meant achieving his life-long dream of playing MLB and if it allowed him to make millions and millions of dollars.[16] If performance-enhancers have negative side effects, and it can be clearly established that young athletes are taking them to be like elite athlete role models who take them, banning such substances from competitive sport should be considered.

Cook[17] claims that even if athletes knew for certain that they would have long-term health problems, many would continue to use performance-enhancing substances. Cook[17] also asserts, with certainty, that athletes will use performance-enhancing substances if they have a chance to make a fortune in a short period of time, have a fabulous lifestyle in their 20s and 30s, and set up their children and their children's children for life.

The Influence of Fans on Banning

If fans are against the use of performance-enhancing substances in sport, they can exercise various options to influence their removal. Fans can boycott events known to be inundated with performance-enhancing substances, and players and upper administrators of leagues will likely act on the will of fans. Fans play a vital role in the financial success of sport and thus have leverage over such controversial issues as performance-enhancing substances. A fan boycott of professional games would result in revenue losses for teams, owners, and leagues, which would motivate upper administrators of sport to rid sport of performance-enhancing substance users.

Fans, however, usually do not collectively take stands against sport issues, including performance-enhancing substances. Furthermore, based on the continued attendance of fans at athletic contests, fans seem willing to continue to watch sports despite the widespread belief that performance-enhancing substances are a part of many sports. Apparently, fans would rather witness extraordinary athletic feats than take a stand against performance-enhancing substances by boycotting events that are enhanced by players taking substances. And, some fans may simply not be opposed to the use of performance-enhancing substances in sport.

Fairness and Earned and Unearned Advantage

Some advantages are considered earned, whereas others are considered unearned. Depending on the circumstances, individual characteristics such as intelligence, personality, body composition, and athleticism may all be considered advantages that are unearned.

Has a person who is born with attractive physical features earned those features? Being physically attractive quite possibly gives one an advantage in the "looks-conscious society" of 21st century America; yet, this advantage, to a large extent, is unearned. Some people are simply born good-looking; their genes play a pivotal role in making them attractive. Even if genes were manipulated for the purpose of improving one's physical features, the societal advantage these individuals receive and the attention they garner would still remain unearned. It is true that physical appearance can be improved naturally, but only to a point. For example, exercise will not turn the body of someone who is naturally overweight into a lean, chiseled physical specimen. Nor can it be shown that reading will improve a persons' intelligence quotient from average to genius.

In a performance- and reward-driven society, people are constantly searching out ways to enhance their performances. In nearly every walk of life, persons prefer enhanced performances. For example, people strive to be better human beings and citizens, better friends and lovers, better parents and neighbors, better students and teachers, and better followers of faiths. The student strives to know more, the soldier to shoot more accurately, the vocalist to sing more musically, the chess-player to play with greater mastery, and the athlete to run faster.[4] Methods of enhancing one's performance include but are not limited to working hard, acquiring more knowledge, having access to better equipment, and the sometimes controversial method of taking performance-enhancing substances.

Substances are available that will enhance one's performance in most every performance-related area desired. An office employee may start the day with coffee as a way to wake up and be more alert during meetings. Students may take substances to help them focus and concentrate on their studies and test taking. Actors may take certain substances to help themselves become more animated. A pianist might take nerve-steadying substances before performing. Airline pilots may take substances to prevent drowsiness while flying. Soldiers may take mood-altering substances to increase their aggression. And sprinters may take muscle-enhancing substances to increase their speed and lower their sprint times.

Some persons, on the other hand, are naturally strong, fast, and have a high capacity for endurance without the aid of substances to boost their performance. When a person is born with physical characteristics that provide him with an advantage over others, it is considered fair and appropriate. These natural, genetic physical differences among athletes are beyond their control. Generally, athletes who are born with unearned physically superior skills are applauded, but when less physically skilled athletes try to enhance their skills by using performance-enhancing substances—also unearned—they are frowned upon.

Beyond the naturally different physical skills that exist among athletes are other differences, such as those related to money which provides some athletes with advantages over others. For example, some athletes may grow up in economically deprived areas where sophisticated training facilities cannot be afforded, thus putting them at a disadvantage compared with athletes who live in affluent areas and have access to state-of-the-art training facilities.

Sometimes funds are provided to athletes to help overcome economic disadvantages and help them gain access to better coaching, facilities, and equipment. The IOC, for example, gives money to poorer nations for the purpose of enhancing the training of athletes. From a team perspective, leagues such as the NFL have taken measures to help teams that are at an economic disadvantage. The NFL has instituted revenue-sharing plans and salary caps to keep economic "haves" from gaining too great an advantage over the "have-nots."

If performance-enhancing substances are believed to provide an unacceptable or unfair advantage, should rules and regulations be formed and implemented to deter their use? Gardner notes that, "It is not the advantage per se that we object to but the action or circumstances that have created the gained advantage."[18(p60)] There is not an objection to superior physical characteristics that people are born with that may give them an advantage over persons born with average physical characteristics. Objections do, however, arise when athletes gain advantages through the use of performance-enhancing substances.

Objections have been widespread over MLB's Barry Bond's breaking of Henry Aaron's all-time home run record in MLB. Court testimony indicated that Bonds was using steroids, whereas it is believed that players such as Aaron and long-time home run leader Babe Ruth achieved their performances without the aid of substances. Respect for the history of the game and protection of records that were set by players who did not take steroids are other reasons that some oppose the use of steroids in sports. The guardians of the game are concerned that records from previous eras cannot be compared with current day performances if today's athletes are using performance-enhancing substances. When the basic tenants of fair play are dismissed, the integrity of the game is undermined.

In deciding whether to ban performance-enhancing substances from sport, the overall onus of proof remains with those who contend performance-enhancing substances do not provide users with an unfair advantage. The majority of athletes, coaches, administrators, and society must be convinced that specific performance enhancers do not give those choosing to use them an unfair advantage over those who choose not to use them. Until then, the current bans will likely be perceived as justified.

Sometimes overlooked in the quick rush to judgment against those taking performance-enhancing substances is the fact that despite their use, athletes must still work extremely hard to reap the benefits of most substances. Someone who takes steroids must be involved in a rigorous weight lifting regimen to gain the maximum muscle mass and strength that steroids can potentially provide. And, athletes who blood dope must still engage in rigorous cardiovascular training in order to advance to a higher level of performance as a result of blood doping. In short, most performance-enhancing substances are not magic pills; athletes still must work extremely hard and be extremely gifted athletically to reap the performance outcomes that can come from performance-enhancing substance use.

"The Blood Doping Cross-Country Skier"

As the Ski-Hard High School cross-country ski team was getting ready for practice, several of the guys were engaged in a passionate debate related to performance-enhancing substances. One of the skiers, Evan, openly spoke out about blood doping and how he believed it was okay to blood dope. Evan spoke passionately about the topic, saying, "Blood doping should not be banned since no one is being hurt except me when I blood dope." Evan's teammate, Jacque, immediately voiced his disagreement, replying, "Evan, you are absolutely wrong. I am being hurt, as are your other clean teammates, because you will have a better chance than the rest of us of being noticed by the United States Olympic Committee because of your blood doping-enhanced performances."

Questions
1. Do you agree with Evan's argument that blood doping should not be banned because it is harming no one else but himself? Explain your answer.

"The Blood Doping Cross-Country Skier" (*Continued*)

2. Do you agree with Jacque's argument that Jacque and his teammates are, in fact, being hurt by Evan's blood doping because Evan will have a better chance of being noticed by the United States Olympic Committee? Explain your answer.
3. Do you believe Evan's blood doping is harming him? His teammates? The sport? Explain your answers.
4. As a coach of the Ski-Hard High School cross-country team, would you implement procedures to deter or eliminate performance-enhancing substances? If not, why not? If so, what procedures would you implement and how would you implement them?

> **drug testing:** the process by which athletes are screened—commonly through a urine or blood test administered by their governing body, such as the National Collegiate Athletic Association, the International Olympic Committee, and Major League Baseball—to determine whether they have taken a performance-enhancing substance; drug testing takes place to help ensure not only a fair and level playing field for athletes, but also the safety of the athletes.

> **invasion of privacy:** in the case of drug testing athletes, infringing on their 4th Amendment rights through the implementation of testing procedures that are an intrusion on an athletes' person, that is, athletes being required to produce urine samples in less-than-private conditions.

Ethics of Drug Testing

When athletes make the choice to participate in organized sport, they are bound by the rules and regulations established by that sport's governing body. Even if they disagree with these rules and have valid arguments against them, athletes must still abide by the rules the governing body has implemented. This responsibility pertains to all rules, including those requiring athletes to be randomly drug tested for their sport. Is it fair for sports to have mandatory **drug testing** policies? Should athletes who believe drug testing is an **invasion of privacy** have to submit to testing?

"Signing Away Rights to Play"

It was the first day of practice, and before practice could begin, Coach Clean had to take care of the beginning-of-the-year administrative duties. As always, one of those duties called for athletes to sign a waiver giving up their right to refuse drug tests. Usually athletes just signed the waiver without reading it, but in rare cases, an athlete would actually read the waiver. Today, Coach Clean ran into one of those rare cases. Darlene, a stickler for details, read the entire document and was taken aback by what she read. "Are you kidding me? This piece of paper is asking me to give up my right to not have my privacy invaded. Anyone who knows me knows that I *have* never taken and *will* never take any banned substances. Furthermore, I am personally insulted by this piece of paper and will not sign it." Coach Clean sat down beside

---

"Signing Away Rights to Play" (*Continued*)

Darlene and calmly explained to her that he could not allow her to practice or play in games until she signed the waiver. Darlene angrily shouted, "Who is behind the waiver anyway? It is completely unfair and coercive!"

Questions

1. If you were Coach Clean, would you try and convince Darlene to sign the waiver? If so, how would you try and persuade her to do so? If not, why not?
2. Do you believe it is fair that athletes must sign a waiver giving up their right to refuse drug testing before they can participate? Why or why not? Provide a rationale supporting your answer.
3. In your opinion, is requiring athletes to sign the waiver coercive? Why or why not?

Disagree as athletes, coaches, fans, and others might, the arguments against drug testing are often stifled by the fact that athletes can exercise their option not to participate and, hence, are not unfairly subjected to rules with which they disagree. Athletes have the right to choose not to participate in a sport if they strongly disagree with rules requiring that they be drug tested or with rules of any other kind. In regard to drug testing programs, Anderson states that "participation in athletics and other extracurricular activities at the interscholastic level is a privilege and not a right."[19(p3)] As outlined by Meyers,[20] the Supreme Court held that the NCAA's drug testing program was justified, and even though consent to drug testing must be given as a condition to compete, consent does not make it involuntary because athletic competition is neither a government benefit nor an economic necessity that would render consent involuntary.

Legal Issues

From a legal perspective, sport organizations exercise their will to establish rules for their games, whereas athletes and others have limited abilities to initiate change. Athletes can choose not to participate in a sport at any time, but is this choice an open one or one of soft coercion? Open decisions are made autonomously and are not forced. Generally, if athletes disagree with drug testing or its procedures, their only choices are to remove themselves from athletic competition or to go along with the testing policies in place. It seems that athletes are, thus, presented with an ultimatum—adhere to the drug testing policies of their sport or become ineligible—rather than a choice.

Simon questions whether athletes should be required to take drug tests and points out that generally in our society, "Individuals are to be left free and undisturbed unless a reasonable case can be made to show that particular persons are guilty of some infraction." [8(p88)] Simon also questions whether forced drug testing might cause drug users to incriminate themselves, which may be a violation of constitutional guarantees against self-incrimination.[8]

Although it does not resolve unsettled legal issues surrounding drug testing programs, a statement included in the American Council on Education Guidelines provides a common sense approach that balances the interests of colleges and universities with the interest of students who are subjected to drug testing. This statement is as follows: "The drug testing program should require students to give their written consent to the program prior to their participation in any intercollegiate athletic program."[21(p908)] Written consent does take place in NCAA intercollegiate athletic competition. When, however, athletes give their written consent to drug testing for the sole purpose of remaining eligible, they are not genuinely supporting the notion of drug testing, but rather agreeing to it only to remain eligible for participation in their sport. In reality, the athletes are required to provide their written consent to drug testing to both be awarded an athletic scholarship and to be allowed to participate.

In a study that surveyed NCAA Division I and Division III male athletes, it was found that the majority of the athletes said that they viewed participation in intercollegiate sports as a privilege and that they saw drug testing as an acceptable part of that privilege rather than a violation of privacy.[22] Athletes most frequently cited the privilege of playing intercollegiate sport and their responsibilities as representatives of their universities as reasons that they supported drug testing in intercollegiate athletics.[23]

Circumvention of Testing Procedures

The specific drug testing procedures of sport leagues and organizations have also come into question over the years. According to Brennan,[24] it is a fact that urinalysis testing alone cannot catch every instance of illegal drug use, because there are too many ways to circumvent testing procedures. Athletes use masking agents—substances designed to hide the presence of certain performance-enhancers—and concoct new substances that urinalysis cannot detect to circumvent these procedures.

To head off potential cheaters, it has become part of urine collection procedures for drug testing officials to be present while athletes produce their samples. On the surface, this intrusion may seem to constitute an unnecessary invasion of the athlete's privacy. There is evidence, however, that the presence of an official is necessary as a further deterrent for those who would attempt to tamper with samples.

Despite the best efforts by governing bodies, athletes still try to beat the tests. For example, in August of 2004 during the Athens Olympic games, IOC officials said that Robert Fazeka of Hungary had been caught attempting to switch a urine sample during dope testing following his participation in the discus competition. Officially, Fazeka was stripped of his Olympic gold medal for refusing/failing to submit a urine sample.[25]

Without an official being present in the room in which the athlete produced the sample, the process is not difficult to circumvent. A friend could provide the athlete with a urine sample and the athlete could conceal the "clean" sample in a jacket pocket as he or she walks from the outside into the private testing area. Once in the private testing area, the athlete could then pour the friend's urine into the athlete's cup prior to exiting the private testing area and delivering it to the official. The athlete would then be assured of testing negative, even if he or she had used banned substances. Circumvention of drug testing procedures, such as the one described above, has contributed to the modification of procedures, so that they are more intrusive and infringe on personal privacy. A case in point was in 1998, when Irish three-time Olympic gold medal winner Michelle de Bruin was charged with deliberately tampering with her urine sample during an out-of-competition drug test.[26]

Is a greater good achieved by invading athletes' privacy to deter the use of performance-enhancing substances? If people could be reasonably sure that drug testing and its procedures have rid athletics of performance-enhancing substances—and if it were agreed on that performance-enhancers should not be a part of sport—then the argument for sacrificing athletes' privacy in the interest of safe and fair athletic competition might be stronger. Unfortunately, regarding drug testing, it seems that many if not most athletes who are using performance-enhancers are not getting caught and are succeeding in their efforts to improve their performances with substances. By and large it seems that even though athletes are being tested for drugs, many athletic achievements that have been at least somewhat unearned have gone undetected, while athletes' right to privacy has been invaded.

"Only Two Tested Positive for Steroid Use"

After two years of public pressure—the public pressure began when two high school football players committed suicide after having "gone off of" steroids—the Commissioner of the Professional Football Guild (PFG) implemented a comprehensive drug testing program. The emphasis of the program was to test for anabolic steroids and designer steroids. After the testing was complete, the commissioner of the PFG arranged a press conference for the express purpose of announcing the results of the drug testing program. At the press conference, the commissioner proudly announced: "Well, the test results are in and I am happy to announce that of the 72 athletes randomly selected for drug testing, only 2 tested positive for steroids. We must be doing a great job of keeping our league drug-free!" Because the press conference took place during the PFG season, PFG players throughout the country were watching it on television. Many of the players were astounded that even two players were caught. One player said, "That just goes to show you that a couple of the rookies have not yet learned how to either take the undetectable drugs or mask the drugs that are being tested." Smiling, the player continued, "Oh well, maybe next time we can make it through without anyone getting caught."

Questions

1. Do you believe the commissioner should have been proactive in setting up a drug testing program instead of waiting for public pressure? Why or why not?

"Only Two Tested Positive for Steroid Use" (*Continued*)

2. Do you believe the commissioner's drug testing program was effective? Why or why not?

3. What are some characteristics of the most effective drug testing programs?

4. If you were the commissioner, would you continue the drug testing program? If so, what changes might you make?

Justification for Testing

How can governing bodies morally justify the perceived invasion of athletes' privacy through drug testing? Here, governing bodies might turn to teleological moral theory to provide the foundation for their assertion that drug testing is necessary. Two goals of drug testing are to keep competition safe and fair for the athletic community. Thus, governing bodies could emphasize the values of beneficence and fairness in an effort to justify the invasion of the athletes' privacy that drug testing entails. This claim could gain further strength if it could be substantiated that most athletes do not want performance-enhancing substances to be a part of sport. Additionally, governing bodies could lean on the values of respect and compassion to rationalize drug testing to deter those using performance-enhancing substances. Under this line of reasoning, it might also be said that those who break rules against the use of performance-enhancing substances do not respect the rules and have no compassion toward the persons who may be negatively affected by the use of performance-enhancing substances.

The teleologist, however, might also use a values-oriented approach to not support drug testing. It could be argued that drug testers are violating the value of trust—trust that persons involved in sport will compete fairly—when administering drug tests. The value of respect can also be questioned because it might be considered disrespectful to expect someone to adhere to the invasive procedures called for in drug testing.

Confidentiality Issues

Are the results of positive drug tests, in fact, remaining private when **confidentiality** has been guaranteed? If not, then a re-examination of some sports policies ensuring confidentiality is warranted. Supporting the notion that measures designed to ensure confidentiality have been ineffective is the fact that human beings, in part, are responsible for carrying out drug testing procedures, which allows for the potential of human error in regard to keeping information confidential. In fact, in politically charged environments, confidentiality "leaks" might even be calculated political strategies. Confidentiality in the world of drug testing may be equally prone to

confidentiality: a state of keeping information classified or private or not communicating it to others; in the area of drug testing in sport, keeping the results of an athlete's drug test between the testing agency and the athlete.

leaks, and the probability of an athlete's identity being revealed increases when more than one person has access to test results.

Is it reasonable to believe that when an athlete fails a drug test and is subsequently suspended for "undisclosed reasons" that teammates, fans, and others close to the team and sport will not find out why? Human curiosity and willingness to provide knowledge for personal and professional gain will render the well-intended notion of confidentiality ineffective. But should leagues or teams provide guarantees of confidentiality when it comes to drug testing? Some might argue that no such policies should be in place, and that positive results should be disclosed to the public to deter athletes from using performance-enhancing substances. Many believe that the fear of public exposure might effectively influence athletes to refrain from banned substance use. According to Dempster (as cited in Antonen, Bodley, Johnson, & Weir[27]), public humiliation is the strongest deterrent to steroid use. Former Los Angeles Dodgers' Manager Tommy Lasorda (as cited in Antonen, Bodley, Johnson, & Weir[27]) noted that MLB's new policy of making public the names of players who test positive for steroid use has strengthened the league's drug testing plan. Thus, a consequentialist who applies utilitarianism might argue that the good that accompanies disclosure outweighs the good that is associated with confidentiality in this situation.

A deontological theorist, on the other hand, might find this issue more difficult to resolve. In developing universalizable principles, the deontologist would have to ask whether confidentiality is something that should be maintained in all cases, or if all athletes who are caught using performance-enhancers should be publicly identified. Presumably, one could devise conditions under which the universalizing of confidentiality or public disclosure would not be in everyone's best interest. Hence, it may be better to follow the consequentialist's reasoning and favor public identification in this case, especially if it does indeed act as an effective deterrent for performance-enhancing substance use.

Should paying fans have the right to know the results of players' drug tests, or should drug testing results be kept confidential? Fans might make the case that when a player is suspended for failing a drug test, they, as paying fans (including season ticket holders), should have the right to demand a refund. This argument is strengthened if the fans can make a case that they purchased season tickets for the exclusive purpose of watching the player that was suspended.

What if a Baltimore Orioles' fan based his or her season ticket purchase on wanting to watch Rafael Palmeiro play throughout the MLB season? Palmeiro was suspended for 10 days during the 2005 season after an uncontested positive result of his drug test was revealed. Or, what if a biathlon fan based his or her attendance at the 2006 Torino Winter Olympics on wanting to watch the performance of Russian biathlete Olga Pyleva, who was suspended midway through the games for testing positive for the banned stimulant carphedon? Are fans entitled to a refund in such cases? After all, the athletes obviously broke a rule to which they previously agreed. The resulting punishments of a suspension and an expulsion affected teammates as well as fans because the athletes were not allowed to perform during their designated punishment periods. Interestingly, in the Palmeiro[28] and Pyleva[29] instances, they both claimed to have not been aware of putting the banned substances in their system.

Effectiveness and Expense of Drug Testing

In the case of many non-profit sport organizations, such as high school organizations, deciding whether to drug test is often a moot point due to insufficient funds. There are instances, however, in which high school athletic organizations, such as Oceanside High School in California, have made the elimination of drugs a priority and are spending large sums of money on drug testing of athletes. Oceanside High School, with the help of a federal grant, committed to a stepped-up program of randomized drug testing of athletes and cheerleaders. Having conducted drug testing in the past, Oceanside welcomed the opportunity that the grant provided to make the drug testing program more widespread. The grant provided resources to enable Oceanside to increase the number of those tested from one-third to approximately one-half of the school's 2000 athletes.[30]

Organizations that can afford the expense of drug testing are often able to do so because of the revenue generated from their sport or organization. The NCAA, with its enormous profits from the Division I men's basketball tournament and football bowl games, can afford to randomly drug test athletes. Other revenue-generating leagues, such as the NFL, have access to funding for the purpose of drug testing their athletes. The IOC also requires that their athletes adhere to drug testing policies.

In a society and world that has had real difficulty making significant progress in its war on drugs, a realistic attitude and approach to the difficulty in ridding sport of performance-enhancing substances must be taken. If it is agreed that performance-enhancing substances should be monitored or banned, decision makers should seriously analyze the effectiveness of the use of funds for drug testing. The success of drug testing in deterring banned substances should be examined. It is possible that reductions in performance-enhancing substance use by athletes could be achieved through means other than drug testing.

The question should be asked as to whether money spent on drug testing could be better spent on other means of deterring the use of performance-enhancing substances. For example, are leagues or teams missing out on opportunities to finance comprehensive drug education programs that outline the positive and negative effects of performance-enhancing substances? Are leagues failing to recognize opportunities to fund research on more **natural training techniques**—training techniques that do not include artificial practices such as taking steroids and other unnatural substances—to enhance athletic performance?

> **natural training techniques:** methods of working out that do not include artificial practices; that is, lifting weights to gain muscle mass is a natural training technique, whereas taking steroids to gain muscle mass is an unnatural training technique.

Could the money spent on the improvement of drug testing go toward helping socio-economically disadvantaged amateur athletes? How should leagues and teams prioritize such needs? Which issues, if any, deserve a higher prioritization? And how

BEATING THE NEW DRUG TEST

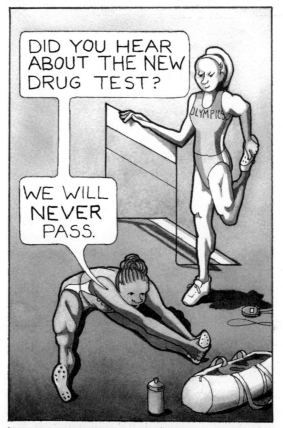

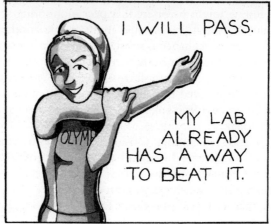

might funding be used to bring about the greatest good for the greatest number of people inside the realm of sport as well as outside of sport?

The Influence of Profit Goals on Efforts to Catch Users

Is it possible that, in the interest of money, teams, leagues, and organizations may not have a genuine desire to catch performance-enhancing substance users? Might they fear that if superstar athletes were to be suspended or expelled from professional or major college teams that attendance and television ratings could drop? Such decreases might, in turn, stifle other streams of revenue, including gate receipts, television contracts, and team apparel. Furthermore, if an athlete's performance is enhanced by banned substances to the point that he or she achieves superstardom, would it be in the best financial interest of organizations to catch and suspend that athlete? The above questions lead to one further question: Are drug testing policies true attempts to catch banned substance users, or are they calculated attempts to pacify public outcries against the use of performance-enhancing substances by athletes, with no genuine intentions to expose, incriminate, and punish users?

If money influences those in leadership positions to compromise their values, the already difficult challenge of catching and punishing athletes who are doping becomes even more difficult. Money can be a tremendous motivator and might cause one to lose sense of their moral values and principles. To ensure that leagues operate ethically, leaders of sport leagues and organizations should be selected based on their virtuous moral character. The practice and expectation of good moral values by sport leaders are critical in promoting the practice of good moral values by sport organizations.

Peer Management by Athletes

As discussed previously, if sport governing bodies continue to fail in their attempts to stop, or at least curb, performance-enhancing substance use, what solutions other than drug testing might be offered? A peer monitoring system by athletes might be one solution; that is, athletes would monitor one another. All aspects necessary to prevent performance-enhancing substance use in sports would be carried out by athletes. Such aspects would include the development and implementation of rules, as well as the carrying out of punishments for those breaking rules. Even if a system is not exclusively monitored by athletes, input from athletes could be included in the strategies chosen to address issues pertaining to performance-enhancing substance use in sport today.

Organizations, including those in higher education, have used peer-based models of management. In higher education, professors evaluate fellow faculty members on the most important areas relating to their jobs: teaching, scholarship, and service. Sometimes, the faculty members of a department elect their peers to a committee that will evaluate them for purposes of pay raises, promotion, and tenure. After a faculty member's peers render a personnel decision, the upper administration often has the opportunity to override the decision, but more often than not endorses it.

The peer-management system in higher education has operated effectively throughout the United States for years. No one is in a better position to evaluate faculty members than faculty members themselves. In evaluating each other, faculty members have an excellent knowledge of which faculty members are excelling and producing and which ones are not. When one is managed by those with whom one works closely, efforts must be made to play by the rules because peers are watching each other at all times.

A peer-management system might also be effective for sport organizations. Given the lack of success that governing bodies have had in stopping performance-enhancing substance use, new strategies such as peer-management might prove to be more effective in the battle against doping. Athletes would establish and enforce banned substance policies for their respective teams, leagues, and organizations. Teams could vote into place a committee that determines who gets tested, when they get tested, and what the resultant punishment would be for those testing positive. Athletes know better than anyone who the banned substance users are in their sports and have a vested interest in seeing to it that their peers do not get away with infractions. Athletes who are known by their peers to be doping, might even be required to accept punitive measures imposed upon them by their peers.

Because those in power typically do not like to relinquish power, a peer management model probably would attract significant resistance from the leaders and members of sport governing bodies. Resistance or not, the challenge of eliminating, or at least reducing, performance-enhancing substance use should be addressed. Administrators are not acting in the best interest of sport if they are not at least receptive to new ideas proposed for the purpose of curtailing the use of illegal performance enhancers.

For example, Don Catlin has proposed that a volunteer drug deterrent program be implemented. Although not exclusively implemented and monitored by peers, Catlin's volunteer drug deterrent program would place the initial onus on the athletes to volunteer to be tested. Prior to competing at the elite level, athletes would volunteer for the program and be given a battery of tests measuring their biochemistry. Athletes in the program would not be tested as often as other athletes, just have their levels checked occasionally. If the levels of the athletes in the program change they would be decertified (removed from the volunteer program) and subject to the aggressive testing for the athletes not in the volunteer program.[31]

peer-managed system: a supervisory structure that is controlled not by a superior but by those who are equal to one another; in the case of deterring drug usage in sport, a peer management system would primarily rely on the athletes to assume the responsibility of policing one another.

A **peer-managed system** including a volunteer system would, of course, be confronted with the same legal challenges that current systems face. Athletes have legal rights, as discussed previously, and those rights must be honored. Organizations should, however, examine peer management as a strategy for deterring the use of performance-enhancing substances in sport and consider implementing the aspects of it that will work within the legal system.

Conclusion

Many issues surround the use of performance-enhancing substances in sport. The risks for the athletes who use such substances are real and are passed down to the peers who try to keep up with them and the young athletes who mimic them. The advantages gained through the use of performance enhancers are also ethically questionable in that they give athletes an edge that is, at least to some extent, unearned. And although current testing procedures have their problems regarding privacy and confidentiality, testing does appear to be warranted based on the fact that athletes and other members of sporting communities generally agree that they do not want performance-enhancing substances to be a part of sport training and competition. Views regarding performance-enhancing substance use may change over time, as more knowledge is gained about them and more thought is given to the issues examined above. For now, if athletes do not want illegal performance-enhancing substances and techniques in sport, they should use aspects of peer management systems and seek assistance from governing bodies to minimize the presence of banned substances and the role they play in deciding athletic contests.

References

1. Committee on Sports Medicine and Fitness. Use of performance-enhancing substances. American Academy of Pediatrics Policy Statement. *Pediatrics* [serial online]. 2005;115: 1103–1106. Available at: http://pediatrics.aappublications.org/cgi/content/full/115/4/1103. Accessed March 27, 2008.
2. Millman RB, Ross BA. Steroid and nutritional supplement use in professional athletes. *Am J Addict* 2003;12:S48–S54.
3. Federman DG. "Bulking up" with steroids: advise against? *J Musculoskeletal Med* 2003;20 (6):268.
4. A Report by the President's Council on Bioethics. Beyond therapy: biotechnology and the pursuit of happiness. The President's Council On Bioethics Web site. Available at: http://www.bioethics.gov/reports/beyondtherapy/2003. Accessed on June 1, 2006.
5. Evans NA. Anabolic steroids: answers to the bigger questions. *J Musculoskeletal Med* 2004;21:166–178.
6. Conseco J. Juiced: *Wild Times, Rampant 'Roids, Smash Hits, and How Baseball Got Big.* New York: Harper Collins, 2005.
7. Puma M. Not the size of the dog in the fight. ESPN Web site. Available at: http://espn.go.com/classic/biography/s/Alzado_Lyle.html. Accessed April 21, 2007.
8. Simon RL. *Fair Play: The Ethics of Sport.* 2nd ed. Boulder, CO: Westview Press; 2004.
9. Fost N. Steroid hysteria: unpacking the claims. *Virtual Mentor* [serial online]. November, 2005. Available at: http://www.ama-assn.org/ama/pub/category/15633.html. Accessed June 1, 2006.

10. Dawson RT. Drugs in sport—the role of the physician. *J Endocrinol 2001*;170:55–71.

11. Zillgitt J. Double standard in singling out Bonds with asterisks. USA Today [serial online]. June 2, 2006. Available at http://www.usatoday.com/sports/columnist/zillgitt/2006-05-31-zillgitt-bonds_x.htm. Accessed April 21, 2007.

12. Chairman's message. World Anti-Doping Agency Web site. Available at: http://www.wada-ama.org/en/dynamic.ch2?pageCategory.id=254. Accessed April 14, 2007.

13. The testimony of Dr. Don Catlin. U.S. Senate Committee on Science, Commerce, and Transportation Web site. May 2005. Available at: http://commerce.senate.gov/hearings/testimony.cfm?id=1511&wit_id=4278. Accessed April 14, 2007.

14. Amendments to the sentencing guidelines. United States Sentencing Commission Web site. Available at: http://www.ussc.gov/2006guid/Finalamend2006.pdf. Accessed May 11, 2007.

15. Lydic R. Performance-enhancing substances present a double-edged sword. *Anesthesia Patient Safety Foundation Newsletter* [serial online]. Spring 2005. Available at: http://www.apsf.org/resource_center/newsletter/2005/spring/03drugs.htm. Accessed June 1, 2006.

16. Kenda R. Pressure to find an edge is heavy. *USA Today* [serial online]. 2002. Available at: http://www.usatoday.com/sports/bbw/2002-07-11/special-steroids.htm. Accessed June 1, 2006.

17. Cook R. Testing won't stop steroid use. *Post-Gazette* Web site. 2002. Available at: http://www.post-gazette.com/sports/columnists/20020604cook0604p1.asp. Accessed May 31, 2006.

18. Gardner R. On performance-enhancing substances and the unfair advantage argument. *J Philosophy Sport* 1989;16:60–73.

19. Anderson PM. The Supreme Court sets the standard: drug testing at the interscholastic level. *Texas Review of Entertainment & Sports Law* 2003;4(1):1–82.

20. Meyers JF. Hill v. NCAA: California adopts a new standard for invasion of privacy. *Employee Relations Law Journal* 1994;20(1):73–84.

21. Yasser R, McCurdy JR, Goplerud CP, Weston MA. *Sports Law: Cases and Materials*. 5th ed. Cincinnati, OH: Anderson Publishing Co.; 2003.

22. Diacin MJ, Parks JB, Allison PC. Voices of male athletes on drug use, drug testing, and the existing order in intercollegiate athletics. *J Sport Behav* 2003;26:1–16.

23. Coakley J. *Sports in Society: Issues and Controversies*. 8th ed. New York: McGraw-Hill; 2004.

24. Brennan C. Anti-doping agency taking right steps. *USA Today*. June 10, 2004:11C.

25. Discus champion loses gold. BBC Sport Web site. August 24, 2004. Available at: http://news.bbc.co.uk/sport1/hi/olympics_2004/athletics/3595006.stm. Accessed April 23, 2007.

26. Ferstle J. World Conference on doping in sport. In: Wilson W, Derse E, eds. *Doping in Elite Sport*. Champaign, IL: Human Kinetics; 2001:275–286.

27. Antonen M, Bodley H, Johnson C, Weir T. Baseball confronts "big" question: Who's juiced? Spring brings size under scrutiny. *USA Today* Web site. February 18, 2005:1C.

28. Bodley H. Palmeiro suspended for steroids policy violation. *USA Today* Web site. August 1, 2005. Available at: http://www.usatoday.com/sports/baseball/al/orioles/2005-08-01-palmeiro-suspension_x.htm. Accessed April 23, 2007.

29. Russian biathlete claims ignorance in Turin doping scandal. MOS News Web site. February 16, 2006. Available at: http://www.mosnews.com/news/2006/02/16/dopingnews.shtml. Accessed April 23, 2007.

30. Parmet S. Drug testing measures will return to Oceanside. *Union-Tribune* Web site. June 15, 2005. Available at: http://www.signonsandiego.com/news/education/20050615-9999-1mi15drugs.html. Accessed April 23, 2007.

31. Lieber Steeg J. Catlin is looking beyond drug testing. *USA Today* Web site. February 28, 2007. Available at: http://www.usatoday.com/sports/olympics/2007-02-28-beyond-testing_x.htm. Accessed April 23, 2007.

Steroid Use in Big Time Baseball

With the recent successes of two superstar Big Time Baseball (BTB) players, rumor has it that the use of steroids in BTB is rampant and players are "juicing" without regard for fair play or physical harm. Players seem to be willing to assume the physical risk associated with steroid use in favor of achieving improved statistics with better on-field performances.

The following notion seems quite credible: players who take steroids hit more home runs, and more fans are willing to pay money to see these outstanding performances, which provides a larger pool of money for players as well as owners. Even players who may be unwilling to assume the risks associated with taking steroids often feel pressured to do so, just to be able to compete for contracts with the players who are taking steroids.

Tragically, recently the perceived dangers of steroid use among teenage athletes became a reality when two high school baseball players, from different parts of the country, committed suicide on the same day. Both of these young athletes (one was 15 years old and the other 17) had been diagnosed as suffering from clinical depression caused by steroid use. Even though the diagnoses were made by different professionals, the findings were nearly identical, directly linking the boys' depression to steroid use. The parents of both boys have become outspoken against the use of steroids by athletes, not only at the middle and high school levels, but also at the professional level. To some degree, these parents blame their sons' initial use of steroids on BTB's lack of a policy against steroid use. The parents believe their sons were initially motivated to take steroids because they aspired to be like star players in BTB who are known to have taken steroids.

Given the circumstances surrounding the use of steroids, this has obviously become a complicated and extraordinarily serious issue for the commissioner of BTB. The commissioner knows he must do something but is not sure where to even begin.

Critical Thinking: Finding Common-Sense Solutions

1. If you were a player and steroid use was illegal, would you turn in a teammate whom you knew was using steroids? Explain your reasoning.

2. If you were a parent of one of the high school baseball players who committed suicide, would you blame your son's death on star players of BTB who are known to have taken steroids? Why or why not?

3. If you were the commissioner of BTB and were charged with the development of a steroid abuse policy, to what extent, if any, would you consider the financial effects that a steroid abuse policy might have on the league?

Critical Thinking: Moral Theory-Based Decision Making

4. If you were the commissioner of BTB and preparing to deal with the steroid issue, which of the following theories would you primarily use as the foundation for your decision: consequentialist, deontological, or teleological? Explain your answer.

5. If you were the commissioner of BTB and were basing your actions concerning the steroid problem on fostering the *integrity* and *morality* of baseball, what actions would you take? Explain how these actions are related to the *integrity* and *morality* of baseball.

6. If you were the commissioner of BTB, in what ways would you consider *fairness, equity,* and the *safety* of players, owners, and fans when planning your strategies to address the steroid problem?

7. If you were the commissioner of BTB, what emphasis would you put on your *own good* versus *the good of others* when deciding how to solve the steroid problem in BTB?

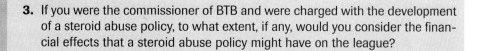

The Hall of Fame Dilemma

It is the year 2010, and voters for the Hall of Fame of the World Baseball League (WBL) are faced with a difficult decision. This is the first year that players who have either admitted to taking steroids during their careers or been implicated by others are on the Hall of Fame ballot. Steroid use remains illegal, and a stronger testing policy instituted by the WBL and its players' union has helped reduce steroid use significantly. Although the WBL and many of its fans recognize that the players' offensive records are impressive accomplishments that resulted primarily from remarkable talent and dedication, the "steroid players" are known to have been "juicing" during their most productive seasons. Furthermore, when asked if they had done so, these players either refused to admit they used steroids or lied about using them. Many former players, Hall of Fame sportswriters, and fans believe that these players should not be allowed into the Hall of Fame because they cheated and then lied about cheating.

Further complicating matters is the fact that baseball great Roderick Measures is still banned from the game. Measures, the WBL's all-time hits and batting average leader and one of the best players in the game during his career, was banned from the sport for betting on WBL games while he was manager of the Backland Bucks in 1991. Measures did not cheat during his career and did nothing to disgrace the game as a player. He only began gambling after his WBL playing career was over. Although many people believe that Measures' ban is fair and just because his actions brought into question the integrity of the game, other people believe that he has served his time and should be recognized for his accomplishments as a player, accomplishments that were not aided by the use of steroids. Given the fact that steroid players may be inducted into the WBL's Hall of Fame, Commissioner Trevor Valley must now decide whether to continue to uphold Measures' ban or reinstate him and allow him to be added to the Hall of Fame ballot for the upcoming vote.

Critical Thinking: Finding Common-Sense Solutions

1. If you were one of the voters for the Hall of Fame, under what conditions, if any, would you vote for players who had used steroids? Explain your rationale.

2. If Commissioner Valley does not reinstate Measures for the upcoming ballot, should he do so if some steroid players are inducted into the WBL's Hall of Fame? Why or why not?

3. If you were a Hall of Fame voter, would you vote for a reinstated Roderick Measures to be inducted into the Hall of Fame? Explain your rationale.

Critical Thinking: Moral Theory-Based Decision Making

4. As a Hall of Fame voter, explain whether you would vote for the steroid players and why you would or would not vote for them if:

   a. you were reasoning as a teleological ethical theorist.

   b. you were reasoning as a deontological ethical theorist.

   c. you were basing your reasoning on consequentialism.

5. If you were Commissioner Valley, would you reinstate Roderick Measures given the fact that the steroid players are on the Hall of Fame ballot? What values or principles might guide you in this case?

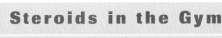

Steroids in the Gym

Ron had been a fitness and strength trainer for the last 20 years. His clients were primarily adolescent and adult athletes looking for a competitive edge. Two years ago, Ron was approached by Tony and Mark, two young men who wanted him to help them train for football. Their primary objective was to bulk up and gain strength that would enhance their defensive line play. Mark, 15, was attending high school with the hopes of earning a football scholarship to a Division I college. Tony was already a college football player who had aspirations of a professional career.

Ron began training the two of them in January, and by March, Tony and Mark were making remarkable progress, a little too remarkable in Ron's professional opinion. He soon realized that the two were experimenting with steroids. As a strength trainer and drug-free bodybuilder, Ron strongly objected to this decision but chose not to confront them on the matter. He knew the steroids were working: Tony and Mark had both put on 30 pounds of muscle and both were training enthusiastically for their upcoming seasons. Both Tony and Mark experienced break-out seasons that fall. Their performances soon prompted teammates interested in increasing strength and performance to ask who was responsible for their training programs. Tony referred them to Ron, who was soon in great demand and suddenly stood to gain status and money from the success of his wayward pupils. Teammates, however, were not the only ones seeking information about Tony and Mark's training regimens. Coaches and scouts called Ron, asking if the two were on steroids or if their strength gains could be attributed solely to their hard work and training methods.

Further complicating matters was the fact that Tony, who was having trouble financing his steroid use, had begun to sell illegal steroids to college students. He even had Mark drumming up interest in purchasing them in high school. Upon discovering this, Ron knew he would have to do something to keep the situation from getting further out of control. But what could he do?

Critical Thinking: Finding Common-Sense Solutions

1. Should Ron have recommended a program for Tony and Mark to make them aware of the dangers of steroids? What should the strength coach have done to help Mark and Tony realize the risks and problems they might encounter?

2. Should Ron have informed Tony and Mark's parents, coaches, athletic directors, and/or counselors about their steroid use? Why or why not?

3. Should Ron accept Tony and Mark's teammates as clients? If so, under what conditions should he do so?

4. When questioned by coaches and scouts about Tony and Mark's training routines, what information should Ron reveal about them?

Critical Thinking: Moral Theory-Based Decision Making

5. Did Ron do the right thing by not confronting Tony and Mark about their steroid use? If you were Ron, would you have confronted them and/or stopped training them? What moral values or principles would you have used in your reasoning?

6. Should Ron tell the police that Tony and Mark are using or selling steroids? Why or why not? What moral values or principles would you have used in your reasoning?

The Narcoleptic Gymnast

Juan, the director of the International Gymnastics Guild (IGG), is faced with a difficult decision. As director of this governing body, he has the tie-breaking vote when the IGG's Rules and Competition Committee is undecided about how to proceed in particular situations. The committee is currently split over whether to grant Cindy, a world-class American gymnast with narcolepsy, an exemption that would allow her to use her banned medication during the upcoming World Championships.

As a narcoleptic, Cindy has to take her medication, the stimulant dextroamphetamine, to function normally. Without it, Cindy has trouble staying awake and can fall asleep even during competition. Since dextroamphetamine is the only medication she can currently use, she must either use it in competition or withdraw. The United States Gymnastics Guild (USGG) has granted Cindy an exemption that allows her to use dextroamphetamine at the doctor-recommended dosage. The exemption was given because, in the USGG's view, this medication was not a performance enhancer for Cindy but a performance enabler—a substance that gave her the ability to compete.

The USGG also stated that, although a banned substance, dextroamphetamine's status as a performance enhancer for gymnastics was somewhat unclear. Although gymnastics requires explosive movements that might be aided by the use of a stimulant, it also requires exact movements that might be hindered by such use. Given this equivocation and Cindy's special circumstances, the USGG decided that it was in everyone's best interest to give her an exemption and allow her the right to compete in USGG-sanctioned events using her medication. Through participation in these events, she earned a spot on the United States Gymnastics Team that will be competing in the IGG World Championships next month in Prague, Czech Republic.

Although the IGG has chosen to ban dextroamphetamine, Juan himself has wondered whether it is a performance enhancer for gymnasts. He has also wondered whether Cindy's performances have been enhanced by her medication. The time has come for him to cast his vote. What should he do?

Critical Thinking: Finding Common-Sense Solutions
1. Should the IGG and USGG have banned dextroamphetamine? Why or why not?

2. How should governing bodies decide whether a substance should be banned? What should they take into account in making this decision?

3. Should one person's vote be allowed to decide a committee's decision on an issue? Justify your answer using moral values and principles.

Critical Thinking: Moral Theory-Based Decision Making

4. Should Juan grant Cindy the exemption? Refer to moral values and principles in justifying your answer.

5. Would Juan allow the exemption if he were reasoning as a consequentialist? As a deontologist? As a teleologist?

Key Terms

coercion—compulsion by force; force or the power to use force to secure compliance. In the context of competitive sport, coercion makes reference to athletes who are pressured to take performance-enhancing substances.

confidentiality—a state of keeping information classified or private or not communicating it to others; in the area of drug testing in sport, keeping the results of an athlete's drug test between the testing agency and the athlete.

drug testing—the process by which athletes are screened—commonly through a urine or blood test administered by their governing body, such as the National Collegiate Athletic Association, the International Olympic Committee, and Major League Baseball—to determine whether they have taken a performance-enhancing substance; drug testing takes place to help ensure not only a fair and level playing field for athletes, but also the safety of the athletes.

harm issues—in athletics, issues related to the potential for injury resulting from taking performance-enhancing substances; of primary concern is the taking of performance-enhancing substances by athletes who would prefer not to, but feel the need to do so to compete with athletes who are taking them.

invasion of privacy—in the case of drug testing athletes, infringing on their 4th Amendment rights through the implementation of testing procedures that are an intrusion on an athletes' person, that is, athletes being required to produce urine samples in less-than-private conditions.

naturally talented athlete—a player whose athletic abilities are not the result of the use of artificial substances; a player who is born with above-average physical abilities, such as speed, jumping ability, and strength.

natural training techniques—methods of working out that do not include artificial practices; that is, lifting weights to gain muscle mass is a natural training technique, whereas taking steroids to gain muscle mass is an unnatural training technique.

overt coercion—in sport, an open form of force or pressure applied to players to take performance-enhancing substances by those who have an interest in the enhanced performance of players.

peer-managed system—a supervisory structure that is controlled not by a superior but by those who are equal to one another; in the case of deterring drug usage in sport, a peer management system would primarily rely on the athletes to assume the responsibility of policing one another.

side effects—the unintended or adverse physical, psychological, and emotional effects that result from taking performance-enhancing substances.

soft coercion—in sport, the self-imposed pressure to take performance-enhancing substances to remain competitive with those who are already taking them.

5 Violence in Sport: Ethically Acceptable Boundaries

Learning Outcomes

After reading Chapter 5, the student will be able to:

1. Describe the relationship between societal and sport violence.

2. Differentiate between in-game violence and peripheral violence.

3. Provide examples of violence inherent in sport.

4. Compare arguments for and against using sport as a catharsis to reduce violence that takes place in non-sport environments.

5. Describe ways that athletes, coaches, and administrators can break the cycle of violence in sport.

6. Explain how the glorification of winning can encourage violence in sport.

7. Identify some examples of and contributing factors to spectator violence.

8. Describe ways that player/spectator violence can be reduced.

Violence is a visible part of today's sport scene. Whether because of increasing violent incidents in and surrounding sports, increasing attention from the media when violent acts occur, or a combination of both, violence is more prevalent in sport today than in years past. Undeniably, the use of violent tactics, fights among athletes and between athletes and spectators, post-game riots, and hazing incidents make headlines with increasing regularity. Given the prevalence of increasingly aggressive behavior and outright violence in sport, and the concern that sport-related violence might extend beyond the playing field, the question arises as to just what are ethically acceptable boundaries regarding sport and violence. Is all violence and aggression related to sport unethical? Is it ever ethical? Or should we apply moral reasoning on a case-by-case basis to determine whether or not particular acts of sport-related violence are ethical or unethical? What can we do, participant and spectator alike, to combat violent and aggressive behavior in sport? And can reduced violence in sport lead to reduced violence in society in general?

This chapter seeks to answer those questions in a moral context. We will examine sport-related violence, the factors that influence it, and the ways in which sport participants and spectators can apply moral reasoning to incidents of sport violence. Readers will thus become acquainted with the different kinds of violence that occur within and around sports and learn ways to eradicate it based on the application of moral analysis.

 ## Societal Violence

Violence has always been part of human nature. We see it all around us, in our homes, our schools, our communities, from historical times to the present. Modern society is bombarded daily with violent images, through war coverage in the media, shootings on campuses, shoot-outs with the police, and movies and videogames that seem to glorify violence and murder. And we see acts of **aggression** and violence increasingly in sports. Competitive sport understandably involves a certain amount of aggressive play, but acts of true violence cross a line that should never be crossed. Sadly, it is a line being crossed with distressing frequency. Some athletes employ violent tactics as a way to injure or intimidate an opponent, and there are some coaches who use violence as part of their overall strategy for defeating an opposing team. Spectators unwittingly demonstrate their support of violent behavior when they cheer as a brawl breaks out on the field between players. But just what is sports violence, and are some sports inherently violent?

> **aggression:** behavior intended to cause psychological or physical pain or harm.

In-Game Violence

> **competitive objectives of sport:** goals within competitive sport that are formally established and known by all; for example, gaining yardage, tackling, and scoring are three competitive objectives in the game of football; teams that are the most effective in attaining the competitive goals of sport usually achieve victory.

Terry and Jackson define sports violence as "behavior which causes harm, occurs outside of the rules of the sport, and is unrelated to the **competitive objectives of sport.**"[1(p2)] Coakley defines it as "the use of excessive physical force, which causes or has the potential to cause harm or destruction."[2(p202)] A tragic example of Terry and Jackson's definition of sports violence occurred during team practice for the Oakland Raiders of the National Football League (NFL). On August 24, 2003, linebacker Bill Romanowski punched 27-year-old teammate Marcus Williams in the face.

Romanowski's crushing blow broke Williams' eye socket, caused brain damage, and ended his NFL career.[3] Romanowski's actions are the very definition of violence in sport: his behavior caused harm, occurred outside the rules of sport, and was unrelated to the objectives of his sport. Although you could argue that Romanowski intended to intimidate his competition by punching Williams in the face, his violent act did not provide him with a direct advantage to gaining yardage, tackling, or scoring—three competitive objectives of the sport of football.

Actions such as Romanowski's would find difficulty gaining support from the three moral reasoning models presented in Chapter 1. From a teleological perspective, it is difficult to find any values that support such behavior. It is unlikely that a deontologist would prefer that Romanowski's behavior be universalized as acceptable to all. And certainly, if applying consequentialism from a utilitarian viewpoint, the consequences of Romanowski injuring Williams did not result in a greater good.

> **in-game violence (sport violence):** within sporting contests, unjust or unwarranted exertion of intense physical force, often resulting in injury.

As its name indicates, **in-game violence** is violence that occurs during the course of play, such as the use of violent tactics to harm opposing players or fights that break out between players. An example of in-game violence is one from the 2004 National Hockey League (NHL) season. In an act of retaliation for an incident that took place three weeks previously, the Vancouver Canucks' Todd Bertuzzi, at 6'3", 245 lbs., assaulted the smaller 6'1", 210 lb. Steve Moore of the Colorado Avalanche. Bertuzzi approached Moore from behind, grabbed his jersey with one hand, and punched him with the other, knocking Moore unconscious. Bertuzzi then shoved the unconscious Moore into the ice as he was falling. As a result of Bertuzzi's assault, Moore suffered a broken neck, spinal ligament injuries, a concussion, and facial cuts and bruises.[4]

From a deontological perspective, would those involved in the game of hockey be willing to universalize Bertuzzi's behavior? This scenario is interesting because from some perspectives, it was not necessarily Bertuzzi's *actions* that drew attention but the *result* of those actions. When examining Bertuzzi's act of retaliation against Moore, hockey players might support the act as part of an unwritten code in hockey that lets players 'police' dirty hits by fellow players by retaliating with even more vicious hits. Thus, Moore's injury aside, players might universally accept Bertuzzi's hit, especially had it been more face to face instead of an attack on Moore's blind side.

Many sports have inherently violent aspects. In football, for example, blocking and especially tackling are often done violently, sometimes to intimidate or 'send a message' to the ball carrier. One violent aspect of the game of hockey is the physical contact that comes from body checking, which is using the shoulder or hip to knock an opposing player against the ice or boards. Hockey's most extreme form of violence, however, is the actual fighting between players that for all intents and purposes is accepted as part of the game. Scrums in rugby include elements of violence also, and boxing is clearly violent in that it consists exclusively of punching an opponent in an attempt to earn victory by causing enough physical harm to knock the other person unconscious.

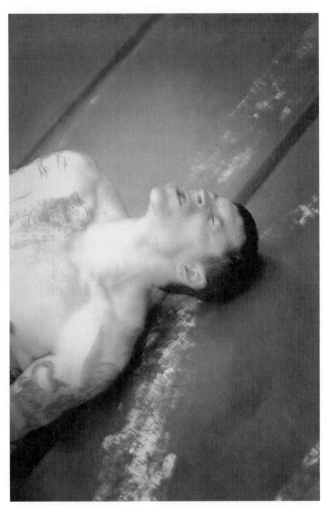

5-1 *A sport such as ultimate fighting is designed with elements of violence included.*

Few sports are more violent than ultimate fighting, however. In 1997, ultimate fighting was forced off television and eventually banned by most states because of its brutality. Ultimate fighting was brought back in 2001 largely because of the sport's rule changes that were supposed to soften the punching, stomping, kneeing, and elbowing so prevalent in the sport.[5]

Spectators and Violence in Sport

Society as a whole seems to have long embraced sports that are violent in nature or that have violent elements. Fans cheer after a violent hit in football, believe they have received their money's worth when ultimate fighters beat their opponents into submission, and are ecstatic when a boxer knocks out an opponent. When discussing the morality of ultimate fighting using the utilitarian method of moral reasoning, we should attempt to determine the amount of happiness that the sport of ultimate fighting brings to not only those close to it but also members of society. If more people are happier with the sport than without it, support from a utilitarian perspective is evident. If, however, more people disagree and are unhappy with ultimate fighting because of its relatively high level of violence, a case could be made to ban the sport or to change its structure to decrease its more violent aspects.

Certainly, fan attendance is an indicator of the popularity and enjoyment of a particular sport. There were 20,455 spectators at the heavyweight boxing title bout between Joe Frazier and Muhammad Ali on March 8, 1971 at Madison Square Garden. Referred to as the "fight of the century," both boxers maintained a pace that was more like lightweights.[6] Frazier attacked with sweeping left hooks while Ali flashed jabs followed by left-right combinations. To the delight of thousands of fans in attendance and those watching on television, Frazier won this fast and furious fight by a decision highlighted by him knocking down Ali in the 15th round.

Exemplifying a perverted sense of enjoyment that some fans seem to receive from violence is an incident that took place at Philadelphia's Veteran Stadium during an NFL game between the Philadelphia Eagles and the Dallas Cowboys in 1999. The incident occurred when Cowboys receiver Michael Irvin landed awkwardly on his head after catching a pass. For 20 minutes, Irvin lay motionless on the turf as he was tended to by his trainers. When the Philadelphia crowd of 66,669 realized Irvin was hurt, many cheered and continued cheering when paramedics removed him from the field on a stretcher.[7] That fans took pleasure in someone else's potentially life-threatening injuries shows a deficiency in the values of beneficence and compassion. It may be that fans dismissed these values in favor of winning at all costs. Irvin performed splendidly against the Eagles on numerous occasions, which made it difficult for them to achieve victory. The cheering by the Eagles fans might have been an indication of their extreme desire to win football games, believing their chances for victory would improve if Irvin was injured and unable to return to the game.

Attempting to identify moralistic rationale on the part of the Eagles fans is challenging. Cheering when someone on the opposing team is injured is not supported teleologically by moral values. It is unlikely to be supported deontologically, since most people probably would not want people around them cheering if they were seriously injured. From a consequentialist perspective, if we were to use utilitarianism as a guide, the happiness or pleasure brought to the fans who cheered was probably not powerful enough to support the act of cheering. It is doubtful that the most amount of people were made happy, since it is likely that many fans throughout the country were disappointed with the actions of Eagles fans.

Despite the fact that society enjoys these violent sports, if it can be demonstrated that violent sports perpetuate violence in society, organizers should assume the responsibility for removing violence from games. If a reduction of violence in sport can contribute to the larger goal of decreasing violence in society, organizers should examine ways to make sport less violent.

Sport as a Catharsis for Violence

As previously mentioned, elements of violence are inherent in certain sports. Physical force and even assault are part of sports like football, boxing, and rugby. Outside of sport, tackling or punching someone would be considered assault, yet in the previously mentioned sports it is incorporated within the rules of the game. Thus, using Terry and Jackson's definition of violence in sport,[1] since the behavior is within the rules of the game, tackling in football would not be considered violent; but, using Coakley's definition of violence,[2] since these sports have the potential to cause physical harm they are, in fact, violent.

Certain violent actions that take place within the framework of the rules of the game are an assumed risk that competitors accept when they agree to compete in a particular sport. Typically, from a liability perspective, "injuries incurred in athletic participation are not of tortuous origin, but they occur rather as a result of the normal risks associated with participation in the sport."[8(p656)] If, when making the decision to participate in sport, participants are assuming the risk that comes with violent sport, in a sense they are adhering to deontological moral theory in that they are not only accepting the violent aspects of sport for others but also accepting it for themselves. In other words, if you support violent aspects of sport for its participants, and you, as a participant, also willingly accept those same violent aspects, you are operating under a deontological foundation. Recall that deontology is not selective in establishing behavior but instead universalizes it to all.

Given the elements of violence in some sports, it seems plausible that violent sport is a stage for **cathartic aggression** in that athletes are able to unleash violence in a more controlled environment against other athletes who have agreed to accept the rules of a sport and the violent conditions of the game. Gill restricts the term aggression to "behaviors intended to harm or injure others."[9(p196)] Also recognizing intent as being an element of aggression, Coakley defines aggression as "verbal or physical actions grounded in an intent to dominate, control, or do harm to another person."[2(p203)] Gill further contends that it is difficult to label aggression as inherently desirable or undesirable because it is open to the interpretation of the observer.[9] Furthermore, if intent is part of the definition of aggression, only the person committing the act truly knows whether or not they intend to harm someone.

> **cathartic aggression:** in sport, the release of violence or hostility while participating in sport.

One example of aggression in sport is the vicious head butt by French midfielder Zinedine Zidane during the 2006 World Cup soccer final. Prior to Zidane lowering his head and ramming Italy's Marco Materazzi, knocking him to the ground, the two had exchanged words. Zidane, the most valuable player of the World Cup, received a red card and was ejected from the game for his act of aggression.[10] Zidane's behavior meets both Coakley's and Gill's aforementioned definitions of aggression; it certainly seems that Zidane's head butting was grounded in an intent to do harm to Materazzi.

In one scientific research study, the belief that observing violent sports leads to a reduction in aggressive urges was examined, and it was found that those with a high level of involvement in aggressive sports can lower their level of aggression (symbolic sport catharsis), particularly if the sport is viewed in person.[11] Acts of aggression in sport, however, are potentially driven by egoistic thinking. In other words, aggression may not take place for the purpose of providing others with pleasure, but for the purpose of providing oneself with pleasure. If aggression is minimized, altruism and beneficence may surface. Important to note, however, is that the literature does not universally affirm the notion that aggression is reduced in those who participate in more aggressive sports. It might be that aggressive people seek out aggressive or violent sports and remain aggressive despite participation.

Players who compete in violent sports may have an affinity for violence and thus are attracted to violent sports. It could be argued that some persons are violently predisposed and are simply attracted to violent sports. These individuals would not become violent because of their participation in violent sports but because of their violent natures. If this is true, an argument could be made that the sport serves the purpose of allowing a violent person to behave violently in a controlled sport setting.

"The Violent Sport As a Catharsis Controversy"

Mr. Tony Tussle was committed to helping teenage boys stay out of trouble. Once a troubled teen himself, Mr. Tussle grew up on the rough side of town and often found himself in the middle of street fights, and he did not want other teenage boys to find themselves in similar dangerous situations. After much thought, Mr. Tussle decided to offer free boxing lessons to teenage boys in the neighborhood. By offering these lessons at the local gym, Mr. Tussle believed that he was performing a service to the community in that he was getting these boys off the street and into the gym. Interestingly, some adults in the community were challenging Mr. Tussle's efforts because they believed he was creating street thugs by teaching teenage boys how to fight. Mr. Tussle defended his boxing lessons by claiming that when the boys were involved in his lessons, they would be venting their violent energies in the gym instead of on the street.

Questions
1. What moral values, if any, might Mr. Tussle be basing his decision on to offer free boxing lessons to teenagers in the neighborhood?
2. What do you believe are the moral values of the community members who are against Tony Tussle's free boxing lessons?
3. Discuss the potential consequences of Mr. Tussle's decision to provide free boxing lessons to the teenagers in the neighborhood.

More specifically, sports that include physical contact might serve as an outlet in which some participants can release their violent tendencies. And if sport serves as a catharsis for violent persons, it might, to some extent, reduce violence in society. There is currently no evidence to confirm this, of course, but hypothetically speaking, it could be argued that more violently disposed individuals might find some sort of release through participation in more aggressive, even violent, sport.

Public Acceptance of Violent Sports

For better or worse, violence is an accepted, even expected, part of many sports. If blame were to be assigned for the perpetuation of violent sports such as boxing and football, there is plenty to go around. Society can be blamed for reinforcing violence not only through their attendance at violent sporting events, but also through their own violent behaviors at those events. Gary Bettman, the commissioner of the NHL, is acutely aware that his league's fan base believes fighting is intrinsic to the game of hockey.[4] Given that many fans expect and enjoy violence in hockey, the leaders of hockey are thus likely to continue supporting fighting in the sport.

Television networks could be blamed for broadcasting violent sporting events. Despite the potentially negative social value that ultimate fighting brings to society, fighters now enjoy star-like status thanks to media coverage. And the violence sometimes extends off the field. As evidence that ultimate fighting's violence extends beyond the ring, cages are installed around the ring not only to keep the fighters within the designated boundary but also to keep violent fans from entering the ring.[4] Governing bodies could be blamed for not changing the violent nature of games under their jurisdiction. Competitors could also be blamed for merely participating in these sports.

Obviously, violent sport is supported and reinforced by a wide range of persons and groups. Why, then, should we be concerned with ridding the sporting world of its violent games? Using the tenants of utilitarianism as a guide, the case would have to be made that violence in sport leads more to short- and long-term happiness than to unhappiness. And to meet the utilitarian standard of bringing the most amount of good to the most amount of people, the most amount of good must be brought to those directly and indirectly affected by the violent aspects of sport. In other words, if the participants are the only ones happy with violence in sport, the utilitarian standard would not support violence in sport. However, if more people, overall, are affected in a good way because of violent aspects of sport (such as a vicious hit in football), the utilitarian standard would hold.

Cycle of Violence in Sport

If society disagrees with the notion that sports have to be violent and is interested in creating more peaceful games, we may need to look beyond sport to understand underlying factors that contribute to the creation and support of aggressive and

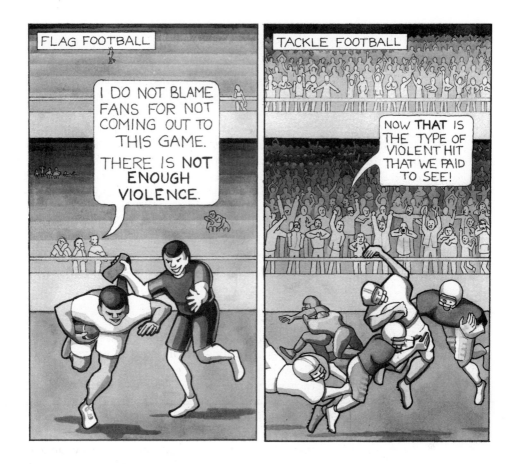

violent games. For instance, masculinity is thought to be a contributing factor. Historically, boys generally have been raised to be tough and manly. Demonstrations of toughness might include winning schoolyard fights or remaining stoic in the face of physical pain. Violent sport is one avenue that exists for boys and men to explore and demonstrate their toughness.

Team moral atmosphere is also strongly related to athlete aggression.[12,13] Stephens found that team norms—an important aspect of moral atmosphere— were the strongest predictor of a player's likelihood to play aggressively.[14] When coaches and teammates condone and show support for aggressive or violent behavior, such behavior is more likely to occur. **Team culture** may also be a factor that influences athletes to commit acts of violence outside of sport. Coakley asserts that common targets of such violence include women and others in the community who publicly challenge an athlete's "assumed status and privilege," what he referred to as "hubris."[2(p173)]

team culture: the general ways of living that are associated with sports teams; team cultures may influence athletes to commit acts of violence outside of sport.

"The Four-Corner Tough Drill"

Coach Young decided his high school team needed some 'toughening up' so he called his former high school coach, Coach Tough, to ask for advice. Thirty years Coach Young's senior, Coach Tough immediately responded with what he referred to as the perfect drill to develop extraordinary toughness in players. The drill was quite simple to set up and execute: Four players are positioned at the corners of a 10-yard by 10-yard square and the player who is to be toughened up is required to stand in the center of the square. When the coach blows the whistle, all four corner players run as hard as possible and inflict vicious simultaneous hits on the player standing in the center. Coach Tough explained that even though serious injuries may result from this drill, the fact that players will be toughened up makes it worth the risk. The four-corner tough drill, according to Coach Tough, had been passed down from previous generations of coaches and over the years has proven its effectiveness through the display of toughness by the teams that used it. Now it is up to Coach Young to decide whether or not to use the four-corner tough drill in his practice.

Questions

1. If you were in Coach Young's position, using moral reasoning what points would you consider when deciding whether or not to implement the four-corner tough drill?
2. In deciding whether or not to use the four-corner tough drill, which decision-making model—consequentialism, teleological, deontological, or strategic reasoning—would you be most inclined to utilize and why?
3. Is it possible for Coach Young to incorporate a level of toughness in his players yet still be compassionate and caring?

Violence in sport is deeply rooted in locker rooms, coaching staffs, and administrations.[15] It frequently continues after athletes retire from competition and assume leadership roles with sport teams and organizations. When they accept positions as coaches, sport managers, and broadcasters, many former players continue supporting the same violent tendencies they experienced as participants. When Vancouver Canucks player Todd Bertuzzi delivered a vicious blow to Colorado Avalanche's Steve Moore, instead of roundly condemning the incident, Canucks president/general manager Brian Burke referred to Bertuzzi as a "quality hockey player who made a mistake."[4(p64)] Statements like Burke's do nothing to help break the cycle of sport violence.

What can be done to break this cycle? How can athletes, coaches, and administrators minimize, if not eliminate, violence in sporting contests? To accomplish this task, everyone must consider what their specific role is in reducing violence. Applying teleological moral theory might be helpful in this endeavor, since it is a brand of moral theory that would require athletes, coaches, and administrators to consider the values they should have and uphold to be morally good. The teleological perspective emphasizes values such as sportsmanship, respect, beneficence, and compassion—values that leave no room for violence in sport. Using a teleological approach, athletes would discipline themselves to not take part in violent behavior, coaches would avoid teaching violent strategies, and administrators would establish rules and sanctions to minimize in-game violence. By emphasizing key moral values, sports people might begin to break the cycle of violence that haunts sport on so many levels.

Teaching Violent Strategies

Playing sports and working for the win is a lesson that is as hard for some adults to learn as it is for young people. Coaches who teach violent strategies usually have a personal rationalization for doing so. Common reasons include the notion that "everyone else is doing it"; the claim that it is the job of the officials to enforce rules that prevent violent practices; and the pressures placed on coaches to win is so great that they develop win-at-all-cost philosophies that sometimes include teaching violent strategies.

If some coaches are gaining an advantage by teaching violent strategies to their players, other coaches may feel compelled to do the same. The pressure to keep up with the competition and to win might be, in the minds of many coaches, justification enough to teach violent strategies to gain an advantage or to keep up with those coaches who are already teaching such practices. And the reinforcement of aggressive behavior by coaches influences aggressive reoccurrences.[16] One possible solution is for officials to enforce the rules that are in place to prevent in-game violence. A prohibition on in-game violence can reinforce values such as integrity and respect for opponents. Although the legislation and enforcement of rules against fighting may not bring about genuine respect among opponents, it reinforces the notion that fighting is considered inappropriate by governing bodies and officials. In other words, game officials and referees can play an instrumental role in preventing the teaching of violent strategies and practices by diligently enforcing rules designed to stop it.

Players and coaches normally modify their decisions and actions throughout a game, depending on how officials interpret and enforce rules. Game #4 of the 2006 National Basketball Association's (NBA) Championship series between the Miami Heat and the Dallas Mavericks serves as an example of how officials can control potentially violent situations. When Jerry Stackhouse of the Mavericks flagrantly fouled Shaquille O'Neal of the Heat, tempers flared, making for an atmosphere poised for violent retaliation. The officials, however, controlled the environment by calling fouls for even slight physical contact until the players regained their composure.

If officials allow aggressive and violent play, players and coaches may become more violent in an effort to gain an advantage. Coaches may even instruct players to play more violently in games in which an official(s) has a reputation for not enforcing rules that prevent violence. However, most scoring prevention strategies that coaches can teach their players can improve their chances of winning without resorting to violence. Thus, it is important that officials enforce rules established by governing bodies that disallow dangerous/violent strategies. For example, it is against the rules in basketball for a defensive player to undercut an offensive player. Undercutting is a technique in

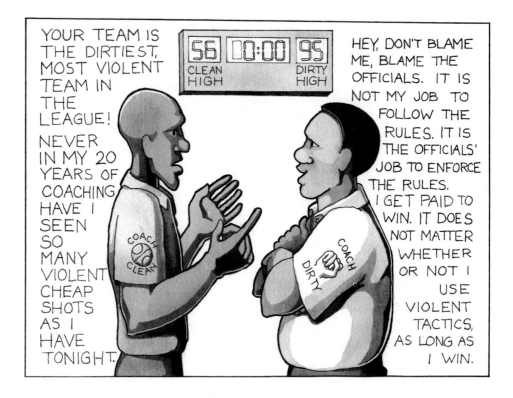

which a defensive player initiates contact against an air-born offensive player—usually as he is driving in the lane and attempting to score—rendering the offensive player helpless in trying to control his landing. Players rarely land on their feet when they are undercut; usually they land face first or on the side of their body. Making undercutting even more dangerous is the fact that the offensive player is usually traveling at a high rate of speed and is elevated well off the ground at the time of impact. Undercutting is a flagrant foul of the rules of basketball, and if officials aren't vigilant in enforcing it, coaches might teach it to their players as a strategy to defend against scoring.

Given the philosophy of win-at-all-costs that exists in some sporting circles, it should come as no surprise when coaches teach and encourage aggressive or violent tactics. Thus, using deontological moral theory, is the teaching of violent tactics acceptable in a win-at-all-costs environment? If those involved in the sport are willing to accept the same infliction of violence on themselves as they inflict on others, in effect they are meeting the universalization standard of deontology. They are acting toward others in a way that they are willing to accept as a way for others to act toward them. Unfortunately, this win-at-all-cost philosophy often leads to and reinforces the type of unethical aggressive behaviors that impact negatively and destructively on the development and well-being of young athletes and on society in general.[17] But, with the pressures to win, can we realistically expect players and coaches to follow rules to the letter, to not circumvent them in some way? This question might draw mixed responses from coaches. Coaches who value sportsmanship and compassion will teach their players to play safely and within the rules of the game, whereas coaches who emphasize strategic reasoning often will teach their players violent tactics that are outside the rules.

As a way to control aggression in young athletes, Nucci and Young-Shim[16] recommend that coaches should not be promoted or fired based solely on their win–loss record. If coaches act under the theory of psychological hedonism, they would seek out the actions that bring them pleasure or those that would help them elude painful consequences. If getting fired is a painful consequence of losing, coaches might go to extreme measures to win. When having to choose between losing or winning through the teaching of violent tactics, the latter may cause less pain and more pleasure for a coach since getting fired could be a painful consequence of losing.

Abiding By the Rules to Prevent Violence

If coaches have agreed to be part of games that have preexisting guidelines and rules, it seems reasonable to expect them to operate within those parameters. If coaches circumvent these rules and officials do not enforce them, the game will change and might even take on the personality of a different sport. For example, at what point do violent strategies and tactics turn basketball into a game more similar to football? If a sport is to maintain the challenges and skills that make it unique, coaches, players, and administrators should also assume the responsibility of abiding by the rules that help define their sport. And officials must diligently enforce those same rules. From a teleological perspective, abiding by the rules that govern the game, including those that prevent violence, reinforce the values of respect and honor for the game. The integrity of the game is maintained when rules are well thought out and are adhered to by everyone involved.

"Taking the Violence Out of Boxing"

The organizers of professional boxing have decided that boxing must be made less violent because it increases violence in society. In other words, when fans watch boxing, they become more violent and are more likely to get into fights. The organizers have decided the best way to take the violence out of boxing is to no longer allow boxers to punch each other. Instead of punching live opponents, the boxers will be scored on how hard they hit heavy bags and how quickly they hit speed bags. Officials will measure the percussion of 100 hits to the heavy bag. Hits to the heavy bag will consist of left and right jabs, crosses, and uppercuts. The boxer who hits the bag the hardest will score the most points. Boxers will also be scored on how many times they can hit the speed bag in two minutes. The highest combined score of the heavy bag and speed bag will be the winner. In other words, much like golf, a winner in boxing will be determined without inflicting any physical pain or violence against an opponent.

"Taking the Violence Out of Boxing" (*Continued*)

When long-time heavyweight boxing champion Barney, "the brutal butcher," heard of the changes, he screamed at the top of his lungs, "Are you kidding me?! Boxing is all about contact! I want to hit someone, and if I get hit, so what? If I did not want contact, I would have decided to play golf or badminton. If you organizers change the rules of boxing, you will also have to change the name of the sport, because it will no longer be boxing!"

Questions

1. Do you agree or disagree with Barney's opinion regarding the newly proposed rules of boxing?
2. If evidence exists that proves boxing does increase societal violence, do you think boxing should be made less violent? Explain your answer.
3. Make a moral argument from a consequentialist, teleological, or deontological perspective that supports *keeping,* as part of boxing, the most violent aspects, such as punching opponents in the face.
4. Make a moral argument from a consequentialist, teleological, or deontological perspective that supports *removing* from boxing the most violent aspects, such as punching opponents in the face.

The Glorification of Winning and its Perpetuation of Violence

Try as those directly affiliated with sport might, external influences make it extremely difficult to lessen or eradicate violence in sport. An argument can be made that it is the glorification of winning and its accompanying rewards that cause the violent rules infractions that frequently occur. Materialistic rewards such as money, trophies, and prizes, along with non-materialistic rewards such as praise, recognition, and adulation motivate athletes to win. Does the probability of athletes engaging in illegal tactics and violent rule-breaking behavior increase as the value of the reward for winning increases?

If we removed the rewards associated with victory, would violent incidents be as prevalent in sport? For example, would an athlete be driven to win at all costs if the competition took place out of the public eye, without any external recognition or rewards? Some people might argue that the removal of strong extrinsic motivators would reduce the occurrences of violence in sport. A sports person who reasons strategically, reasons egoistically and is focused on personal gain. An athlete, coach, or general manager who reasons strategically might very well base his/her actions on gaining external rewards. On the other hand, many athletes and non-athletes are naturally competitive, regardless of whether or not the setting is sport related. Such individuals may commit acts of violence during sport competition out of frustration when they believe they are not achieving their goals. That is, acts of violence in sport may be spontaneous and not based on any form of moral theory.

Pappas, McKenry, and Catlett[17] acknowledge that frustration may stimulate aggressive behavior in athletes, which may partially explain sport aggression. The frustration that accompanies the failure to achieve a goal often increases the likelihood of aggressive acts.[18,19] For example, poor play in an important contest such as a rivalry game, playoff, tournament, or championship match might influence an athlete to react violently when fouled or contacted aggressively. This reaction may have nothing to do with the extrinsic rewards that accompany victory, but instead be simply the frustrated response of a highly competitive athlete.

Does Eliminating Violence Eliminate the Game?

As discussed in the previous section, rewards and the glorification of those who win can perpetuate violence. A win-at-all-cost approach that results in violent behavior might be restrained if the sport had no fans to applaud or jeer, no trophies to win, and no recognition to be gained. However, removing the fans and the rewards and the accolades would not eliminate violence completely from sport. By definition, athletes are highly competitive, some more aggressively so than others, and there is an element of aggression in most sports. Given the commercial interests, finances, and capitalistic forces involved in the structure and operation of many sporting endeavors, it is probably unrealistic to entertain the notion of sport without fans, recognition, and rewards. The purpose of most sports, at least at the elite level, is as much about revenue generation as it is about displays of athletic prowess. Of course, that is not to say that sport as a moral endeavor should be sacrificed to greed.

The person who supports the reduction of violence over the generation of revenue might be more interested in the best available state of affairs for sport, which is a consequentialist way of thinking. The consequentialist who is guided by utilitarianism could argue that reducing violence in sport is the best available state of affairs for all involved in sport. Conversely, if revenue is necessary to continue to be able to operate a sport and/or sport league, utilitarianism might support the generation of revenue for the purpose of being able to continue to provide the good that sport generates.

Another possible option for minimizing in-game violence would be to eliminate the violent part of each particular sport. It is the rules and conventions of games like football and ice hockey that leave room for violence within these sports. Why not simply change the rules and disallow the violent acts that have become part of the game? Is it possible to do so without changing the game itself? Removing the violence from inherently violent sports would drastically alter their very traditions and popularity. Such actions would certainly meet opposition from the athletes, coaches, administrators, and spectators who value sports that have aggressive or violent aspects. Those who support violent sports could argue that altering contact sports by removing the violent aspects would take away the very same traits that partially define the game. For example, if fighting was no longer allowed in American hockey, the game may need to be renamed as something other than hockey since professional hockey in the United States is known for and partially defined as, a sport that includes fighting.

What arguments might advocates of violence-prone sports make to support violence in their games? A deontologically based argument might well serve such advocates. If a deontologist believes that the violent aspects within a game are appropriate for others, he must also believe those same violent-like aspects are appropriate for him. Deontologists must be willing to make general law the principles to which they adhere. In other words, violent aspects of the game may not be supported by all who are involved, but if someone has a deontological perspective, he or she must believe it to be appropriate to be exposed to the same in-game aspects of violence as all of the other participants.

Reducing some of the most violent aspects might be a realistic modification of some violent sports, but making wholesale changes that eliminate all violent aspects is unlikely, as is banning a sport completely because it is too violent. But, if banning a sport because of violence is unlikely to be supported by those affiliated, is there an acceptable compromise? How can in-game violence be reduced or eliminated without also eliminating the very things that make contact sports desirable enterprises? These are questions that sport-governing bodies will need to address as they oversee sports and the future of sports.

Peripheral Violence

Peripheral violence in sport can be loosely described as violence that is related to a

peripheral violence: violence resulting from sport by those other than sport participants during the game. Violence by fans and hazing are examples of peripheral violence.

sporting event but is not directly part of the game itself and does not involve fighting among players. It occurs at all levels of sports and athletics, from youth leagues to professional leagues, and also includes the practice of hazing. Examples of peripheral violence include violence between players and fans, fans fighting with other fans, post-game rioting, and violent hazing. An example of player/fan violence occurred in the NHL in 2001, when Tie Domi of the Toronto Maple Leafs pulled a Philadelphia Flyers fan into the penalty box and started fighting with him.[20]

A more violent example of peripheral violence is the riot that ensued outside of Major League Baseball's (MLB) historic Fenway Park after the Boston Red Sox defeated the New York Yankees in the 2004 American League Championship Series. Boston police used pellet-like guns in their attempt to subdue a crowd outside the ballpark estimated to be between 60,000 and 80,000. Police were trying to stop riotous fans from overturning cars, starting fires, vandalizing cars and stores, and climbing the "Green Monster" wall. Tragically, one of the projectiles from an officer's gun hit an innocent bystander in the eye and killed her.[21]

Another incident of peripheral violence was the rioting after Togo took a lead in a World Cup soccer qualifier game against Mali. Officials stopped the game after fans at the 70,000-seat sold-out stadium rushed the field. As the rioters took to the streets, dozens of people were injured as fans set cars ablaze, looted shops, destroyed monuments, and burned down a multi-story building housing the local Olympic committee.[22]

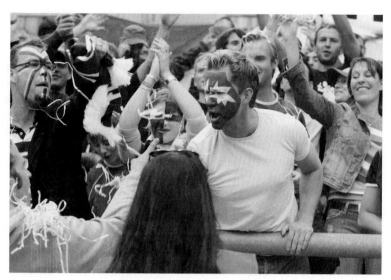

5-2 *Fan violence is an example of peripheral violence.*

Acts of peripheral violence are somewhat difficult to rationalize using the three deontological moral theories presented or using strategic reasoning. From a strategic reasoning perspective, it is difficult to explain a real advantage that is gained through peripheral violence. The player who goes into the stands to fight a fan who threw a cup of beer at him gains no real game advantage. The same could be said for post-game rioting. Although the rioting might be linked to fan emotion after a championship victory, no real game-related advantage can be identified based on the action of rioting.

Spectator Violence

There are many varieties of spectator violence in modern sports. Fans often verbally abuse and fight one another in the stands. Cassandra Johnson, the wife of Dallas Maverick's head coach Avery Johnson, was involved in an altercation in the stands during a 2006 NBA Western Conference finals game against the Phoenix Suns. Allegedly, Mrs. Johnson became belligerent after complaining that two Phoenix Suns season ticket holders were standing too much. Witnesses said that Mrs. Johnson took three swings at a female fan, but missed and instead hit her fiancée.[23]

Fans also attack coaches. Kansas City Royals first base coach, Tom Gamboa, was attacked during the 2002 MLB season. A 34-year-old male fan and his 15-year-old son charged onto the field and tackled Gamboa. Fortunately, Royals players quickly intervened, restraining the two crazed fans, and Gamboa escaped with only minor cuts and bruises.[24] A chilling incident of peripheral violence took place in Dallas, Texas, at Canton High School in April of 2005, when the parent of a ninth grade football player, upset at his son's lack of playing time, shot his son's football coach/athletic director in the chest. Fortunately, the coach survived the attack.[25] Perhaps unsurprisingly, game officials have long been targets of abuse, from spectators and participants alike. Referees are often verbally abused or threatened when they make what others see as a bad call or don't make a call at all. Some referees have even needed police escorts after highly charged games.[26]

Unruly fan behavior is often linked, perhaps not surprisingly, to alcohol consumption.[27] Fans often begin drinking at tailgate parties and local bars long before game time and are intoxicated when they enter the ballpark. College football is especially representative of the kind of overindulgence that leads to disturbing, riotous, celebratory alcohol-fueled incidents following games. After the Ohio State football team defeated arch rival Michigan in 2002, the celebration in Columbus made its way from the stadium to the streets, where eventually it turned riotous. Fans drank and urinated in the streets, assaulted one another, and committed acts of vandalism, including overturning cars and setting them on fire. Students kept the fires burning by fueling them with furniture from their apartments. Columbus police were unable to restore order until the early hours of the next morning, using riot gear and tear gas.[28] Incidents like these have contributed to limiting or even banning beer sales at many sports events. By stopping beer sales at a designated time—such as the end of the 7th inning in baseball and the end of the 3rd quarter in football—the belief is that fans will have time to sober up before leaving the facility, decreasing the likelihood of alcohol-fueled violent behavior.

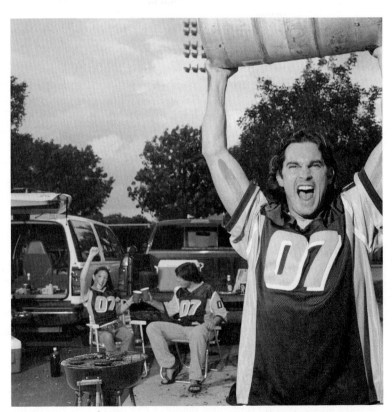

5-3 *Peripheral violence on the part of fans is sometimes fueled by alcohol consumption.*

"Beer Sales and Violence"

The general manager of the Redbirds minor league baseball team, Martin Manager, is considering eliminating alcohol sales at the Redbirds' ballpark. Martin has become convinced that alcohol was the cause of last week's post-game parking lot riot between Redbirds fans and rival Bluebirds fans. Police had to be called to restore order; several fans suffered serious injuries and dozens more were arrested when the riot spread to surrounding neighborhoods. However, two owning partners of the Redbirds are pressuring Martin to continue selling alcohol at the ballpark because it is a significant revenue generator for the franchise.

Questions

1. If you were the Redbirds general manager, what *factors* would you consider when arriving at your final decision regarding banning or continuing alcohol sales at the Redbirds ballpark?
2. As the general manager of the Redbirds, using teleological moral theory, what *values* would you consider when arriving at your final decision regarding banning or continuing alcohol sales at the Redbirds ballpark?
3. In whose best interest is it to ban alcohol sales? In whose best interest is it to continue alcohol sales?

From a moralistic perspective, it is difficult to defend unruly fan behavior. It is doubtful that most fans would welcome violent behavior to be directed at them (a deontological perspective). It is also doubtful that the most amount of good for the most amount of people results from unruly fan behavior (a utilitarian perspective). And moral values such as respect and honor are not practiced when fans behave violently (a teleological perspective).

Post-Game Rioting

Post-game rioting that breaks out in neighborhoods surrounding sport facilities or college campuses is destructive, dangerous, and gives sports as well as local communities a bad name. It often involve setting fires, overturning cars, and fighting in the streets. Although post-game riots seem to occur most frequently following championship games, they sometimes occur after rivalry games or any other regularly scheduled game. Many times, the people involved are not even sport fans; they are people from the area who take a perverted pleasure in celebrating or partying in a destructive manner. Over the years, riots have taken place in major sports cities following professional championships. There was rioting in Chicago following the Bulls' NBA world championships and in Los Angeles when the Lakers won the NBA championship. Although a byproduct of some

> **post-game rioting:** violent disorder by people following a sporting contest; post-game rioting by fans sometimes occurs after their team wins a championship.

high-stake events such as rivalry games in certain sports, post-game rioting is difficult to justify morally when applying the moral decision-making models of consequentialism, teleology, and deontology.

It is difficult to see any moral value in such violent activities. Aside from the waste of community resources and money needed to combat rioting, the senseless acts of vandalism and personal injury that accompany rioting are morally problematic. If respect for people and their belongings is important in American society, such acts of vandalism should not be tolerated. This point must be emphasized in campaigns aimed at preventing post-game rioting. If moralistic approaches can be encouraged that emphasize practicing good values, respecting others as we would respect ourselves, and understanding the effect that our actions have on others, post-game violence and rioting might be deterred. Society should assume a position of responsibility and practice the morals it preaches, lead by example, and act in morally good ways. Morally good actions on the part of society could help decrease violence that sometimes results from high-stake events in certain sports.

Spectator/Player Violence

Altercations between spectators and players disrupt the essence of sport, which should be a safe and fair contest between like-skilled competitors. These altercations can be precipitated by fans who overstep their boundaries by insulting players, threatening them, throwing bottles, batteries, or other objects at them, or jumping fences and attacking them. During the 2006 MLB season, a fan tossed a syringe at San Francisco Giants slugger Barry Bonds as he came off the field between innings at San Diego's Petco Park.[29] Bonds has undergone intense public and media scrutiny regarding his rumored use of steroids to boost his performance. Bonds' efforts to become the all-time MLB home run leader over Hank Aaron and Babe Ruth has been overshadowed by his alleged use of steroids. Throwing a syringe at Bonds was probably symbolic of the animosity many baseball fans have for Bonds, believing he is breaking home run records unfairly.

The way an athlete responds to an abusive fan can be indicative of his or her moral values. For instance, a player operating from a teleological perspective would not retaliate against an abusive fan. The player who does retaliate is not practicing the moral values of respect and honor, of beneficence and altruism. Unfortunately, players with less self-restraint sometimes let their emotions get the best of them and have gone into the stands after their tormenters or have thrown objects at them. During spring of the 1922 professional baseball season, Ty Cobb of the Detroit Tigers jumped over a guard rail and ran up 12 rows to punch, kick, and gash (with the spikes on his shoes) a heckling fan.[30] In a more recent incident, during the 2004–2005 NBA season, Ron Artest of the Indiana Pacers went into the stands to attack a fan who tossed a beer at him.[30] Professional leagues and their governing bodies now mete out strong punishments to players who go after spectators, as evidenced by the 73-game suspension handed out to Artest. Stiff fines and suspensions hopefully deter other athletes from such undisciplined actions in order to preserve the long-term best interests of the game, a consequentialist point of view.

Can anything be done to reduce the incidents of spectator/player violence? Increasing security at sporting events and limiting the sale of alcohol are good preventative measures, but they will not entirely stop such incidents from occurring. Nor will the threat of tougher penalties stop some players from retaliating against abusive fans. Athletes and fans alike must treat each other with respect; if they look upon one another as fellow human beings rather than as enemies, they will be less likely to verbally insult or physically assault one another. To adopt a teleological approach would mean to practice the moral values of respect, honesty, trust, and beneficence, an approach that would benefit not just sport participants and spectators, but perhaps society in general.

Granted, expecting athletes to be ruthlessly competitive on the field yet non-violent off the field is often easier said than done. Some athletes have difficulty balancing the demands placed on them. Retired Oakland Raider linebacker Bill Romanowski described the difficulty in being both a family man and a football player in the NFL.[3] And given the frustration that athletes and fans of poorly performing teams frequently experience, it can be difficult to behave as a humanitarian when potentially explosive moments arise in the heat of competition. Those who train themselves teleologically to act out of compassion and beneficence rather than anger and frustration will be better equipped to deal humanely and rationally at moments when violence is an option. Those who decide to not act violently because they would not want others to act violently toward them are basing their actions on deontological moral theory. Those who are aware of the negative long-term consequences of violent behavior are acting under consequentialism and the overall good that comes from a utilitarian approach.

Youth Sport Violence

It is unsettling enough when fans of professional and college sport teams act violently toward other fans, officials, and players. It is more unsettling when parents behave violently at their own children's sporting events. Youth sports are not immune to violence. Sometimes parents and fans take out their ire on officials, who often are local community members volunteering their services or trying to make a few extra dollars. Those people who act out violently are not considering the long-term best interests of youth athletes, who model their behavior on the adults and the environment around them.

At times arguments break out between opposing fans or even parents or fans of children on the same team. Violent outbursts of this kind have led many youth leagues to require parents to sign codes of conduct in order to attend their children's games, restrict spectator viewing areas in a way that prevents spectators from getting close to the playing surface, and even enforce bans against cheering. Wakefield and Wann recommend the following remedies to control fan behavior: (a) award points or match points to opposing teams when unruly fans disrupt play; (b) ban or suspend fans guilty of disruptive or violent behavior; (c) prohibit signs, clothing, or verbal assaults that denigrate rivals and ban such offenders from games; and (d) limit attendance in terms of total restrictions or by segments (adults, parents, students) likely to cause disruption.[31(p181)]

Policies and procedures that are well thought out can help curtail violent incidents, but it is the value of respect that is most crucial. If people recognize that they are dealing with other people and not things, they are more likely to think twice before using violence against one another. Practicing good moral values because you are compelled to do so could be more effective in preventing violence in sport than not behaving immorally for fear of policy-based punishment. To act teleologically, parents must make a conscious effort to practice good moral values such as compassion, respect, and honor. It is highly doubtful that parents would want other parents to act violently toward them or their children; therefore, a deontological point of view does not support violent behavior by parents.

Hazing and Violence

The definition of hazing addresses several specific ways in which hazing can occur. In the **Hazing Prohibition Act of 2003,** hazing is defined as "any assumption of authority by a student whereby another student suffers or is exposed to any cruelty, intimidation, humiliation, embarrassment, hardship, or oppression, or is required to perform exercises to excess, to become sleep deprived, to commit dangerous activities, to curry favor from those in power, to submit to physical assaults, to consume offensive

> **Hazing Prohibition Act of 2003:** the United State's first piece of proposed federal anti-hazing legislation introduced by Rep. Diane Watson (D-CA) on March 11, 2003.

foods or alcohol, or the threat of bodily harm or death, or the deprivation or abridgement of any right."[32(p1)]

Often hazing is directed by a team's leaders and actions are performed on, or required of, persons aspiring to be members of the group. Prospective members who successfully undergo hazing are unofficially or officially recognized as members of the group. Hazing is not restricted to sport; it takes place within many groups and in various forms. Hazing often includes acts that are embarrassing or humiliating to the person being hazed. Minor and serious injury can and does result from hazing.

The general application of moral theories to examples of hazing might be helpful in making good decisions related to hazing. Using deontological moral theory, would those who engage in hazing willingly accept that they be hazed? From a deontological perspective, unless someone is willing to be hazed they should not haze others. Using teleological moral theory, if hazing is usually humiliating and disrespectful to the person(s) being hazed, you should not engage in hazing. Using the utilitarian form of consequentialist moral theory, you would have to make a case that hazing produces the best available state of affairs and the greatest amount of good possible, which seems unlikely. Thus, if applying any of the three theories of moral reasoning discussed in this text, you would find little support for hazing.

Grievous injury as a result of hazing does occur and serves as a sobering reminder of the seriousness of the act. Historically, common forms of hazing in sport have included forced consumption of alcohol to the point of vomiting or losing consciousness, physical abuse that is often tortuous, acts of humiliation, and sexual abuse. Hazing has gained widespread attention thanks to the Internet. As Internet usage grows and events are easily recorded by anyone with a cell phone or other device equipped to capture pictures or videos, more and more accounts of hazing are being recorded and shown online. Hazing incidents are also uploaded to websites like face-book.com and badjocks.com.[33]

In 2006, numerous websites included photographs of hazing from more than a dozen colleges. The photographs showed what appeared to be initiation scenes in which athletes were drinking excessively, wearing degrading costumes, caught in sexually suggestive poses with strippers and fellow athletes, and leading a blind-folded woman, with her hands tied behind her back, down a staircase. The Internet postings led to disciplinary action against some of the schools, including the baseball team at Elon University in Elon, North Carolina, and the women's soccer team at Northwestern University in Evanston, Illinois.[34]

Acts of hazing are problematic to sport. According to Hawes, college athletes have been forced to engage in the following hazing acts: drink Tabasco sauce concoctions and run with cookies wedged between their buttocks, get tattoos, have their athletic supporters or sports bras coated with Cramer's Icy Hot, run a mile or play a game of soccer in the nude, be kidnapped, be tied to a teammate, be tied naked to benches in locker rooms, be blindfolded and forced to find their way across campus, and forced to urinate on each other.[35] In the worst hazing cases in sport, some athletes have been spanked, beaten, branded, and sodomized with brooms wrapped in athletic tape or with frozen bananas or hot dogs.[35]

Equally disturbing is that some authority figures in sport actually support such types of hazing. Sometimes adults affiliated with athletic teams and programs, such as coaches and athletic directors, turn a blind eye to hazing. Coaches sometimes even become actively involved in the hazing of players. Such was the case in 2000 when the basketball coach at Winslow High School in Arizona was indicted on three felony counts of child abuse for a hazing-related incident.[36]

From the examples described above, it may be difficult to discover any good that results from hazing. But although hazing is generally perceived as negative, it would be irresponsible to at least not examine the possibility of potential good that can result from the practice. Recall that an act can be supported morally in utilitarianism if more good than bad results from an act. Is it possible that the good that comes from non-violent hazing is greater than the bad that comes from violent hazing? Can hazing have positive effects? Researchers in one study, in which 2000 undergraduate students were surveyed, found that participation in hazing behavior was perceived to be fun, a positive team builder, and encouraged group cohesion.[37] When rookie teammates go through the same initiation that veteran players went through, the new players are recognized as part of the team since they 'survived' the same initiation as the veterans. Those undergoing the ritual of initiation thus do so to earn respect from their more established teammates and to display their loyalty to their new team.

Is it the initiation itself or is it the degree of the uniqueness or danger of the initiation that creates team bonding and camaraderie? In other words, do more dangerous forms of hazing create stronger team bonds? Irrespective of the answer to this question, it does seem somewhat preposterous to argue that engaging in dangerous and life-threatening hazing for the purpose of team bonding and camaraderie is morally justifiable, and there are many people who want hazing prohibited. People opposed to its practice are up against those who believe hazing is nothing more than harmless fun that builds character.[38] But even if hazing does build character, which is debatable, should the enhancement of character supersede the moral value of respect? Can character be developed through acts of hazing that are embarrassing, humiliating, and degrading?

At first glance, hazing may seem like harmless nonsense or a rite of initiation that draws members of a team closer together.[38] If it can be proven that some good does come from hazing, then instead of dismissing all forms of hazing it may be more prudent to dismiss only those acts that are dangerous and life-threatening. From a consequentialist viewpoint, exercising non-dangerous forms of hazing for the purpose of gaining benefits such as team unity and cohesion may be acceptable. The level of humiliation suffered by those who are hazed is an important consideration from a moral perspective. Deontological moral theorists might ask if non-dangerous forms of hazing like carrying the team's equipment or singing songs in public are acts that could be reasonable from a moral perspective for all team members. Teleologists might ask if morally good teammates would request that new team members do these things. If the level of humiliation for those being hazed is low or negligible, then perhaps such actions would be ethically acceptable from deontological, teleological, and consequentialist perspectives.

It would be helpful to understand whether or not there is a distinction between hazing and initiations rituals. Initiation usually includes steps that individuals must take to be admitted into an organization. Initiation is considered hazing if it contains the elements of hazing that include but are not necessarily limited to cruelty, intimidation, humiliation, embarrassment, hardship, or oppression. Hazing involves acts that are potentially painful, harmful, humiliating, and deadly. In a study examining hazing, researchers considered—based on their university's definition of hazing—the following activities to be hazing: participating in a drinking contest/games; being deprived of sleep; being kidnapped or transported and abandoned; acting as a personal servant to others; destroying or stealing property; being tied, taped up, or confined; engaging in or simulating sexual acts; being hit, kicked, or physically assaulted in some form; and making body alterations such as branding, tattooing, and piercing.[37]

Initiation rituals, on the other hand, are positive events in which team unity is celebrated in an atmosphere of respect for one another and for the team or school to which team members belong. Initiations include such things as teammates receiving their uniforms at a special ceremony honoring them for making the team. If initiation does foster the moral values of honor and respect, then this type of initiation is supported by teleological theory. As Hawes points out, initiation is often tradition based, necessary, and often in need of adult supervision; as long as responsible adult supervision is a part of initiation, those being initiated will most likely reap positive benefits.[35] An evening of initiation might also be an opportunity to introduce players to team history and explain the pre-game rituals that many teams develop over time. Other things can be added, but the focus of the evening should be on unity and the important bond between teammates. New players should be made to feel welcome and that they are becoming a part of something special. Initiations do not include acts of humiliation. Deontological moral theory calls for persons who are honoring and respecting others through initiation ceremonies to expect the same conditions of honor and respect if and when they are initiated.

Hazing is an ongoing cycle of repeated behavior and is often continued over the years, based on statements like, "I had it done to me, so you have to have it done to you," or "I did it so you have to do it." Statements like these that do not follow any logical line of thought or reason, but rather a "monkey see, monkey do" mindset, are ineffective in demonstrating the good that may result from hazing. Deontologically, the claim that first-year athletes should have to endure hazing because other teammates, who most likely disliked it, had to endure it does not hold up morally. If hazing is not something you would want to go through yourself, then it is not something you would want everyone to go through. Hence, it is not an ethically acceptable act according to deontological moral theory.

"Coach and Captains Debate Hazing"

One of the first agenda items for the new hockey coach, Coach Cease, was to meet with the three senior team captains and make clear his position on hazing. Coach Cease began by saying that he was against all forms of hazing and that if they worked together, Coach Cease and the captains could put an end to the cycle of hazing that has been a part of the hockey team for many years. Coach Cease continued by saying that he did not want to ban hazing completely without input from his team captains. In describing their positions on the issue, the team captains recalled how they did not enjoy being hazed three years ago but believed it was helpful for team camaraderie and team building. After patiently listening to the team captains, Coach Cease pointed out that they should seize this opportunity to rid the hockey team of the dangerous practice of hazing and gain the respect of the community for doing so. Coach Cease further explained that schools that do not put an end to hazing will continually be faced with hazing-related lawsuits.

Questions
1. Regarding their positions on hazing, do you side with Coach Cease or the three captains? Provide reasons for your answer.
2. Using deontology as a foundation, point out reasons in support of Coach Cease's position to ban hazing.
3. Using strategic reasoning, point out reasons to support the three captains' position to continue the tradition of hazing.

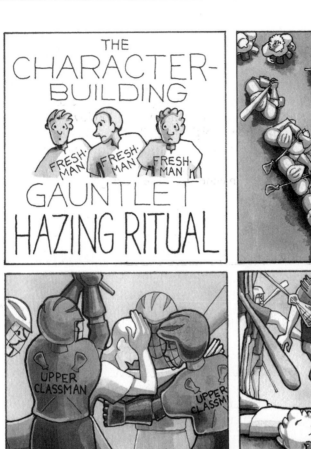
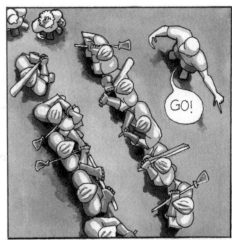
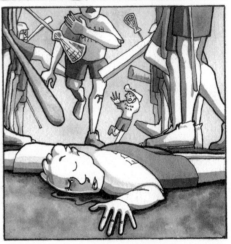
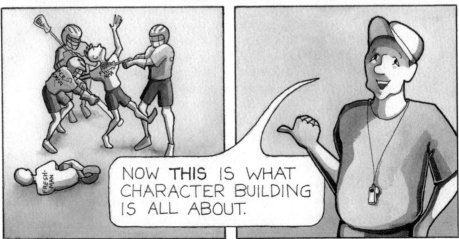

Because of the seriousness of hazing, federal legislation has been proposed against it, but can legislation guarantee the eradication of violent hazing and the serious injuries and deaths that sometimes result? Are laws adequate in their detailing of unacceptable behaviors and correlative punishments? Or do others, including athletes, coaches, sport managers, and parents, have a moral responsibility to put an end to hazing? Everyone involved in sport, including society as a whole, can have a positive impact by becoming vigilant against hazing. This approach might be similar to neighborhood watch groups. Understanding the difference between hazing and positive initiation rituals, and recognizing that loyalty often follows respect can perhaps help eliminate the practice of hazing and improve sport's image as an endeavor that encourages and rewards good moral character along with athletic prowess.

Conclusion

The numerous in-game and peripheral violence issues discussed in this chapter should be of concern to anyone who wishes to reduce unnecessary violence in sport. Athletes, coaches, administrators, and fans alike must come together and acknowledge the violence surrounding sports and collaborate on ways to reduce or eliminate it. It is the moral responsibility of everyone involved in sport to create a safe environment for the enjoyment of participants and spectators alike. By understanding the factors that contribute to unnecessary violence, sporting communities can take proactive steps to safeguard their environment and preserve its integrity.

References

1. Terry PC, Jackson J. The determinants and control of violence in sport. *Quest*. 1985; 37(1):176–185.
2. Coakley J. *Sports in Society: Issues and Controversies*. 8th ed. New York, NY: McGraw-Hill; 2004.
3. Associated Press. Romanowski testifies in fight lawsuit. *WJLA* website. http://www.wjla.com/headlines/0305212285html. Accessed June 23, 2006.
4. Kindred D. The NHL must clean up its bloody act. *Sporting News*. March 22, 2004;228 (12):64.
5. Chua-Eoan H, Neuman C, Poole GA, et al. The new rules of fight club. *Time*. September 26, 2005;166(13):66–67.
6. The fight of the century. *The International Boxing Hall of Fame* website. Available at: http://www.ibhof.com/ibhfhvy1.htm. Accessed June 20, 2006.
7. CNN/Sports Illustrated. Philadelphia fans criticized for reaction to Irvin injury; October 14, 1999. *CNN Sports Illustrated* website. Available at: http://sportsillustrated.cnn.com/football.nflnews/1999/10/11/philly_fans_ap/. Accessed June 20, 2006.

8. Yasser R, McCurdy JR, Goplerud CP, et al. *Sports Law Cases and Materials.* 5th ed. Cincinnati, OH: Anderson Publishing Co.; 2003.

9. Gill DL. *Psychological Dynamics of Sport.* Champaign, Il: Human Kinetics;1986.

10. FIFA to investigate Zidane's head-butt; July 11, 2006. *CBC* website. Available at: http://www.cbc.ca/news/story/2006/07/11/fifa-investigation-zidane.html. Accessed May 4, 2007.

11. Wann DL, Carlson JD, Holland LC, et al. Beliefs in symbolic catharsis: the importance of involvement with aggressive sports. *Social Behavior and Responsibility.* 1999;27(2): 155–164.

12. Stephens D. Predictors of likelihood to aggress in youth soccer: An examination of coed and all-girls teams. *Journal of Sport Behavior.* 2000;23(3):311–325.

13. Stephens D. Predictors of aggressive tendencies in girls' basketball: An examination of beginning and advanced participants in a summer skills camp. *Research Quarterly for Exercise and Sport.* 2001;72:257–266.

14. Stephens D. Moral atmosphere and aggression in collegiate intramural sport. *International Sports Journal.* 2004;8(1):66–77.

15. NCAVA website. *Prevention Programs.* Available at http://www.ncava.org/prevention.html. Accessed March 11, 2008.

16. Nucci C, Young-Shim K. Improving socialization through sport: An analytic review of literature on aggression and sportsmanship. *The Physical Educator.* 2005;62(3):123–129.

17. Pappas NT, McKenry PC, Catlett BS. Athlete aggression on the rink and off the ice: Athlete violence and aggression in hockey and interpersonal relationships. *Men and Masculinities.* 2004;6(3):291–312.

18. Baron RA, Richardson DR. *Human Aggression.* New York: Plenum Press; 1994.

19. Berkowitz L. *Aggression: Its Causes, Consequences and Control.* Philadelphia: Temple University Press; 1993.

20. Previous examples of fan violence. *Sports Illustrated* website. Available at: http://sportsillustrated.cnn.com/baseball/news/2002/09/19/fan_violence/. Accessed June 19, 2006.

21. Police 'devastated' by Red Sox fan's death; October 22, 2004. *KOAT* website. Available at: http://www.koat.com/news/3841878/detail.html. Accessed June 24, 2006.

22. Associated Press. Mali soccer fans burn cars, riot after World Cup qualifier. *USA Today* website. Available at http://www.usatoday.com/sports/soccer/world/2005-03-28-world-cup-roundup_x.htm. Accessed June 19, 2005.

23. Watkins C. Avery's wife finds trouble; 2006. *Dallas Morning News* website. Available at: http://www.dallasnews.com/sharedcontent/dws/spt/basketball/mavs/stories/053106dnspomavswife.17cf4b14.html. Accessed: June 19, 2006.

24. Associated Press. I was stunned. *CNN/Sports Illustrated* website. 2002. Available at: http://www.sportsillustrated.cnn.com/baseball/news/2002/09/19/royals_whitesox_ap/. Accessed: June 19, 2006.

25. Lavandera E. Coach shot at Texas high school; 2005. *CNN* website. Available at: http://www.cnn.com/2005/us/04/07/canton.shooting. Accessed: June 30, 2006.

26. Estroff-Marano H. The last referee. *Psychology Today.* Jan/Feb 2006;39(1):31.

27. National Collegiate Athletic Association. Safety of student-athletes, officials, fans focus of NCAA group studying postgame crowd control issues; April 14, 2006. *NCAA* website.

http://www.ncaa.org/wps/wcm/connect/NCAA/Media+and+Events/Press+Room/News+Release+Archive/2006/Miscellaneous. Accessed: March 11, 2008.

28. Football, tailgating parties, and alcohol safety; 2005. *The NCADI Reporter* website. Available at: http://www.health.org/newsroom/rep/2005/football_alcohol.aspx. Accessed: June 19, 2005.

29. Chronicle News Services. Fan throws syringe near Bonds; 2006. *Houston Chronicle* website. Available at http://www.chron.com/disp/story.mpl/sports/3768985.html. Accessed June 19, 2006.

30. Hudson H. Brawl games; 2004. *Roanoke Times* website. Available at: http://www.roanoke.com/printer/printpage.aspx?arcID=15274. Accessed June 20, 2006.

31. Wakefield KL, Wann DL. An examination of dysfunctional sport fans: Method of classification and relationships with problem behaviors. *Journal of Leisure Research.* 2006;38(2):168–186.

32. Scott P. H.R. 1207, the hazing prohibition act of 2003: A legislative analysis. *Washington Insider* website. Available at: http://www.clhe.org/lawpolicyquarterly/H.R.%201207.pdf. Accessed June 20, 2006.

33. O'Toole T. Internet revives hazing issue. *USA Today.* May 19, 2006:9C.

34. Teicher SA. Online photos put hazing in spotlight again. *Christian Science Monitor.* June 14, 2006;98(139):16.

35. Hawes K. Athletics initiation: Team bonding, rite of passage or hazing? 1999. *NCAA News* website. Available at: http://www.ncaa.org/news/1999/19990913/active/3619n03.html. Accessed June 22, 2006.

36. Nuwer H. Unofficial clearinghouse for hazing and related risks in the news. Available at: http://hazing.hanknuwer.com/. Accessed June 22, 2006.

37. Campo S, Poulos G, Sipple JW. Prevalence and profiling: Hazing among college students and points of intervention. *American Journal of Health Behavior.* 2005;29(2):137–149.

38. Rosellini L. The sordid side of college sports; 2000. *U.S. News and World Report* website. Available at: http://www.usnews.com/usnews/edu/articles/000911/archive_012912.htm. Accessed June 22, 2006.

High School Hockey Brawl From a Player's Perspective

This past Saturday night, our hockey team, Fairplay High School, had a home game scheduled against Cheapshot High School. This game had special meaning since it would affect our sectional tournament seedings. The last time we played Cheapshot High, they beat us 4–2. As a result, we were bound and determined not to be defeated again. As the game began, Cheapshot High was playing overly aggressive to the point that they were living up to their name. The one penalty called against Cheapshot in the first period helped us, as we scored a power play goal with five minutes remaining in the period to take a 1–0 lead.

The second period started off the same as the first. Cheapshot High kept taking cheap shots, and the referees seemed to ignore them, not calling any penalties. During the 12th minute of the second period, one of Cheapshot High's players, Hitman Hank, slammed into our goalie, Goaltender Gregg, who retaliated by punching him. Goaltender Gregg was given a five-minute major penalty for fighting, yet Cheapshot High's player was not penalized. After it became apparent, in our team's view, that the referees were not calling enough infractions against Cheapshot High, our mindset changed. If Cheapshot could inflict what we perceived to be cheap shots without being penalized, then we could fight fire with fire and retaliate in kind. This was an important game and we were not going to be pushed around.

During Goaltender Gregg's major penalty, Cheapshot High scored two quick goals, putting them up 2–1 at the end of the second period. Five minutes into the third period, Cheapshot High's Slasher Sam slashed our star forward, Sammy Star, causing him to fall down, injured. Sammy Star was later diagnosed with a grade one contusion. Slasher Sam's actions resulted in a bench-clearing brawl. To our surprise, the referees cancelled the game after the fight. Even more surprising, the next day at a team meeting our coach told us that the district decided to cancel the rest of our season, including sectionals. I was shocked. This was my senior year and I had my heart set on winning sectionals. My temper was at a boiling point because I was not talented enough to play hockey in college. The tournament was all I had left, and it was being taken from me. To make matters worse, I was not even a participant in the fight.

That night I went home angry and told my parents what had happened. They already knew that the season had been canceled because it was broadcast on the news. At dinner I tried to explain my frustrations, but my Dad wasn't on my side. He also said that some of my teammates should be glad they did not get arrested for committing assault. My dad then suggested that I go to the school board meeting the next day to voice my opinions. Although I do not like speaking in public, this was too important to me to not get involved. To keep my season from ending, I had to succeed in my goal of convincing the school board to not punish the entire team.

Critical Thinking: Finding Common-Sense Solutions

1. As a coach, what would you do if, in your opinion, the referees were calling an uneven game and placing your players in danger?

2. What could the referees have done differently, if anything, to prevent this fight?

3. As a player, what factors do you believe should be considered when deciding how to deal with the actions of Hitman Hank? Slasher Sam? The referees? The team as a whole? What factors would you consider as the coach? As the athletic director?

4. Do you believe the entire team should be punished, even if not all team members were involved in the fight? Why or why not?

5. As an athletic director, would you have suspended the team or the players involved in the fight if the district had taken no action?

6. If you were responsible for developing district policy, would you treat all fighting the same, or would you address fighting on an individual, case-by-case basis? Explain your answer. What would you include in your policy?

Critical Thinking: Moral Theory-Based Decision Making

7. Is fighting in hockey ethical from the point of view of either deontological or teleological moral theory? Why or why not?

8. Identify one of your above answers as one that is based on moral reasoning. Describe some characteristics of moral reasoning and demonstrate how your answer is, in fact, based on these characteristics of moral reasoning.

9. Identify one of your above answers as one that is based on strategic reasoning. Describe some characteristics of strategic reasoning and demonstrate how your answer is, in fact, based on these characteristics of strategic reasoning.

Hazing Julie

Julie was a freshman on the women's college basketball team and had just finished participating in a captains practice (a practice without the presence of any coaches). Although pleased with her basketball performance, there were a couple of non–basketball-related issues that confused and disturbed Julie. One was the fact that the returning players constantly called Julie and the other first year players "rookies" rather than by their names. Julie also could not understand why, at the end of practice, the first-year players were ordered by the returning players to pick up all the basketball practice equipment and put it away.

Captains practices continued over the next two weeks and the returning players were still berating the first-year players by referring to them as rookies and making them pick up equipment. One day the returning players on the team told Julie and the other first-year players that they would be required to go through an initiation. The first-year players obeyed the orders and met the returning players at the center of campus at noon on Saturday. The returning players, led by the captains, were waiting with smiles on their faces as the first-year players arrived.

They then told the first-year players they were going on a scavenger hunt and, in preparation for the hunt, ordered them to dress in costumes. Even though the first-year players were embarrassed and knew they would be humiliated, they acquiesced to the demands.

As the captains handed out the list of items to be found, the first-year players began to hunt for the items. Julie and the other girls were not happy about the way things were going, but felt like they had to go along with the scavenger hunt since it was explained as part of the women's basketball tradition. The girls searched endlessly and somewhat fearfully since they were told that if they did not come back with every single item on the list they would be punished. Exhausted, Julie and the other girls found all of the items and made their way back to the center of campus to meet the captains. The captains were standing beside their cars waiting with duct tape. One by one, the captains taped the first-year players' mouths shut and put them in the trunks of their cars. Julie knew this was wrong but went along with it since she, like the other girls, was too tired, mentally and physically, to even consider resisting.

Approximately 30 minutes later, they arrived at the home of one of the captains and were led inside, where they were forced to drink shots of tequila every 10 minutes. The returning players continued calling them rookies and again explained that since it was tradition, they had to go along with it. Once the first-year players were intoxicated, they were put in front of the boy's basketball team and told they had to take their clothes off and dance for the boys. Julie knew that this was completely wrong but went along with the others because she no longer had the willpower to resist.

After that terrible night, Julie spent most of the next by herself, crying and feeling a sense of helplessness. She was unsure what to do, but also felt a sense of closeness with the other girls who had been subjected to the hazing. As difficult as it was, Julie decided to go to the next day's practice. Upon their arrival, the captains instructed Julie and the other first-year players not to talk about what had happened.

Critical Thinking: Finding Common-Sense Solutions
1. As the head coach, would you have allowed the captains to conduct preseason practices without your presence? Explain your answer.
2. As the head coach, would you have allowed your returning players to refer to your first-year players as rookies? Why or why not?
3. Do you believe this was an incident of hazing or initiation? Explain your answer.
4. If you were one of the first-year players, would you have notified your coach of this situation?
5. If you were one of the first-year players, would you have gone to the police? Why or why not?

6. Do you believe that Julie and the other first-year players will gain anything positive from this experience? If so, explain how. Do you believe they will suffer in any way from the experience? If so, how?

7. If you were the coach or athletic director and Julie came to you with the entire story, what actions, if any, would you take?

Critical Thinking: Moral Theory-Based Decision Making

8. As the athletic director, do you believe these actions *betrayed the integrity of the sport* in any way? Explain your answer. Do you believe these actions *fostered the morality of the sport* in any way? Explain your answer.

9. If you were one of the returning players on the team and were basing your actions on *deontological theory,* how would you have reacted to the treatment of the first-year players?

10. As the coach of this team, do you believe the actions of the returning players toward the first-year players were in the *best interest* of the team? The returning players? The first-year players? The opposing teams? The fans? The athletic department?

Football Hazing Death

It was just another early Sunday morning at Pineville University for head football coach, Coach Flash, as he sat in his office breaking down game film after a Saturday night victory. Coach Flash's heart jumped when his phone rang at 2:00 a.m. He picked up the phone and listened nervously as the voice on the other end introduced himself as the Pineville chief of police, Chief Blunt. Chief Blunt informed the coach that the traditional rookie party the previous night had ended in the death of his top two recruits, Eddy, a running back, and CJ, a cornerback. The cause of death was alcohol poisoning.

Chief Blunt informed Coach Flat that his three senior captains, who had been at the party, were being held at the local jail. Quenten, Lionel, and Ron all lived in the house (known informally as the Football House) where this year's rookie party took place. The three captains took responsibility for throwing the party and for organizing the deadly drinking games. The rookie party was known as a type of initiation to formally welcome all the new players into the football program. A central element and tradition of rookie parties always included an evening filled with drinking games, in which large amounts of alcohol were consumed in a short amount of time. At last night's party, new players were involved in a contest to see who could be the first person to finish an entire bottle of vodka. To the delight and cheers of those at the party, both Eddy and CJ guzzled an entire 750-mL bottle without taking a breath. Little did anyone know that this would be the last night that Eddy and CJ would ever breathe again; both were dead a few hours later from alcohol poisoning.

The tragic deaths of these two young players has shattered not only personal lives but also professional lives. As a highly successful coach at Pineville for the past 11 years, Coach Flash was expecting this year to be his best year ever. The coach was quoted back in August during a two-a-day practice session as saying, "Given our talent-laden freshmen class along with our senior leadership, we should make a run for a national championship this year." Also in serious question now are the careers of the three captains. Quenten and Ron had been contacted by professional scouts and both have aspirations of playing professionally at the quarterback and running back positions, respectively. With a 4.0 grade-point average, Lionel still has aspirations to attend medical school.

The local media have received early word that the city prosecutor's office will press charges against the three seniors for the deaths of Eddy and CJ. Instrumental in deciding the athletic fate of these three players is Pineville's current athletics director of 10 years and former football coach of 15 years, Mr. Jones. Coach Flash is in the unique position in that he may also play a role in determining the fate of his three senior captains, yet others, including Mr. Jones, will determine his fate as the head coach at Pineville.

Critical Thinking: Finding Common-Sense Solutions

1. If you were Mr. Jones, what punishments, if any, would you mete out to the three captains who were responsible for the drinking initiations at the rookie party?

2. If you were Coach Flash, would you take accountability for Eddy and CJ's deaths by submitting your resignation? Why or why not?

3. If you were Coach Flash and were required to provide examples of positive initiation rituals, what would you provide? How would you make the distinction between acceptable initiation rituals and unacceptable (hazing) rituals?

4. Who, ultimately, should be held accountable for Eddy's and CJ's deaths, and why?

5. If you were Mr. Jones, what would you have done to try and prevent the events that led to the deaths of Eddy and CJ? What would you have done if you were Coach Flash? If you were the parents of Eddy or CJ?

Critical Thinking: Moral Theory-Based Decision Making

6. If you were Mr. Jones and you were using *teleological moral theory* to guide your reasoning, what values would you rely on in determining your actions, or lack thereof, toward Coach Flash and the three team captains?

7. If you were Coach Flash, explain how you might use *consequentialist moral theory* to create policies that would prevent an incident such as this one from occurring again.

8. If you were Coach Flash, explain how you might use *deontological moral theory* to create policies that would prevent an incident such as this one from occurring again.

Mascot Violence

Oceanfront High School's men's basketball team hosted its annual home game versus city and conference rival, Beach High School. Each year, the gym at Oceanfront is filled to capacity with students, parents, and members of the community, and this year was no exception. Unfortunately, however, this game was marred by a violent incident that made it different from past games. The game was in the second half, with Oceanfront working to maintain a 4-point lead. On the visitor's side of the gym, the Beach High mascot (a student dressed as a crab) was trying to rally the team's fans. On a dare, two Oceanfront students walked over to the opponent's section down on the floor and began to verbally torment the crab. After a minute or two of this, the two young men pushed the mascot to the ground and began beating on him to the delight of the Oceanfront crowd. Police officers responded quickly, grabbing the two students and removing them from the gym before any further violence erupted. The students were escorted out of the school and taken to the local police station, where they were held for aggravated assault. Ultimately, however, no charges were pressed against the students and they were set free later that evening.

As respected school officials, Oceanfront principal Albert and athletic director Berrant were expected to address this situation on an administrative level. The two boys had nearly incited a riot with their actions, and although no one had been seriously injured, the two administrators knew that they were fortunate that no other violence had resulted from the students' shenanigans. Further complicating matters was the fact that one of the young men, Matt, was a member of Oceanfront's highly ranked and respected men's soccer team. Although this team was not in its season, athletic director Berrant was faced with a dilemma. Should Matt be suspended for part of the next soccer season as part of his punishment for his actions? Should he be suspended from off-season training and conditioning programs and banned from the use of training facilities? Or should his punishment not be related to his athletic participation?

Critical Thinking: Finding Common-Sense Solutions

1. What aspects of this incident should be considered when determining the actions to take against the two students involved in the assault on Beach High's mascot? Explain your answer.

2. What steps should athletic director Berrant take to ensure that an incident like this does not happen again?

Critical Thinking: Moral Theory-Based Decision Making

3. Should principal Albert suspend the two students for attacking the Beach High mascot? Justify your reasoning by referring to moral principles and values relevant to the situation.

4. Under what conditions, if any, is it ethical to suspend a student athlete for part of his or her season for actions occurring during the off-season? Justify your reasoning by referring to relevant moral principles and values.

5. Should athletic director Berrant punish Matt, the soccer player, for his part in the attack? If so, what punishment should be imposed on Matt? Justify your answer.

Key Terms

aggression—behavior intended to cause psychological or physical pain or harm.

cathartic aggression—in sport, the release of violence or hostility while participating in sport.

competitive objectives of sport—goals within competitive sport that are formally established and known by all; for example, gaining yardage, tackling, and scoring are three competitive objectives in the game of football; teams that are the most effective in attaining the competitive goals of sport usually achieve victory.

Hazing Prohibition Act of 2003—the United State's first piece of proposed federal anti-hazing legislation introduced by Rep. Diane Watson (D-CA) on March 11, 2003.

in-game violence (sport violence)—within sporting contests, unjust or unwarranted exertion of intense physical force, often resulting in injury.

peripheral violence—violence resulting from sport by those other than sport participants during the game. Violence by fans and hazing are examples of peripheral violence.

post-game rioting—violent disorder by people following a sporting contest; post-game rioting by fans sometimes occurs after their team wins a championship.

team culture—the general ways of living that are associated with sports teams; team cultures may influence athletes to commit acts of violence outside of sport.

6 Race Equity in Sport

Learning Outcomes

After reading Chapter 6, the student will be able to:

1. Recognize traditional and more recent forms of racial and ethnic discrimination.

2. Explain possible solutions to racial problems plaguing sport today.

3. Formulate equitable decisions, using moral theory as a basis, that could help resolve instances of racial and ethnic discrimination in sport.

4. Discuss discrimination as it relates to the process of selecting and hiring sport personnel, along with strategies to achieve equity in the process.

5. Compare and contrast sport as a meritorious working model of equity versus sport as a dysfunctional model of race equity.

6. Evaluate sport organizations' adherence to standards of racial equity.

In the minds of many, sport is a meritocracy—a venue in which people advance because of talent and hard work rather than because of politics or cultural ideology. Unfortunately, the meritocratic view that holds that athletes, coaches, and sport managers always earn their jobs, salaries, and status through disciplined effort and not as a result of the color of their skin or ethnic background is only somewhat true.

Although participants often do earn their positions based on achievement, even in modern times race and ethnicity play a role in both advancing and impeding a sport person's participation and advancement. On the surface, at least, it is encouraging that racial and ethnic discrimination in sport has been reduced over the last 60 years, but it is also discouraging that less blatant forms of racism still exist in some sport leagues and organizations.

In this chapter, racism in sport in its traditional and more recent, subtle forms will be identified and examined against a broader perspective of the history of racial discrimination. In gaining a better understanding of racial discrimination in sport, hopefully all involved in sport endeavors will be better able to act in ways to stop it. After reading this chapter, students should be able to first recognize and then fairly and equitably resolve discriminatory situations in sport using the various decision-making models first described in Chapter 1.

Author's Note: It should be noted that given that the preponderance of literature related to racial discrimination in sport addresses African-Americans, the content of this chapter thus centers primarily on examples and analysis of racial discrimination issues related to African-Americans. This emphasis in no way implies that other races, ethnicities, or people of non-mainstream sexual orientations do not face discrimination challenges in sport.

Race Issues in Sport

Racial discrimination is the practice of treating people unfavorably or unfairly because of their race or skin color. Kivel notes that discrimination "varies in form and ranges from mild to severe depending on one's skin color, ethnicity, level of education, location, gender, sexual orientation, physical ability, age, and how white people and white-run institutions respond to these factors."[1(p37)] Inequality among races exists when opportunities are not the same for various races. When a person, based on his or her race, is not provided with the same privileges, status, or rights as other races, he or she is being treated inequitably. Examples of inequities in the world of sport include player personnel decisions made on the basis of race, underpayment of minority players, and the circumvention of fair hiring practices that give African-Americans a fairer chance to earn coaching and administrative positions in sport organizations.

Coaching and Racism

In the coaching profession in major college football, employment is generally based on who you know. Given the tendency of athletic directors to use extremely subjective criteria in evaluating potential coaching candidates, president of Arkansas Baptist College, Fitzgerald Hill, recommended that specific hiring criteria for coaching positions should be implemented.[2] But should the use of specific measurable criteria be required when hiring coaches? Or could an argument be posed that supports the use of subjective criteria instead? Strategically speaking, coaches who benefit from established personal relationships with athletic directors might argue that it is acceptable to use subjective criteria when hiring coaches. In other words, coaches who have gained employment through networking rather than superior skills might support networking as the primary means to gain employment for themselves as well as for others. Athletic directors might argue the same since they could then pick and choose whom they want to hire for a coaching job based on who they know. But wouldn't picking and choosing a coach or athletic director based on subjective criteria open the door for racial discrimination, since some people might subjectively decide to hire only a certain race?

Would a teleologist support the use of subjective criteria for hiring coaches? Teleologically, the moral value of fairness could be questioned if subjective criteria were used to hire coaches. Would it be fair to hire a friend simply because he is a friend, and not because that person is the most skilled? Would it be not only unfair but also discriminatory to hire a friend for a position based on race? Contrarily, if a person has worked hard at networking, could it be perceived as unfair to hire an unknown candidate when that candidate did not work to establish a rapport/personal relationship with, say, the athletic director?

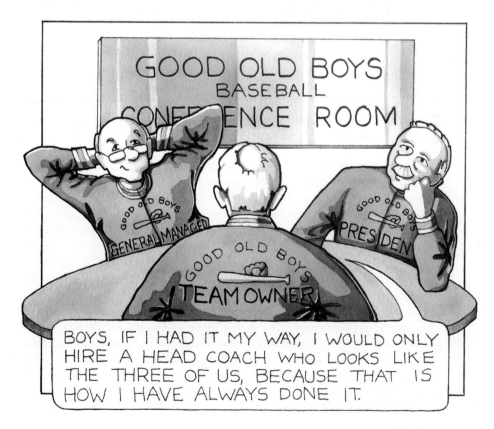

History and Racism

Racial discrimination in sport represents only a fraction of the overall problem of discrimination in the world at large. The daunting challenge of reaching and maintaining racial equity in sport might be better appreciated against the backdrop of the widespread and various forms of discrimination that have existed throughout the history of humankind. According to Bell-Fialkoff, "Discrimination and prejudice provide the thread that ties together the long history of religious and ethnic cleansing."[3(p120)] The earliest known examples of ethnic cleansing took place between 745–727 BC.[3] Being cognizant of the effects of ancient and more recent past racist acts in society helps us anticipate and prevent the potential for and the effects of racism in sport today. But to overcome some of the deep-seated racial hatred and animosity that has existed for thousands of years, it must first be acknowledged. Only then can a state of racial equity begin to exist and be practiced not just in sport but in society at large.

Why does racial discrimination take place? Discrimination is often a way for those in power to maintain a higher social status than those they discriminate against. This, in turn, gives the discriminators greater access to the limited opportunities, wealth, and privileges that might be available. Discriminatory practices against specific races are often passed on from generation to generation, commonly from parents to children. Racism has persisted over time and seems to be enmeshed within the fabric of many societies around the world, making it incredibly difficult to overcome but not impossible. Thanks to the dedication and sacrifices of those involved in the Civil Rights Movement in the United States, many of the most blatant back-of-the-bus bylaws of bigotry have been overturned. That is not to say that racism has been eradicated in this country; in many cases, it's simply been diverted. And sadly, racial inequity in sports is still a problem, both in the United States and abroad.

Europe has its share of problems with racism, as was evident during the World Cup in 2006. At times, in Germany and in several other European nations, the crowds showered minority players with racial insults. To help ensure their safety, German officials even warned non-white players not to wander into parts of eastern Germany, which has a strong reputation of racism toward non-whites.[4] Several of the U.S. team's African-American players who compete professionally in European leagues claimed they had been targets of discrimination and verbal and even physical abuse because of their race, both on and off the field.[4] Such was the case with defender Oguchi Onyewu, an African-American from Olney, Maryland, who was expected to be one of the United States' breakout stars in the 2006 World Cup. According to Onyewu, in March of 2006 fans of rival Club Brugge attacked the car he was in by shaking, spitting on, throwing food at, punching, and kicking it. He was punched in the face and heard monkey chants. Even though Onyewu played in France and in Belgium for four years prior to the 2006 World Cup, it was only during the 2006 season leading up to the World Cup that he experienced such overt acts of racism.

Interest Convergence

Interest convergence may help explain the progress in racial equity that has been made in sport. In interest convergence, the interest of blacks in achieving racial equity is met only when it converges with the interests of whites. If it is in the interest of whites, establishment of laws and social policies that remedy racial injustices will take place. In other words, the economic interests of middle and upper class whites usually have to be met for judicial relief for racism to occur.[5] In sport, it is the upper class whites who have an economic interest and most often hold the positions of power, such as owners and general managers of professional teams, commissioners of leagues, and athletic directors of teams. When reviewing some of the past actions by whites in power to meet the interest of blacks in overcoming racial discrimination and helping achieve racial equity in sport, interest convergence is apparent. The integration of Major League Baseball (MLB) serves as a classic example of interest convergence.

According to Stricherz,[6] Major League Baseball was the first institution in the United States to desegregate itself willingly, predating racial integration by the U.S. Army, the Supreme Court, and public schools, which were not desegregated until the **1964 Civil Rights Act.** The desegregation of Major League Baseball even predated legislative attempts to establish more equitable conditions for African-Americans through the 1954 *Brown v. Board of Education* decision. The ruling in this case struck down the doctrine of "separate but equal" facilities for blacks and whites and set in motion the toppling of the elaborate apartheid system known as Jim Crow that separated Southern blacks from Southern whites in nearly all walks of life, including schools, workplaces, buses, hotels, restaurants, and movie theaters.[7]

1964 Civil Rights Act: (Pub.L. 88-352, 78 Stat. 241, July 2, 1964) landmark legislation in the United States that outlawed discrimination based on race, color, religion, sex, or national origin in voting, employment, and public services.

In 1947, Brooklyn Dodgers owner Walter O'Malley (and Dodgers president Branch Rickey) took what has since been seen as the first step toward racial equity in baseball by accepting Jackie Robinson as the first black player into what until then had been an all-white league. Was O'Malley motivated by an interest in achieving racial equity in Major League Baseball or by an interest in making money through Robinson's extraordinary baseball talent? Knee believes the decision was driven by revenue, not by a desire for racial equity.[8] Prior to Robinson's signing, other baseball owners were also considering signing African-American players because of the increased revenues that could be generated from their talents and playing abilities.

Using a more current interest convergence example, it could be argued that black players are now being recruited to play football and men's basketball to benefit white people. White sport administrators in athletic departments could benefit from increased salaries and bonuses, while white athletes in non-revenue-generating sports could benefit from monetary subsidies to their programs as a result of successful football and men's basketball teams. Coakley explains the situation as one in which in some programs, black males generated revenues that funded the programs and scholarships of white men and women athletes in other sports, and paid for their coaches.[9] Donnor assumes a similar stance when asserting that "black males dominate football, which in some instances generates enough revenue to financially underwrite non-revenue-producing athletic sports such as crew, swimming, tennis, and golf that are overwhelmingly populated by white middle and upper class students."[5(p48)] The sports teams that do not make money, however, generally do not have the same high number of black participants as found in football and basketball. Interest convergence helps explain the limited recruitment of black players to sports teams that do not make money as a result of winning. If the interest of white sport administrators at universities is to generate money, they will select the most talented players regardless of color. Based on interest convergence, if some sports will not make money regardless of whether or not they win, whites will not be motivated to select the best players since their interest in making money will not necessarily be met by doing so.

Looking at this example from a deontological perspective, if the tables were turned and a sport that consists primarily of white athletes generated a surplus of money, would that money be used to support sports generally made up of minority athletes, or would it be used to support sports that are generally made up of non-minority athletes? Based on deontology, it would be expected that if programs that consist primarily of black players subsidize predominately white programs, then the opposite should also be true; that is, programs consisting predominately of white players should be expected to subsidize predominately black programs. From a teleological perspective, the moral value of fairness should be considered when it comes to the selection of players for teams.

If decisions are made for strategic rather than moralistic purposes, is true moral progress being made? Is racial equity genuinely being addressed? When a decision is made strategically as opposed to morally, from a utilitarian perspective it might be questionable as to whether a long-term greater good will be achieved. Although more opportunities might present themselves for minorities in the short run, if a mindset of racism or discriminatory ways of thinking remain unchanged, the real long-term gains in **race equity** might be questionable.

race equity: provision of the same opportunities for all persons, regardless of race.

Regarding collegiate sport in general, Donnor points out that by the end of World War II, the practice of racial exclusion changed as a result of economic factors both inside and outside of college athletics and higher education that led to the integration of football and men's basketball.[5] And Davis states that the commercialization of sport allowed African-American student athletes greater access to opportunities to compete.[10] According to Davis, "while moral desire to end segregation may have prompted many to seek the integration of organized collegiate sport, the economic interests of others may have been of primary importance."[10(p100)] Rader also notes that the desegregation of sports arose from a combination of pressures, including quests for additional profits by sports entrepreneurs."[11] Despite the many apparent efforts to achieve racial equity in sport, however, racist attitudes and behaviors in sport persist today in less obvious forms.

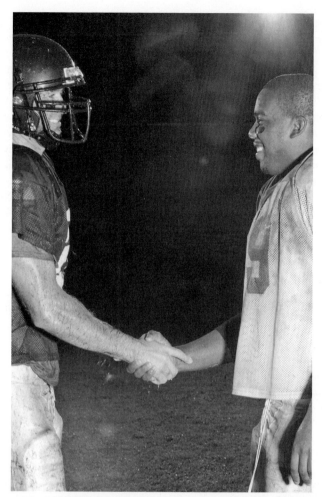

6-1 *The integration of sport has served a moral good as well as the economic interests of some sport leaders.*

"Boycotting the All-Star Game"

Marvin Mann was the captain of the Professional League Baseball (PLB) All-Star team that happened to be composed primarily of minority athletes. After thinking long and hard, Mann decided it was time to use his influence over his fellow teammates to make inroads in the hiring of minorities in professional baseball front office positions. The PLB was at the height of its popularity and was being televised globally for the first time in its history. Mann understood the power of money and knew that if he could convince his teammates not to take the field for the opening pitch of the PLB All-Star Game, he

"Boycotting the All-Star Game" (*Continued*)

might be able to force the commissioner into agreeing to two minority hiring actions. The first minority hiring action would start in the commissioner's office. The commissioner would be required to hire a percentage of minorities to management positions in his office that is equal to the percentage of minority players that are on the team. In this particular case, of the 20 players on the team, 5 are minorities, which is 25%. The commissioner, in turn, thus would be required to hire 25% minorities to management positions, which in this case would be one since his office has four management positions. The second minority hiring action would be a guarantee to negotiate for a policy requiring a quota system for hiring minorities for front office positions. Given the millions of dollars riding on the televised broadcast of the game, Mann was fully aware of the commissioner's vulnerability and believed the timing was perfect to make inroads for minorities in baseball management positions.

Questions
1. Do you think Mann's idea of boycotting the PLB All-Star Game is a sound approach to gaining equity in management positions for minorities? Why or why not?
2. Do you believe Mann's approach would be effective in the short term? In the long term? Why or why not?
3. Using deontological moral reasoning, discuss whether or not Mann's actions are ethical.
4. What harm might result from Mann's actions?
5. What good might result from Mann's actions?

From a sport perspective, when reasoning strategically, there are instances when it may not be self-serving to discriminate. Jackie Robinson's integration into Major League Baseball serves as a model to support this point. Walter O'Malley knew that he would win more games and, in turn, draw more fans (which would lead to more money) if Jackie Robinson's integration into the all-white league was successful. From an economic standpoint, O'Malley's reasoning may have been strategic in that he was interested in making more money. In all likelihood, Rickey (president of the Dodgers) would not have made as much money had he supported the ban on African-Americans in Major League Baseball.

Sport: A True Meritocracy?

As discussed above, when Jackie Robinson entered Major League Baseball in 1947, it can be argued that he was signed for economic rather than racial equity reasons. If signing Robinson was in fact done for economic reasons, it would appear that Robinson's

meritocracy: a venue in which people advance because of talent and hard work rather than because of politics or cultural ideology; sport is often perceived to be a true meritocracy in that players earn their positions based on skill.

signing is an example of how sport indirectly operates as a **meritocracy.** Winning games makes money for owners, and winning happens by selecting and signing the players with the best playing merits or skills. O'Malley understood that his chances of winning would increase if he selected players based on their playing merits instead of on the color of their skin. The fact that integration of Major League Baseball did not happen sooner than 1947 is an indication of the strong racist views held by society in that time, as is the fact that African-Americans black players who were integrated into MLB teams stayed in hotels separate from their white teammates.

In meritocracies, players attain levels of achievement based on merit instead of on race or politics. Sport operating as a meritocracy is supported from a teleological perspective, since matching one player's skills against another is a fair assessment of talent. The National Basketball Association (NBA) of the 1990s serves as a more recent example of how sport can operate as a meritocracy. Lomasky credits the NBA's enormous popularity among white and black fans alike during this period to its being a "meritocracy that works."[12(p53)] He described the league as one in which the success of players was not contaminated by a suspicion that it was undeserved; one in which positions, players, and salaries were earned on the basis of ability to perform on the court.[12]

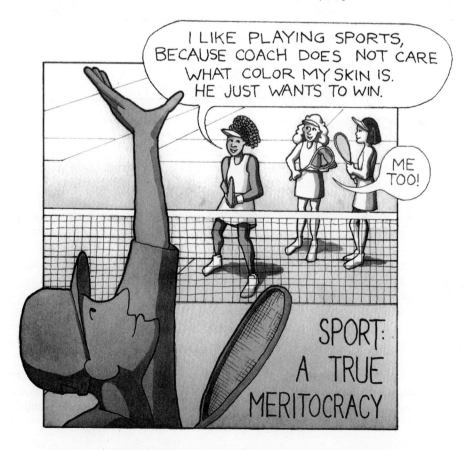

Although it is true that sport can be driven by meritocratic forces, it can also be strongly influenced by racism that stems from various cultural ideologies. MLB's Gary Sheffield states (as cited in Harris) that "back in *the day*, racism was more open, now it's more hidden."[13(p43)] Prior to integration, no secret was made about the fact that African-Americans were not allowed to compete equally for positions on teams because of their skin color. Ansari contends that racism in sport still remains a significant part of the sporting experience, even though sport's meritocratic structure has been partly responsible for black achievement in sport.[14]

Underrepresentation of Minorities in Head Coaching and Administration

Discrimination in sport does not begin and end with players. Minorities seeking head coaching and administrative positions have been discriminated against in the past and are still discriminated against in many sports today. Those individuals racially discriminated against for head coaching and administrative positions have not been judged on their abilities but on the color of their skin. Usually some form of individual gain can be acquired from strategic reasoning, but how can it be in an owner's or upper administrator's best interest to not hire or promote a coach who has the best skills? Using race instead of skills as the criterion to hire or promote a coach or sport administrator does not seem to be in the best interest of sport organizations, because without the most highly skilled employees, overall performance would reflect poorly on the organization and those involved in the hiring. Ultimately, though, through a strategic reasoning mindset, could the hiring of a person of one's own race have an egoistic or individual benefit to the person responsible for the hiring? If a sport employer hires people of his or her same race, the favor may be returned at some point; thus, it might be strategically beneficial to hire someone of the same race.

From a strategic perspective, it does seem that discrimination provides a short-term individual gain for those who are doing the discriminating. However, the long-term strategic gains for those involved in discrimination are questionable. If hiring is based on race and not skill, the sport organization or team may ultimately suffer if they are not acquiring the most skilled players, coaches, and administrators.

Despite the strides made by African-American athletes, racial minorities continue to be underrepresented in coaching and upper management positions in sport organizations.[15] With the exception of the NBA, in which approximately 50% of head coaches are African-American, there are few minorities in coaching and management positions in the four major sport leagues in the United States.[13] Cunningham speaks of similar inequities in intercollegiate athletics,[15] and according to Hill, many well-meaning academic and athletic administrators refuse to admit that race might still be a factor in the employment (or lack thereof) of African-Americans as head football coaches at the college level.[2] The numbers speak for themselves, however. In 2005, it was reported that African-Americans were employed as head coaches at only 5 of the 119 Division I-A colleges and universities.[16] And in 2002 when examining the leadership spots immediately underneath head coaching positions, only 12 African-Americans were offensive and defensive coordinators at the Division I-A level.[16]

The question can always be posed as to whether or not it is inequitable or unfair that there is not an equal distribution of minorities and non-minorities as players on teams and in leagues, and as coaches and administrators throughout leagues. Equity and the moral values of fairness and justice could be used when applying teleological moral theory to demonstrate both fairness and the lack thereof when creating an equal distribution of minorities and non-minorities throughout sport leagues. Without taking talent into account, the least discriminatory and most fair method of placing people in sport positions is through equal distribution based on race. On the other hand, it could also be argued, teleologically, that it is unfair and unjust to dismiss the skill and talent of individuals and to use race as the sole or primary factor in determining which individuals are placed in sport positions.

Private Sport Country Clubs and Race Discrimination

Private country clubs are associations that include an array of social activities for their members, including many sporting opportunities. Although several sports are often featured, golf and tennis are two of the more common ones offered through country clubs. Country clubs can be grouped into two categories: public and private. Whereas public country clubs offer open and equal access to memberships and do not discriminate based on race, some private country clubs have been criticized for excluding minorities from becoming members. In the past it was not uncommon for private country clubs to blatantly exclude minorities. Today, even though it is not as usual to see clubs openly publish and post racist policies as in the past, it is likely that discriminatory practices based on race still take place in private country clubs.

In a *USA Today* study, 129 private, semi-private, public, and resort golf courses hosting tournaments in 2003 were surveyed to see how well they met the non-discrimination guidelines set by their respective tours and organizations. The survey revealed that only 50% of private, member-owned golf clubs had non-discrimination policies.[17] Interestingly, 19% of the member-owned clubs refused to answer questions that would reveal whether or not they actually had non-discrimination policies in place.[17]

"Putting a Price on Racial Diversity"

The president of Lilly Golf Club (LGC) is confronted with a dilemma. The LGC board of directors has given their president full power to make a decision regarding a policy allowing minority members into the LGC for the first time. From a membership perspective, LGC is divided on this issue, and there have been some heated arguments for and against minority membership. One very affluent member is strongly in favor of minority memberships and has threatened to withhold future monetary contributions

"Putting a Price On Racial Diversity" (*Continued*)

to the LGC if the policy is not changed to allow minority members. The president relies heavily on this member's annual contributions and is not sure whether the LGC can absorb the impact of any potential losses of this member's funds.

Questions

1. If you were the president of the Lilly Golf Club, what decision would you make and on what would you base your decision?
2. If you were to use teleological reasoning to guide your decision regarding minority memberships at the LGC, what factors would you consider and how would you use values as a basis for your decision?
3. In what way, if any, should money be an influential factor in this decision?

Moral Perspectives

What moral views exist relative to the issue of race discrimination and country clubs? Deontological and teleological moral theorists would likely contend that it is unethical to restrict club membership based on race. Deontologists might quickly point out that, if the tables were turned and white people experienced what it was like to be denied membership because of their skin color or ethnic background, they would conclude that such treatment is not something that should be universalized. Focusing on justice, teleologists would also recognize such actions as unjustifiable based on the claim that morally good individuals would not keep others from benefits because of their race or ethnicity. Such unjust treatment would not be accepted by those committed to the values of compassion and fairness, and, hence, would be viewed as unethical by teleologists.

From a moral perspective, if persons should not be excluded from private clubs based on race, should it then also be unacceptable to exclude them based on other criteria? For example, should private clubs be required to place a cap on membership fees since individuals of lower socioeconomic status cannot afford high fees? Or is it acceptable for clubs to have high fees and, thus, effectively discriminate based on personal income or wealth? Numerous other examples of discrimination might be identified when examining the membership criteria of private country clubs.

Legislating Race Equity Policies

If private clubs are found to be discriminatory, should some form of intervention take place requiring the adherence to non-discrimination policies? Should the government intervene in the affairs of private clubs in efforts to minimize or eliminate what might be considered immoral forms of discrimination? What is the likelihood of government effectively legislating morality if there is mixed public support? Is there a point

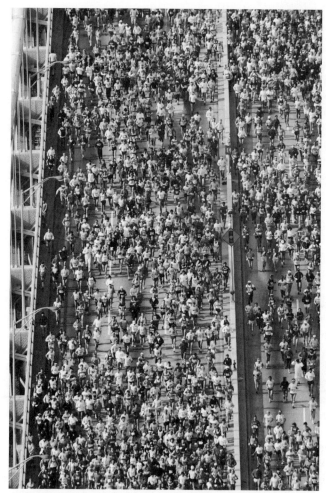

6-2 *A non-discriminatory approach welcomes all for participation.*

at which interventions of this kind become too invasive? For example, since the affairs of families are considered private, should families also be required to welcome and accept all persons into their private homes regardless of race, gender, or other characteristics? Should families also be restricted from establishing criteria by which to determine whom they include in family activities?

Most people would probably see the previously mentioned types of interventions as infringements on personal choice. Similarly then, would it also be an infringement if private country clubs were required to have membership policies that did not preclude persons of a particular race, ethnicity, or economic status from joining? Or, if discrimination is occurring in private country clubs, should these clubs be required to implement membership policies and procedures that would allow equal access to individuals regardless of racial or ethnic background? Generally, governments have not intervened in the business of private country clubs, just as they have not intervened in the affairs of private families.

Whether or not legislation might be an effective way to attain race equity in country clubs and sport organizations might be aided by an examination of moral theories. Looking at legislating equity from a consequentialist view, creating the best available state of affairs is something to consider. To that end, a consequentialist, who chooses to focus on utilitarianism, would require that the number of persons who are resentful of policies be less in number than those satisfied with policies. Keeping peace among as many people as possible should be a factor in creating policy. Legislators and policy makers should also consider moral values that are grounded in teleology. Is it fair, just, and respectful to minorities as well as non-minorities to create race equity policies in private country clubs? Will higher levels of trust and compassion be more prevalent among all races as a result of race equity policies at private country clubs? These and more questions should be discussed when considering legislating race equity policies in country clubs as well as in non-sport organizations.

Consequences of Government Intervention

What might the consequences be if the government decided to intervene in people's private matters? Attempts to legislate non-discriminatory practices might only succeed in pushing such practices underground. Is it possible that outside intervention may cause feelings of resentment and anger against the intervening body and the race or ethnicity on whose behalf it intervened? It could be argued that such anger and resentment might intensify the racist attitudes of members and cause them to become more discreet in their racist practices instead of eliminating them altogether.

Wise political leaders want to create and maintain a civil society and understand that racial discrimination can undermine that goal. According to Bermanzohn,[18] in the mid-1960s violent racists went underground after Congress passed and enforced significant civil rights laws. However, the fact that federal legislation in the 1960s resulted in racists being more careful not to get caught practicing racism should not prevent current and future attempts to curb racist behaviors. It is also necessary to understand the long-term gains against racially discriminatory behavior that accompany intervention. If the long-term result of intervening in the business of private country clubs progresses the cause for racial equity, then the risk of short-term turbulence may well be worth the overall gain.

The challenge of maintaining civility is significant, since racial discrimination is a deep-seated problem that has existed long before sport reached its current level of popularity in the United States. As mentioned earlier, general acts of discrimination can be traced back to at least the Middle Ages. Any progress toward equality and fairness for people from different racial and ethnic backgrounds is important. One form of progress might be a decrease in blatant racist actions; elimination of blatantly racist behaviors is certainly a goal worthy of attainment.

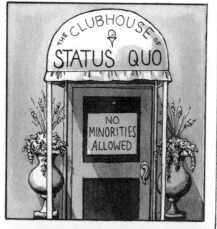

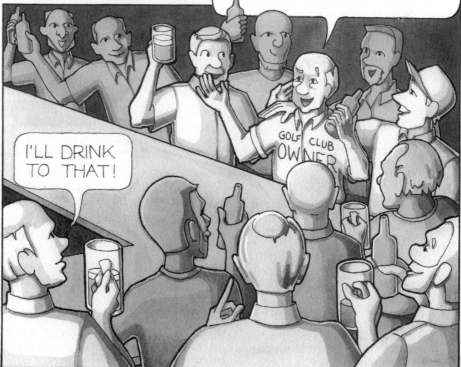

Public Pressure Against Discrimination

In the past, minority groups have attempted to stop racist practices in private organizations by appealing to the public. Public appeals often related to the ability to use revenue as a point of leverage. In 1952, when black golfers Bill Spiller, Eural Clark, and former ex-champion boxer Joe Louis were rejected from entering a Professional

Golfer's Association (PGA)-sponsored San Diego Open golf tournament, they effectively used Joe Louis' popularity to attract national attention to the controversy.[19] Even though the PGA's response did not include the formal elimination of its policy disallowing the entrance of blacks to PGA events, some progress was made in that they allowed blacks to participate in selected events.[19]

Although sanctions and punitive measures against those who commit acts of racism can have an immediate effect, long-term sustained eradication of racism is unlikely. To effectively erode racially discriminatory behavior within private country clubs and society itself, the beliefs, views, and attitudes of those accepting of racism must be modified. This might best be accomplished by educating the public about the long-term detriments of racism to our society and the negative effects to everyone in that society.

From a consequentialist viewpoint, if the public believes that racial discrimination will ultimately have a negative effect on them personally, attitudes toward racist practices might more quickly change for the better. Teleologically speaking, people might come to recognize racist practices as unjust. Through their compassion for others, people might realize that a morally good person will not accept racist practices because of the hurt it causes the person being discriminated against. The recognition that racist practices are wrong might, in turn, influence individuals to take steps toward eliminating exclusionary acts that deny people of different races and ethnicities opportunities to join groups or participate in activities of their choice.

Racial Statements

A basic litmus test to determine whether or not a statement or action is racially discriminatory need not be complicated and can be determined by answering the following question: Does, or could, the statement or action result in an inequality toward another race? If the answer is "yes," the statement or action is racist and should not be made or taken. But who decides whether or not the statement or action does or may result in an inequality for another race? Cause and effect are sometimes difficult to connect, and unless one can accurately link a statement or action to an inequality, determining whether or not an inequality toward a race results from a statement or action can become unclear and controversial.

Although the majority of race discrimination literature in sport relates to African-Americans, by no means are other races immune. Though it exists, Guillermo asserts that anti-Asian racism is still a foreign notion to many Americans.[20] As evidence to support his claim of a lack of respect for Asians, he points out Shaquille O'Neal's comment to a reporter to tell Houston Rocket center, Yao Ming, "ching-chong-yang-wah-ah-so." When asked about the comment later, O'Neal claimed that he had already apologized.[20] According to Guillermo, racism against Asians is held in so little regard that we do not have to look very hard to find people who are considered respectable and good yet promote anti-Asian views.[20]

Intent Behind the Statement

Can a person make racist statements without intending to cause inequities to another race? If a person does not have a full understanding of the hurt that can result from an insensitive comment about someone's race, then, yes, a person can make racist statements without being aware of doing so. It is possible that as a part of someone's childhood they were regularly exposed to racist statements and behaviors without comprehending or having been taught the full negative impact of such statements. But regardless of intent, if the words or actions create or contribute to an inequality, those words and/or actions must be considered racially discriminatory.

After the 1997 Masters golf tournament, Fuzzy Zoeller, a PGA tour veteran of 23 years, made racially insensitive statements to that year's champion, Tiger Woods.[21] Zoeller, who later apologized, first referred to Tiger Woods as "that little boy" and then urged him not to order fried chicken or collard greens for the following year's Champions Dinner.[21] (Masters tradition calls for the current year's champion to select the menu at the following year's Champions Dinner.) Zoeller, who referred to himself as a jokester, said that he meant nothing by the comments and was sorry if the comments offended anyone.[21]

Although certainly problematic, making racially charged statements can be based on ignorance rather than a deep-seated intent to hurt another race, as mentioned earlier. The answer to the question, "Who or who is not a racist?" may not be as important as identifying racist statements and actions and making attempts to eliminate them. Nonetheless, given today's media coverage concerning race, it is more and more improbable that individuals who make racially insensitive comments do so out of ignorance or because they do not know any better. Certainly, if intent to damage another race is the motive behind making racist statements, such statements are indefensible on most all counts.

Applying moral theory to this problem from a consequentialist point of view, if the short- or long-term consequences of such statements have a negative effect, and if the statements are not in the best interest of most persons, the statements are unacceptable. Deontologically, regardless of intent, the statements should not be made if the person making them would not want similar statements made about them. Teleologically, if the statements could result in an inequity, unfairness, or unkindness, they should not be made.

One of the best methods for addressing the issue of racial insensitivities might be through education. According to Moore, educators can play an important role in helping reduce stereotyping, prejudice, and discrimination throughout society, not just in sports.[22] If a person making racist statements is truly ignorant, education is as an effective tool to make them aware of the negative impact that their words can have on another race. We can also teach racial sensitivity to children. According to Woolf and Hulsizer, children who develop biases and prejudicial attitudes are more likely to become adults with these same belief systems.[23] Education related to teaching tolerance and an appreciation for diversity must be provided in schools, religious institutions, and other community organizations. Thus, schools and universities are a natural environment for education about tolerance, diversity, and hate.[23]

Types of Racism in Sport

Racist practices in sport today may not be as blatant as in the past, but they still exist. The practice is just more discreet. And although the discriminatory practice of placing players in positions based on race or ethnicity (stacking) is not as prevalent today as in the past, it also still occurs. Even professional coaches have spoken publicly about how players of a particular race are best suited for a particular sport because of skills inherent to "their" race. Making progress in race equity in sport requires an understanding of the various types of racism, along with the ability to apply moral reasoning to moral dilemmas related to race.

Discreet Racism

The more discreet forms of racism that continue to operate within sporting communities are, as the word *discreet* implies, more difficult to categorize as racial discrimination. One such example can be found in NCAA Division I intercollegiate athletics. The NCAA Division I-A football and men's basketball teams are the only two intercollegiate sports that typically make money and whose participants are predominately African-American. Is it a coincidence that the non–revenue-generating sports teams such as crew, swimming, tennis, and golf often have few if any African-American participants? Although athletics has progressed to a point well beyond laws and rules preventing African-Americans from joining college sports teams, the discreet selection of whites over blacks when winning does not generate revenue is still a concern.

Discrimination By Player Positions (Stacking)

Hawkins describes **stacking** in sport as positional segregation and notes that it is "well documented in the research literature as a major form of discrimination in sport."[24(p147)] Gonzalez defines stacking as the disproportionate relegation of athletes to specific sport positions on the basis of ascribed characteristics such as race or ethnicity.[25] Stacking is viewed as a negative phenomenon because it keeps individuals from playing positions they may desire to play and for which they may be well suited.

stacking: the disproportionate representation of athletes and/or sport administration positions based on characteristics such as race or ethnicity, which can lead to stereotyping and myths, i.e., black men cannot swim and white men cannot sprint. In sport, stacking is negative because it reinforces stereotypes that prevent athletes from playing certain positions that they may be capable of playing.

During early integration of collegiate and professional sports, a strict but silent quota system limited the number of black athletes who could participate and relegated them to a few specific positions. Even though sport integrated rapidly during the 1960s, the proportion of black athletes remained high at these positions and low at others as a result of the practice of stacking.[24] Determining players' positions based on race is discriminatory because it is not an equitable means of deciding what positions players should play on a team. Equitable means that the players are placed in positions based on skill- and talent-related criteria, including tryouts, which provide all players with an equal opportunity to demonstrate how well they can perform at a particular position. Coaches who use race as the basis for placing players in positions either consciously or subconsciously push players into specific positions instead of allowing them opportunities to earn positions through their own talents and abilities. Whether intentional or not, these coaches are unnecessarily discriminating against athletes of different races and ethnicities. If using teleological reasoning, each player should have a fair opportunity to earn a position based on his or her particular sport skills. Thus, the moral value of fairness is not being adhered to when stacking is practiced.

Harrison et al. conducted a qualitative study in which European-American college students who had participated in high school sports with African-American teammates were asked questions related to racial discrimination.[26] More specifically, the questions primarily related to whether or not persons in their lives had steered them away from sport participation and, if so, for what reasons. In most cases, those questioned reported that coaches, both black and white, gave preferences to black athletes, particularly in basketball. One respondent indicated that all the players on the basketball team were black and that the coach did not really give serious consideration to white players trying out for the team. The following statement, quoted by a participant in the study, was made by a European-American coach in humor but it portrays a pervasive attitude of steering particular races away from sport participation. The participant recalls the coach's speech:

> "I remember one instance, our head football coach was talking to us and he was going about, saying how you're man enough to ask the question but are you man enough to hear the answer? And then he looked at one of our white players and told him, he was like, 'Mike, if you come to my office and ask why can't I play defensive back? Well, I'm going to tell you that you are white and slow.' So there were generalizations made that the more skilled positions would be played by African-Americans."[26a(p157)]

In this instance, the coach was placing players in positions because of their race, not for their skills. Deontology calls for consistency in the application of principles. It might be interesting to see if this same coach would prefer that his boss gave him specific duties based on his race, regardless of his talents. If the coach would prefer that he earn a coaching position based on his coaching skills, then he is behaving inconsistently in that he is placing players in positions because of their race and not because of their skills. If the coach would also prefer to be placed in a particular position because of his race and not his skills, then his actions would be supported from a deontological perspective, but only if sound principles were followed.

Harrison et al. also discovered that many participants believed coaches were not only responsible for steering white players away from playing on basketball teams, but also tended to racialize players' positions on the teams by giving certain positions to African-Americans.[26] Harrison goes on to assert that while political correctness is emphasized and efforts to project racial neutrality are made, the underlying reality is that these long-standing and potent stereotypes remain entrenched and strongly influence how we view athletic performance.[26] These coaches are being unfair to the athletes who have the skills and abilities to play positions other than the ones into which they have been stereotyped. They are also being unfair to their teams, which might be strengthened if these individuals were allowed to play a position based on the demonstration of their skills.

"Finding Shooting Guards in the Suburbs"

Coach Stack is the head men's basketball coach at Channel University, and he is intent on finding a high school shooting guard who can come in and start as a freshman. To that end, Coach Stack has decided to send his number one recruiting assistant coach, Coach Catch, to the suburbs to recruit a shooting guard. Upon finding out that he was being sent to the suburbs, Coach Catch asked, "Why the suburbs?" Coach Stack responded, "Because the best shooters are white and the suburbs are where you will find the white players." Not wanting to argue, Coach Catch replied, "Well, I guess if we only look for shooting guards in the suburbs, the suburbs are the only place we will find them."

Questions
1. Is Coach Stack's behavior discriminatory?
2. Is this an example of stacking? Explain your answer.
3. Is Coach Stack subconsciously biased, and, if so, what might have caused the formation of his bias?

Further perpetuating the practice of stacking is the real possibility that youth might only practice for the particular positions they see adults of their same race playing. For instance, prior to the 1990s when the prevalence of black quarterbacks was low, African-American youth may not have considered practicing the skill of passing since they did not see the position of quarterback as one they could achieve at elite levels. As a result, many black athletes may not have developed the skills to become a quarterback, which helped to further perpetuate the myth that African-Americans could not excel at that position. As time passed and African-Americans received opportunities to develop quarterbacking skills and to play the position, the partitions of racism surrounding the quarterback position began to crumble. Today, the myth has been shattered and black quarterbacks thrive at both the collegiate and professional level. Saraceno even argues that the black quarterback has become the prototype for the position.[27]

Even though myths of stacking have been shattered, present-day views that reinforce the generalization of players of a particular race to a position or, even more broadly, to an entire sport still exist. Statements made by former NBA Boston Celtic great Larry Bird serve as an example. Bird stated in 2004 that the NBA is a black man's game and that it would be forever.[28] If NBA front office personnel act on Bird's belief that the NBA is forever a league for black players, they will not be providing fair opportunities for players of all races. From a moral value perspective, it is important to provide fair opportunities for players of all races, regardless of stereotypical statements like Bird's.

Although not as frequently discussed, non-minorities can also be victims of stacking. For example, Caucasian youths may not be offered the opportunity to play the position of defensive back in football since African-Americans predominantly hold this position at the elite level. Non-minorities also face stacking in basketball. Even though the number of players of European descent in the NBA has recently increased, the league still consists primarily of African-American players, especially at the point guard position. This could lead to stacking against Caucasian athletes, since many may perceive that only African-Americans can succeed as point guards in the NBA. There are exceptions, of course. Steve Nash, a white point guard for the NBA's Phoenix Suns, is a phenomenal player who was awarded the league's MVP award for his outstanding performance in two consecutive seasons.[29]

The Token White Players

Rules may no longer preclude people of all races from participating in sport on an equal basis, but can rules in and of themselves eliminate racial discrimination in sport? One example for study might be the claim that NBA teams include a white player or two on their rosters even if other non-white players are more talented. Duster acknowledged this practice 30 years ago when he indicated that the **affirmative action** for whites is to keep the predominantly white fans happy by making sure at least one white player is on each NBA roster.[30] Informally, these players are referred to as **token white players.** Is this practice an example of racism? Fairness and respect are the two moral values that are germane when viewing this question from a teleological perspective. Is it fair and/or respectful to the non-white player who is overlooked for a position on the team because they are not white even though they may be more skilled than the token white player?

> **affirmative action:** a policy or a program that seeks to redress past discrimination through active measures to ensure equal opportunity, as in education and employment.

> **token white players:** including one white player on a sports team even if more talented minority players are available and interested in being on the team; an informal type of affirmative action or quota system for whites.

There has been an outcry against the informal practice of selecting a white player for a team based on the mere fact that they are white. The controversy might lie in the fact that the process of making player personnel decisions involves several factors—not all of which are necessarily talent related—and ends up being subjective. For example, race aside, there may be cases in which players are selected to be part of a team in college because they are from the local area and will help the team draw local fans. Being local has nothing to do with talent but nevertheless might be a determining factor in a coach's or administrator's decision as to who makes the team. If part of the criteria for making a team has to do with an athlete's ability to draw fans, regardless of their physical talent, then other factors become considerations in the process of selecting players to be on a team. The values of fairness and respect may be applied differently if criteria to make the team are not solely based on physical talent and sport-related skills.

Is it inappropriate or racist to select a player to be on a team because their race may lead to increased fan attendance? In 2004, former Boston Celtic's Larry Bird stated that he thought more white players in the NBA would be good for the fan base since the majority of the fans are white.[28] Bird went on say that a couple of white players might get fans a little excited. From a strictly business perspective, it becomes more difficult to label the choices administrators and coaches make as racist if player selections are made strictly from a business perspective. This scenario begs the question as to whether or not basing business decisions on race serves an overall good, or if a greater good would be served by not basing business decisions on race. Personal wealth may need to be sacrificed to serve a greater good to society. Interestingly, with the influx of white players who are coming from Europe to play in the NBA, tokenism related to white players in the NBA is not as evident as it once was.

Minority Advancement or Regression?

Significant participation opportunities have opened up for minority athletes over the past 60 years that did not previously exist. For example, at Washburn University in the early 1950s, whenever traveling in the south, black athletes were housed with black families in the area and could not eat with the team in public restaurants.[31] In Kansas in the 1940s, black students who were barred from joining the Topeka High School basketball team formed their own team, the Rambles.[31] Since that time, evidence of progress in racial equity can be seen in the three major professional sports in the United States. Baseball, football, and basketball have achieved a state in which persons of various races and ethnicities have equal opportunities to compete for positions, playing time, and salaries.

In his 2005–2006 Season Racial and Gender Report Card, Lapchick reported that almost 78% of the players in the NBA were people of color.[32] Although Lapchick's 2005 Major League Baseball Racial and Gender Report Card showed the lowest rate of African-American participation in 26 years (8.5%), Latino player participation increased from 3% to 28.7%.[32] The majority of the players in Major League Baseball during the 2005 season were white (59.9%) while the least number of players were Asian (2.5%).[33] These numbers alone show a representation of minority players in professional sports that were non-existent in the past. But what do these numbers mean in terms of equity? Is it inequitable or unfair if participation rates of particular races are not similar or equal? It would seem that the moral value of fairness can be met if equal opportunities are provided and if all persons are honestly assessed on objective skill-related criteria—even if those opportunities do not lead to positions on a team.

As times have changed, many minority athletes have taken advantage of the opportunities now available, attaining levels of extraordinary wealth and fame through sport participation. Minority advancement in sport, however, has a downside. Although some minorities have achieved fame and fortune, unfortunately many players may have sacrificed their education in favor of placing all of their efforts toward advancing to professional levels.

Low Odds of Playing Professional Sport

Given the limited number of spots available on professional rosters, it is mathematically impossible for more than a few players to realize their dreams of playing professionally. While many athletes excel at the high school level, few go on to make the team and play at the collegiate level, and only a miniscule percentage of players make it to the pros.[34] For example, approximately 3 in 10,000 senior boys playing interscholastic basketball will eventually be drafted by an NBA team.[34] And approximately .02% (1 in 5000) of senior girls playing high school basketball will eventually be drafted by a WNBA team.[34] Given the slim likelihood of playing sport at the professional level, athletes' overall chances for socioeconomic growth and social mobility through sport participation is also low.

Should someone step forward and let aspiring young athletes know the low probabilities of them playing professionally? Youth are easily inspired by and in awe of superstar athletes of their own race or ethnicity to the extent that many of them will sacrifice educational and career opportunities for a chance to play professionally. Should educators and professional leagues and their athletes take responsibility for educating minority youths and their parents about the low odds of making a living in sport? Do educators and professional sport people have a moral responsibility to address these issues with minority youth athletes? Certainly, an honest portrayal of the facts regarding the probability of making it to the professional level is supported by not only teleological moral theory but also deontological moral theory.

"I Know I Can Go Pro"

Ms. Green was excited to discover that 15 of the 20 African-American boys in her second grade class, when asked to write about what they wanted to be when they grow up, wrote extensively about how they wanted to be professional athletes. At first Ms. Green was elated that her boys had such lofty goals, but then she became concerned that they may be setting unrealistic expectations for themselves.

Questions
1. Why do you believe Ms. Green's boys wanted first to be professional athletes and not other professions?
2. Does Ms. Green have an ethical responsibility as a teacher to educate her students on the low probability of them becoming professional athletes?
3. Discuss the positive and/or negative outcomes that might result from the unrealistic expectations of Ms. Green's African-American students.

Knowing the facts about a given situation can help people make decisions that are in their best interest. Perhaps coaches, teachers, school counselors, and administrators should assume the responsibility for educating youth about their misconceptions of the likelihood of playing professional sport and stress the importance of getting a sound education. Professional educators usually have a good understanding of both the high aspirations of youth and the pitfalls they will encounter in the real world. Young athletes who aspire to play professional sport may then use the facts provided to them to make more informed decisions about their education and sporting and non-sporting lives.

Hiring Minorities in Sport

The influence of reward structures in sport may have helped reduce racial discrimination against athletes, but it has failed to significantly reduce discrimination against minority candidates applying for coaching and management positions in many sports. Making coaching and management selections based on talent should be reinforced. Regardless of their racial biases, owners of professional sport franchises and directors overseeing athletics in major programs clearly understand that playing the best players results in a stronger team that will generate increased fan interest and greater revenues. According to Davis, commercialization and the pressure to field winning teams propels colleges to recruit and obtain the services of the most talented student athletes regardless of their color.[10] But when hiring head coaches and general managers, do owners and administrators hire for these positions based on talent and the ability to perform, as they do for players? Owners and athletic directors of major college athletic programs seem more hesitant to apply this same player selection logic when it comes to hiring head coaches and general managers. Often white candidates who seem less qualified for these important positions get hired. Why might this be the case?

One possible reason for discrimination against minority coaches may lie within the job descriptions of head coaching and top management positions. The required and preferred qualifications related to these positions may differ, but experience and past success are two factors that are weighted heavily in owners' decision-making processes. Since minority candidates have not had the opportunities to hold such positions, they often lack the experience and levels of achievement that owners are looking for. This may help in understanding certain instances of apparent discrimination, but it does not explain why white candidates who also lack these qualifications are hired over minority candidates who appear more qualified.

Situations like these are more puzzling, and may indicate racial or ethnic biases of the hiring personnel; however, it is unlikely that discrimination is the sole reason for the lack of minorities in coaching and administration. But, without a visible presence of minorities in coaching and athletic administrative positions, minority youth may not view those positions as realistically attainable. Generally, those who aspire to reach head coaching and administrative leadership positions in elite sport organizations have to begin the process early. Enrolling in educational programs, developing a track record of experience, and networking are all areas that require attention when a person plans and begins his or her career path in coaching and athletic administration. If minority youth do not have role models in this area of sports, they may not begin gaining the education and developing a resume that makes them qualified to interview for those positions when the time comes.

Inequities For Non-Minorities in Sport

The effort to hire minorities goes beyond equity, sometimes, creating a state of inequity for non-minorities referred to as **reverse discrimination.** It could be argued that, in an attempt to achieve fair hiring practices for all, an overemphasis has been placed on the implementation of practices that provide minorities with opportunities not available for non-minorities. It is challenging, to say the least, to achieve equity that is to the satisfaction of all coaches and individuals from various races and ethnic backgrounds. Historically, persons of various races and ethnic backgrounds have all experienced different race-based inequities that may require different present-day solutions to provide a model of equity for all.

> **reverse discrimination:** unfairness against members of a dominant or majority group, especially when resulting from policies established to correct discrimination against members of a minority or disadvantaged group.

"The Minority Hiring Mission"

Mr. Mix, the athletic director at Middle College, could not have been happier with himself. It was the end of the year and he had just hired a third head coach who was a minority. Mr. Mix believed that he put his best foot forward in meeting one of the campus's missions of achieving and maintaining a racially diverse atmosphere in leadership positions. The next day in a meeting of administrators, Mr. Mix proudly stated, "I have successfully hired not one, not two, but three minority head coaches this year. Our sports of football, baseball, and women's soccer are now all under the leadership of head coaches who are minorities. In all three cases, some coaches who were non-minorities looked better on paper and interviewed a bit better, but we were fortunate to have been able to attract three minority candidates who at least met the minimal hiring criteria. I feel great about being able to make our head coaching staff more racially diverse." The reactions from the table of administrators to Mr. Mix's statements were varied; some smiled, some frowned, while others showed no emotion at all.

Questions
1. Do you agree with the mission of Middle College?
2. Were Mr. Mix's methods of hiring three head coaches who were minorities ethical from a deontological perspective? Were Mr. Mix's methods ethical from a consequentialist perspective?
3. Discuss utilitarianism and how the greatest amount of happiness for the greatest number of people might be realized or not realized by hiring these three particular head coaches.

Is it more difficult to determine the best candidate for a particular coaching or management position than it is to determine the most talented players for a team? Are the criteria for a successful general manager less tangible than the criteria that allow scouts and player personnel experts to choose the best athletes? In other words, is it more difficult to empirically identify and select the best coaches and general managers? Despite the criteria that seems to sometimes determine the hiring of coaches and general managers, should owners have to hire the person who is perceived to be the best available coach or general manager to win the most games? Are there cases in which teams are talent laden to the point that they win games not because of their coach but despite their coach?

Establishing Non-Discriminatory Hiring Criteria

What is fair criteria in hiring, and who decides what is fair? For the purpose of attaining program goals, if the impact of coaching skills is secondary to the impact of player skills, the potential to hire a coach based on factors other than coaching skills is likely higher. In other words, if a head coach believes that he or she does not need an assistant coach to help with actual coaching duties, the head coach may simply hire a friend instead of an applicant that has the best coaching skills. Or, if the head coach does not believe his or her job depends on the coaching skills of an assistant, the head coach might be more likely to select an assistant coach based on race instead of on coaching skills. If, however, a head coach's job does depend on assistant coaches and their ability to coach and recruit, the head coach might be more likely to hire an assistant coach based strictly on that person's coaching skills.

If the method for hiring coaches and general managers is not well supported empirically, or if it is not necessary to hire the best coach or general manager to win games, then the potential for racial discrimination may become more likely. Thus, owners and those hiring for sport organizations should continue to do their best to establish job descriptions with a set of required and preferred qualifications that are fair and will best assist them in identifying the best candidate for coaching or management positions. This system should minimize discriminatory hiring practices in sport organizations and give qualified minority candidates a fairer opportunity at open positions.

Discussion about race inequities as related to those directly involved in sport is extensive. Major college sport organizations have been made aware of inequities in their sport, league, and even their own teams. Race inequities must be addressed not only in the selection of players and coaches but also in the treatment of players and coaches once hired. For example, Sagas and Cunningham[35] suggest that head coaches may racially discriminate when it comes to treatment of their assistant coaches. More specifically, head coaches may provide minorities with fewer opportunities or less favorable opportunities for advancement while on the job.[35]

According to Sagas and Cunningham, prolonged discrimination in this manner may limit the mobility and success of minority coaches and also contributes to their absence from leadership positions.[35] For example, if an assistant college basketball coach is provided only with the opportunity to recruit, he or she will not acquire the floor coaching skills that are necessary to advance to a head coaching position. From a teleological vantage point, the head coach who does not offer his assistant coaches the opportunities to gain a broad set of coaching skills is potentially violating several moral values. Most head coaches are not required to develop the skills of their assistants in a way that will help them become head coaches themselves someday, but those who do are acting altruistically. Head coaches who do not help their assistant coaches broaden their skills may not be fully respecting their assistant coaches and their aspirations to become head coaches. Head coaches are being beneficent, or are doing good, when they help their assistant coaches reach their professional goal to become a head coach.

Hiring Minority Sport Media Personnel

Has there been an equal attempt at eliminating racial inequity in professions that are closely affiliated with sport? In looking at the case of sports media personnel, according to Lapchick the answer is a resounding, "No."[36] Racial inequities exist in sport media positions including sports editors, assistant sports editors, columnists, and reporters. Although sport media personnel are quick to point out the racial inequities that exist on teams and front office positions, evidence indicates that the number of minority employees in the Associated Press Sports Editors Association is quite low. Lapchick indicates that more than 85% of those employed at the Associated Press Sports Editors are white males.[36]

If approaching the issue of the disproportionate number of minority sports editors from a deontological perspective, current sports editors would not only have to honestly assess whether or not racially biased hiring took place under a set of principles, but also decide whether or not they would support racially biased hirings that favor a race other than their own. From a teleological standpoint, the hiring criteria and the selection process should be analyzed for fairness; if the hiring process focuses on skill and the race of one applicant is not favored over the race of another applicant, then the hiring process could be considered fair.

The Good Old Boy Network

The **good old boy network,** also known as the "old-boy network," is defined as an informal, exclusive system of mutual assistance and friendship through which men belonging to a particular group, such as the alumni of a school, exchange favors and connections as in politics or business.[37] In the world of sports, the good old boy network is an informal network of males that has developed as a result of shared sport experiences such as playing, coaching, and managing. Previous to integration, minorities were not included in the network, since they could not enter it as players.

The networking of white male candidates within this discriminatory framework led to their hiring for coaching and management positions that became

good old boy network: an informal fraternity of white men who exchange business and political favors with other white males while excluding women and minorities. In sport, the exclusion of women and minorities from the good old boy network has resulted in hiring inequities in sport organizations.

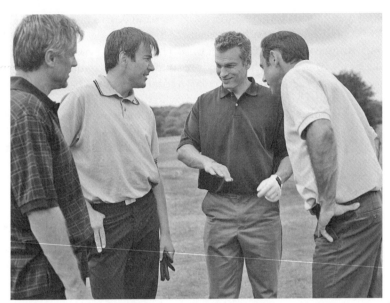

6-3 *Before integration, minorities were not included in the good old boy network, which often helped one another with coaching and sport management positions.*

available in sport. Those not in the network (minorities) did not have an equal opportunity to compete for these positions and, thus, were excluded from consideration. When Tyrone Willingham was fired as the head football coach of Notre Dame, there was no evidence that race played a role in his firing, but as the first black coach of any sport at Notre Dame, Willingham did acknowledge the fact there were only two black head coaches among the 117 Division I-A schools.[38] Based on the near dearth of African-American head coaches in major college football, it would seem that the old-boy network still rules the sport.

Negative Effects of the Good Old Boy Network

Former offensive coordinator Norm Chow of the University of Southern California (USC) football team may have experienced the negative effects of not being part of the good old boy network.[39] Chow, an Asian college football coach, has an outstanding reputation as an offensive coordinator. Known for developing top college offenses and quarterbacks, Chow was passed over for head coaching jobs even after directing the USC offense that was partly responsible for back-to-back national championships in 2004 and 2005. Add the 32 years of overall football coaching experience that is part of Chow's resume, you cannot help but wonder if Chow was not hired because he did not fit the mold of the good old boy network. If applying the best-interests-of-all aspect of consequentialism, in whose best interest was it to pass over Norm Chow for head coaching positions? It was unlikely to be in anyone's best interest if Chow was passed over because of race. According to the greatest happiness standard of utilitarianism grounded in consequentialism, there must be no doubt that a decision makes other people happier and that the world gains by the decision. In the case of passing over Chow in favor of other non-minority coaches, the good old boy network may be happy but minorities are most likely less happy, and society does not gain if the decision to pass over Chow was based on the fact that he is a minority.

Today in sports, even though minorities have become established players, the lucrative positions of coach and general manager that many of them covet after their retirement are often out of reach because of the good old boy network. In some cases, minorities have been proactive in their attempts to gain equality, forming minority sport organizations such as the Black Coaches Association (BCA), which has recently undergone a name change to Black Coaches and Administrators that better reflects their primary purpose of fostering the growth and development of ethnic minorities at all levels of sports, both nationally and internationally.[40]

Hiring Based on Merit

It is fair to ask why organized efforts to promote race equity on behalf of minorities in sport are still necessary in this day and age. Are sports meritocratic to the extent that hiring practices are fair for players but not for managers, coaches, and administrative personnel? Can sport operate as a meritocracy for management the same way it does for players? Lomasky suggests that the NBA operates as a minor meritocracy and that it may promote clearer thinking concerning larger issues such as race equity in management positions.[12] He also points out that the NBA has no affirmative action programs, quotas, or overseers of political correctness.[12] But can minority coaching and management candidates realistically expect fair access to employment opportunities from an organization with no established standards to promote minorities? Without a formal process that allows minorities an equal opportunity for employment, we have to rely on just and fair behavior by those responsible for hiring for these positions. In the past, it was questionable as to whether non-minorities provided minorities with an equal opportunity for employment. Forms of public pressure or the law may motivate employers to hire minorities more than would relying on individuals to use moral values grounded in teleology as part of the process.

Identifying the Merits of Coaches and General Managers

Whereas players' merits are tested daily in the heat of competition, the merits of coaches and general managers are somewhat more difficult to identify over the short and long term. Players' talents and abilities are publicly exposed on a daily basis and directly affect the win/loss record of their teams. If undeserving players receive too much playing time, fans will voice their opinions and might choose not to attend games. Coaches might also make the claim that with inferior player talent, winning at the championship level is out of the question. Without an exceptional quarterback in football, shooter in basketball, or goalie in hockey, can a coach really be expected to produce championship teams? Coaches can create outstanding offensive and defensive schemes, but without at least average talent they will not be able to coach teams to championship levels. Even if coaches succeed in motivating players of below-average talent to perform at their highest possible level, they will not win championships. In other words, a coach's win/loss record may not be indicative of good or bad coaching.

Consider NBA coaching great Pat Riley. In the 1980s, Riley coached the Los Angeles Lakers to four NBA world championships. Playing for Riley on those championship teams were two Hall of Fame players, Earvin "Magic" Johnson and Kareem Abdul Jabbar. Aside from Johnson and Jabbar, during the "show time" years the Lakers had a talent-laden roster from top to bottom. Without question, Riley successfully placed players in the correct positions and managed the dynamics of the team in a way that melded elite individual players into a dominating basketball team. After leaving the Lakers for the New York Knicks, Riley experienced very good success but did not win any championships with what would, overall, be considered very good but not all-time great players. Later in Riley's coaching career, from 1995 to 2001, he took over head coaching responsibilities with the Miami Heat. The same "great" Pat Riley had some good records but he also finished with a dismal 36–46 season in 2001 and a poor 25-57 record in 2002 before stepping aside to become general manager of the Heat franchise. Then, after acquiring, arguably, the best center in the league in Shaquille O'Neal along with a top point guard in DeWayne Wade, Riley came back as head coach of the Heat and led them to a World Championship. Throughout Riley's NBA coaching years, from the beginning to the end, like most coaches he experienced his best coaching years with players that had extraordinary talent.[41]

When it comes to selecting players, the pressure to win and produce a profit, along with other factors, does influence sport to establish and maintain a meritocratic foundation. The good old boy network would likely have a difficult time existing under conditions of true meritocracy. Since teams usually produce greater revenues when they win, the players with the most talent are appropriately rewarded with playing time and money. If the good old boy network decided which players to select based on race, teams would likely be less effective than if players were chosen for their talents and merits. According to Franke, "For all its well-documented faults, big league sports epitomized a wonderful American ideal: that anyone—regardless of race, creed, wealth, upbringing, or zodiac sign—can make it to the top. Just be among the best performers. Period. End of story."[42(p29)]

In the case of coaches and general managers, however, success is measured over the length of a season or over several seasons. Many factors other than their own talents affect their success; hence, it may be more difficult for owners to determine whether they have the best general manager or coach for their franchise, leaving room for discriminatory practices to be established or continue operating.

If there is a candidate pool of minimally competent general managers who have applied for and are capable of managing a sport organization that has superior athletic talent, it may not matter which general manager is hired. Or, if a general manager is responsible for signing talented players, attracting the best players may not have anything to do with stellar recruiting skills of the general manager but instead have to do with being able to offer a superior facility or more money to prospective players. In other words, it might just be that any of several candidates could come in and turn out productive results. In such cases, chief executive officers may be more apt to allow their racial biases to enter into the hiring process since they have equally qualified candidates. If those hiring general managers are truly doing so from a teleological moral perspective, they should engage in a fair and honest process that measures the talent of individuals and not the color of their skin.

Hiring Quotas

What is the best way to eliminate discriminatory hiring practices in sport? Is the establishment of a **quota system,** which requires a certain number of minority applicants to be hired, an effective means of accomplishing this task? Under a true race-based quota system, a specific number of persons of a particular race, regardless of qualifications or lack thereof, might be required to be hired. Interestingly, from a consequentialist and a teleological perspective, the use of quotas might appear to be a blatant example of discrimination—even though the intent is good—since race is the criteria for hiring. Consequentialists could note here that race-based quota systems will create situations in which the best-qualified individuals will not be hired because of their race or ethnicity. Emphasizing fairness, teleologists might point out that morally good sport managers will not deny the best-qualified individuals a job because of their ethnic background or the color of their skin.

> **quota system:** a number or percentage, especially of people, constituting a required or targeted minimum; a system of quotas for hiring minority applicants.

Correcting Past Exclusions

Duster portrayed the basis for programs attempting to provide fair participation practices with the following statement: "Sensitive and progressive persons often acknowledge that there has been a vicious circle of exclusion that has prevented minorities from full participation in the accessible routes to economic and political advantage."[30](p78) The teleologist, if choosing to acknowledge the vicious circle of exclusion that Duster speaks of, might support a quota system as a form of justice for past wrongs that minorities have experienced.

In one case, the National Football League (NFL) has attempted to end these vicious circles of exclusion by requiring organizations to interview minority candidates for coaching positions. The NFL created the Workplace Diversity Committee, which developed what has come to be known as the **Rooney Rule.** The Rooney Rule requires that one minority candidate must be interviewed for all vacant head coaching positions.[43] Teams who fail to follow this regulation face fines or other penalties. Although some people may argue against rules instituting quotas, the NFL and its Workplace Diversity Committee believe that the Rooney Rule will help to eliminate discriminatory hiring practices and help more minorities attain head coaching positions within the league.

> **Rooney Rule:** a rule in the NFL requiring that one minority candidate must be interviewed for all vacant head coaching positions.

Moral Justification Difficulties

Are quotas in and of themselves a form of racial discrimination? On the surface a deontologist may disagree with hiring quotas. As previously mentioned, a true hiring quota based on race will call for the hiring of a candidate even though he or she may not be the most qualified candidate in terms of skill related to the job. If a particular race is being singled out to be hired, the practice of hiring quotas cannot be universalized. In other words, if hiring quotas are in place for the purpose of providing minorities with opportunities based on the mere fact that a person is a minority, non-minorities are obviously not being provided with the same opportunity, which makes the practice of hiring quotas non-universal.

Quota systems may be difficult to justify morally, since they seem to pit one injustice against another—something that deontological moral theory would not condone. Again, deontologists might contend that it is morally wrong to be unjust in particular situations for the purpose of correcting past injustices. In the deontologist's eyes, two wrongs cannot make a right. Teleologists, on the other hand, might find themselves in a dilemma over which value to prioritize, compassion or fairness. The morally good person would not choose to act unjustly, all things being equal. But given the history of discriminatory practices against minorities, *are* all things equal? Prioritizing values might be a way to level the playing field for minorities, who as a whole have historically suffered from discrimination. In an effort to rectify some past wrongs, the teleologist might choose to prioritize compassion over a strict definition of fairness. If a greater good is provided by rectifying past wrongs, the utilitarianism form of consequentialism would be achieved through a quota system. Further debate and analysis is necessary to determine if a quota system that attempts to make up for past injustices does in fact achieve a greater good, in the long run, for society.

As in society itself, there are challenges involved in creating racially equitable employment environments in sport. A quota system is one mechanism that could provide minorities the opportunity to gain employment experiences in front office and administrative positions in sport organizations that currently are underrepresented by minorities. Continued discussion and debate related to moral theory will be helpful in determining the best course of action regarding the establishment of quota systems in sport organizations.

Conclusion

As demonstrated in this chapter, racial and ethnic discrimination still exists in sport leagues and organizations. It is important that the more subtle varieties of discrimination be recognized by athletes, coaches, administrators, and others who have the power to resolve the inequalities these practices bring about. Such individuals have a moral responsibility to examine alleged instances of discrimination and develop and implement policies and procedures that will at least reduce, if not eliminate, the types of racial and ethnic discrimination operating within their leagues, organizations, and teams. If they are resolute in their efforts, discrimination can be controlled, and sport will more closely resemble the meritocracy idealists want it to be—one in which individuals are judged on their merits rather than by their race or ethnicity.

Racism in sport is not supported by teleology because values like fairness, honesty, and compassion would not allow for unequal treatment of people in sport. Nor is racism supported by a deontological line of reasoning. Deontologists would only approve of actions if they believed those actions to be effective when universalized to all, including themselves. It is unlikely that a person, deontologist or not, would expect to be treated unfairly and with prejudice. Even when applying consequentialism to moral dilemmas in sport, racist actions are not supported. More often than not, the consequences are at least negative to those being discriminated against, and in the long run may be negative to the discriminators.

Ultimately, sport personnel must take it upon themselves to exercise moral values like fairness and honesty when dealing with the issue of discrimination in sport. Displaying and acting with a level of compassion for those individuals who are of a race that has historically been the victim of discrimination will be helpful for those individuals who hold decision-making positions in sport.

References

1. Kivel P. *Uprooting Racism*. British Columbia, Canada: New Society Publishers; 2002.
2. Hill F. Shattering the glass ceiling: Blacks in coaching. *Black Issues in Higher Education*. 2004;21(4):36–37.
3. Bell-Fialkoff A. A brief history of ethnic cleansing. *Foreign Affairs*. 1993;72(3):110–121.
4. Whiteside K. Concerns raised over racism during Cup; June 2, 2006. *USA Today* website. Available at: http://www.usatoday.com/sports/soccer/worldcup/2006-06-01-intolerance-cup_x.htm. Accessed May 13, 2007.
5. Donnor JK. Towards an interest-convergence in the education of African-American football student athletes in major college sports. *Race and Ethnicity and Education*. 2005;8(1):45–67.
6. Stricherz M. Baseball and meritocracy. *America*. June 17, 1995:172(21);7–8.
7. Bartolomeo C. AFT: A proud history of fighting discrimination. *On Campus*. May/June 2004:11–12.
8. Knee S. Jim Crow strikes out: Branch Rickey and the struggle for integration in American baseball. *Culture, Sport, Society*. 2003;6(2/3):71–87.
9. Coakley J. *Sports in Society: Issues and Controversies*. 8th ed. Boston: McGraw-Hill; 2004.
10. Davis T. The myth of the superspade: The persistence of racism in college athletics. *Fordham Urban Law Journal*. 1995;22(3):615–698.
11. Rader BG. *American Sports: From the Age of Folk Games to the Age of Televised Sports*. 5th ed. Upper Saddle River, NJ: Prentice Hall; 2004.
12. Lomasky LE. Meritocracy that works. *National Review*. December 5, 1994;46(23):52–53.
13. Harris JC. Yes, racial profiling is alive and well in the world of sports. *The New York Amsterdam News*. March 28, 2002:43–44.

14. Ansari H. Introduction: racialization and sport. *Patterns of Prejudice*. 2004;38(3):209–212.

15. Cunningham GB. Already aware of the glass ceiling: Race-related effects of perceived opportunity on the career choices of college athletes. *Journal of African American Studies*. 2003;7(1):57–71.

16. USA Today. College football fumbles minority hiring. *USA Today* website. Available at: http://www.usatoday.com/news/opinion/editorials/2005-12-29-our-view?x.htm. Accessed: August 10, 2006.

17. Lieber J. Golf's host clubs have open-and-shut policies on discrimination. *USA Today* website. Available at: http://www.usatoday.com/sports/golf/2003-04-09-club-policies_x.htm. Accessed August 10, 2006.

18. Bermanzohn SA. Violence, nonviolence, and the civil rights movement. *New Political Science*. 2000;22(1):31–48.

19. Dawkins D. Race relations and the sport of golf: The African American golf legacy. *The Western Journal of Black Studies*. 2004;28(1):327–331.

20. Guillermo E. Golden stuff tarnished by Tolbert race apology; January 24-30, 2003. *AsianWeek.com* website. Available at http://www.asianweek.com/2003_01_24/opinion_emil.html. Accessed May 6, 2007.

21. CNN. Golfer says comments about Woods 'misconstrued'; April 27, 1997. *CNN* website. Available at: http://www.cnn.com/US/9704/21/fuzzy/. Accessed August 5, 2006.

22. Moore JR. Shattering stereotypes: A lesson plan for improving student attitudes and behavior toward minority groups. *The Social Studies*. 2006;97(1):35–39.

23. Woolf LM, Hulsizer MR. Psychosocial roots of genocide: Risk, prevention, and intervention. *Journal of Genocide Research*. 2005;7(1):101–128.

24. Hawkins B. Is stacking dead? A case study of the stacking hypothesis at a Southeastern (SEC) football program. *International Sports Journal*. 2002;6(2):146–159.

25. Gonzalez GL. The stacking of Latinos in Major League Baseball: A forgotten minority? *Journal of Sport & Social Issues*. 1996;20(2):134–160.

26. Harrison L Jr., Azzarito L, Burden J Jr. Perceptions of athletic superiority: A view from the other side. *Race Ethnicity and Education*. 2004;7(2):149–166.

27. Saraceno J. Some day, hiring will be fair to all. *USA Today*. January 6, 2003:3C.

28. ESPN. Bird: NBA 'a black man's game'; June 8, 2004. *ESPN* website. Available at: http://sports.espn.go.com/nba/news/story?id=1818396. Accessed August 2, 2006.

29. Suns' Steve Nash wins second consecutive MVP award; May 7, 2006. *NBA* website. Available at: http://www.nba.com/news/nash_mvp_05-06.html. Accessed May 15, 2007.

30. Duster T. The structure of privilege and its universe of discourse. *The American Sociologist*. 1976;11:73–78.

31. Beatty R, Peterson MA. Covert discrimination: Topeka—Before and after Brown. *Kansas History*. 2004;27(3):146–163.

32. Lapchick R, Martin S. The 2005-06 Season Racial and Gender Report Card: National Basketball Association. *The University of Central Florida* website. Available at: http://www.bus.ucf.edu/sport/public/downloads/2005_Racial_Gender_Report_Card_NBA.pdf. Accessed August 2, 2006.

33. Lapchick R, Martin S. The 2005 Racial and Gender Report Card: Major League Baseball. *The University of Central Florida* website. Available at: http://www.bus.ucf.edu/sport/

public/downloads/2005_Racial_Gender_Report_Card_MLB.pdf. Accessed August 2, 2006.

34. NCAA. Estimated probability of competing in athletics beyond the high school interscholastic level; February 16, 2007. *NCAA.org* website. Available at: http://www.ncaa.org/research/prob_of_competing/probablity_of_competing2.html. Accessed May 15, 2007.

35. Sagas M, Cunningham GB. Treatment discrimination in college coaching: Its prevalence and impact on the career success of assistant basketball coaches. *International Sports Journal.* 2004;8(1):76–88.

36. Lapchick R, Brenden J, Wright B. The 2006 Racial and Gender Report Card of the Associated Press. *The University of Central Florida* website. Available at: http://www.bus.ucf.edu/sport/public/downloads/2006_Racial_Gender_Report_Card_AP_Sports_Editors.pdf. Accessed July 31, 2006.

37. Dictionary of the American Language. 4th edition. Old-boy network. *dictionary.com* website. Available at: http://dictionary.reference.com/browse/old-boy network. Accessed May 15, 2007.

38. Wilstein S. Old boy network rules in college football; December 2, 2004. *Boston Globe* website. Available at: http://www.boston.com/sports/colleges/football/articles/2004/12/02/old_boy_network_rules_in_college_football?pg=full. Accessed March 18, 2008

39. Wilstein S. High marks for NFL in minority hiring. *Titans Online* website. Available at: http://www.titansonline.com/news/newsmain_detail.php?PRKey=2616. Accessed August 9, 2006.

40. Hendon CS. Membership deadline to vote for BCA name change is July 1, 2006. *Black Coaches Association* website. Available at: http://www.bcasports.org/MiContent.aspx?pn=NewsListings&nid=NewsArticle.1055.xm. Accessed August 5, 2006.

41. Pat Riley. *NBA* website. Available at: http://www.nba.com/coachfile/pat_riley/. Accessed May 13, 2007.

42. Franke G. Quotas undermine NFL's colorblind tradition. *Human Events.* October 13, 2003;59(35):29.

43. Nordlinger J. Color in coaching: How racial games are played in the NFL. *National Review.* September 1, 2003;55(16):25–26.

Hiring Discrimination in the Mid Northern Conference

From the beginning of the Mid Northern Conference to the present time, there has never been an African-American head football coach at any of its 10 major universities. Over the years, head coaching positions have opened and several qualified African-American coaches have applied without success. As a result, fairly or unfairly, the Mid Northern Conference has become labeled as a league that discriminates against blacks when it comes to hiring for head coaching positions.

As a member of the Mid Northern Conference, the Oakadelphia University has a reputation for not only hiring white coaches but also handpicking them from the local area. Last year, however, when the head football coaching position opened up at Oakadelphia, the athletic director decided to conduct a national search. Six months before the start of the season, Oakadelphia's athletic director was pleased to announce the hiring of one of the nation's most sought after coaches, Coach Steel. Unfortunately, Coach Steel's tenure at Oakadelphia was short lived; he was fired two weeks after signing one of the most lucrative contracts in college football. Still celebrating his new job, Coach Steel used an Oakadelphia University credit card to pay for approximately $1500 worth of charges at a neighboring state's gentleman's club. Steel's inappropriate spending spree continued late into the night, when he brought two female dancers back to his room and spent an additional $1000 for expenses that included lap dances and room service.

After learning the nature of his spending, Oakadelphia University promptly fired Coach Steel. Now feeling a sense of urgency since the recruiting season was at its peak, Oakadelphia felt the need to quickly conduct another search and fill their head coaching position with another qualified candidate. After having been turned down just a few weeks ago during the first search and for three other head coaching positions within the Conference, long-time Oakadelphia assistant coach, Coach Tevester, had to think long and hard as to whether or not he would apply again for the same position. An African-American, Tevester was listed in a national college football publication as one of the country's top head coaching prospects. Despite being turned down repeatedly, Coach Tevester was hoping this time would be different.

Given Coach Tevester's many years of experience at Oakadelphia, his astute football knowledge and recruiting skills, and his widespread popularity among members of the university community, he was, again, outstanding during the interview process. But Coach Tevester was once again turned down. The job was instead offered to a white man, Carl Ashen, who came from a professional football coaching family but was much less qualified than Tevester in terms of skills and experience. Many people believed Ashen was offered the job because he was part of the good old boys network that existed in the Mid Northern Conference. When Coach Tevester learned of his latest rejection, he experienced mixed emotions, particularly hurt and anger, as he pondered his coaching future.

Critical Thinking: Finding Common-Sense Solutions

1. If you were Oakadelphia's athletic director, would you have fired Coach Steel? Why or why not?

2. If you were Oakadelphia's athletic director, on what criteria would you have based the hiring of your head coach?

3. After being turned down for the job a second time, if you were Coach Tevester and believed you were discriminated against, would you demand an answer and seek justice in any way? Why or why not? If so, how?

4. If you were the executive director of the governing body of college athletics, would you investigate the perceived discriminatory hiring practices taking place in the Mid Northern Conference? If so, how? If not, why not?

Critical Thinking: Moral Theory-Based Decision Making

5. Using the *deontological theory* as the foundation for your decision, as athletic director would you hire Tevester or Ashen, and why? Through the use of *deontological theory* describe how you arrived at your decision.

6. If you were the athletic director, who would you have hired and how would you have justified your decision based on each of the following moral values: *justice, fairness, honesty, compassion, respect,* and *beneficence.*

7. Is the *integrity of sport* weakened, maintained, or strengthened by the firing of Coach Steel? By the hiring of Coach Ashen?

Professional Football Conference Hiring Quotas

Last month, general manager Mark Money of the Atwater Alligators was fined $200,000 for not complying with the Professional Football Conference (PFC) hiring quotas. According to the diversity enhancement rule, each PFC team with a head coaching vacancy must interview at least one minority candidate. After years of underrepresentation of minorities in head coaching and upper management positions, the PFC enacted the diversity enhancement rule in an attempt to create a more racially balanced workforce. The rule does not allow for exceptions. Simply stated, organizations must interview at least one minority candidate for open head coaching positions.

Interestingly, Money contacted no less than five minority candidates by phone, but all declined to interview. Their refusals to accept Money's invitation was based on knowledge acquired through the grapevine that Money was planning to hire his best friend, Sam Superb, who was currently coaching a team in the PFC. From a rules enforcement perspective, Money's infraction was clear: He did not interview at least one minority candidate, which is why the commissioner of the PFC fined Money and the Alligators. The commissioner also publicly scolded Money and the Alligators organization for ignoring the Conference's attempts to promote racial diversity.

Money responded to the fine and scolding by saying that it was unfair since he invited several minority candidates to interview but they had all declined. Money claimed that his intentions were good and that he made a valid attempt to abide by the diversity enhancement rule; however, he could not force candidates to interview if they chose not to. From his point of view, Money had done everything he could to follow the spirit of the rule. Acting on his belief that the fine was unjust, Money stated that he planned to appeal the fine since it was based on circumstances beyond his control.

Critical Thinking: Finding Common-Sense Solutions

1. In your opinion, do you believe the diversity enhancement rule can effectively create an environment of healthy racial diversity in the PFC? Explain your answer.

2. Should exceptions be granted for the PFC's diversity enhancement rule? If so, as the commissioner of the PFC what might be some of these exceptions and how would you determine these exceptions?

3. Could Money have done more to try and attract a qualified minority applicant to interview?

Critical Thinking: Moral Theory-Based Decision Making

4. Is it possible that Money employed *strategic reasoning* throughout the process of hiring Coach Superb?

5. Do you believe Money's intentions were good? Do you believe Money did, in fact, follow the *spirit* of the diversity enhancement rule?

6. Using the *consequentialist moral theory* to guide your actions, if you were the commissioner of the PFC would you have fined and publicly scolded Money? Why or why not?

7. Do you believe the fine imposed against Money and the Alligators was *just*? Explain your answer

Tryout Tainted by Reverse Discrimination

Coach Thomas is the head men's basketball coach at Willow State, a prominent Division I university. He is facing a difficult decision concerning the final cuts that would round out his roster for the upcoming season. As tryouts are coming to a close, Coach Thomas has all but finalized his team. His only concern is the final roster spot, for which there are two contenders: Steve and Greg. Steve is the kind of player who every coach loves to have on his team—a scrappy player who always gives 100% effort whether in practices or games. Steve is of average height and has decent basketball talent, but his work ethic is by far his strongest asset. While similar to Steve in ability, Greg, on the other hand, lacks Steve's dedication to the sport. Greg does not work hard in practice to improve his game and prefers to rely on the skills he has already developed to maintain his spot on the team.

This seemingly straightforward decision is complicated by the fact that Steve is Caucasian and Greg is African-American. In addition, Greg has told other players that if he is cut, he will go to the Dean of Students, Dean Simmons, and claim he was a victim of racism. The dean is a prominent member of the African-American community and has worked extensively to end racism in the university and local community. Coach Thomas knows that an athlete bringing charges of racism against the head basketball coach will unquestionably draw unwanted negative attention to his program, and that he could even lose his job if Greg is able to substantiate the charges in some way.

After careful consideration, Coach Thomas chose not to speak with the dean prior to making his decision on whom to cut, so as to not bring the issue to her attention. Going against his own beliefs and criteria for choosing his athletes, Coach Thomas decided to cut Steve and retain Greg. When the other players on the team found out about this decision, they were shocked, confused, and felt somewhat betrayed. As the season progressed, the team's overall work ethic declined steeply, and Willow State fell to last place in its conference. When Coach Thomas tried to discipline his players and push them to work harder in practice, he got little to no response from them. Finally, he lost control of the team completely and a player revolt ensued.

Several members of the team walked out of practice the day before a big game against their rival, Oak University. Once Dean Simmons was made aware of this, she called Coach Thomas to her office seeking answers. Frustrated and confused, Coach Thomas proceeded to tell the dean about the decision he made concerning Steve and Greg. He discussed the reasoning behind keeping Greg and his reluctance to approach the dean because of a fear that charges of racism might follow. Although upset that Coach Thomas would make a player decision based on race, Dean Simmons tried to put herself in the coach's shoes and understand his position. The two had a long conversation about the decision and its consequences that afternoon. Not wanting to make any hasty decisions, Dean Simmons informed Coach Thomas that she would take some time to determine whether or not he would be allowed to keep his job.

Critical Thinking: Finding Common-Sense Solutions

1. What factors, skills, and characteristics should coaches take into account when making cuts? What steps should be taken to make sure players understand why they have been cut?

2. Should Coach Thomas have allowed input from the other players on the team regarding his decision? If so, how might he have done so constructively?

3. If you were Dean Simmons, would you fire Coach Thomas given his decision and everything that happened as a result of that decision? Explain why or why not.

4. If Dean Simmons chose not to fire Coach Thomas, what measures would you take to help him mend the relationship with his players and help ensure that such problems would not develop in the future?

Critical Thinking: Moral Theory-Based Decision Making

5. From a *consequentialist* point of view, should Coach Thomas have discussed the Steve and Greg situation with Dean Simmons before making final cuts?

6. What values might help Coach Thomas make a good decision regarding whom to cut?

Key Terms

1964 Civil Rights Act—(Pub.L. 88-352, 78 Stat. 241, July 2, 1964) landmark legislation in the United States that outlawed discrimination based on race, color, religion, sex, or national origin in voting, employment, and public services.

affirmative action—a policy or a program that seeks to redress past discrimination through active measures to ensure equal opportunity, as in education and employment.

good old boy network—an informal fraternity of white men who exchange business and political favors with other white males while excluding women and minorities. In sport, the exclusion of women and minorities from the good old boy network has resulted in hiring inequities in sport organizations.

meritocracy—a venue in which people advance because of talent and hard work rather than because of politics or cultural ideology; sport is often perceived to be a true meritocracy in that players earn their positions based on skill.

quota system—a number or percentage, especially of people, constituting a required or targeted minimum; a system of quotas for hiring minority applicants.

race equity—provision of the same opportunities for all persons, regardless of race.

reverse discrimination—unfairness against members of a dominant or majority group, especially when resulting from policies established to correct discrimination against members of a minority or disadvantaged group.

Rooney Rule—a rule in the NFL requiring that one minority candidate must be interviewed for all vacant head coaching positions.

stacking—the disproportionate representation of athletes and/or sport administration positions based on characteristics such as race or ethnicity, which can lead to stereotyping and myths, i.e., black men cannot swim and white men cannot sprint. In sport, stacking is negative because it reinforces stereotypes that prevent athletes from playing certain positions that they may be capable of playing.

token white players—including one white player on a sports team even if more talented minority players are available and interested in being on the team; an informal type of affirmative action or quota system for whites.

7 Gender Equity in Athletics and Title IX

Learning Outcomes

After reading Chapter 7, the student will be able to:

1. Explain, from a gender equity perspective, why Title IX was legislated.

2. Describe how equality for women in athletics affects society.

3. Using moral theory, list some gender inequities in intercollegiate athletics prior to the enforcement of Title IX.

4. Compare and contrast, from an equity perspective, the dropping of men's sports and adding of women's sports as strategies to comply with Title IX.

5. Establish arguments for and against the online survey as a method to determine the athletic interests of women.

6. Based on moral theory, list points for and against including revenue-generating sports in Title IX's proportionality formula.

7. List moral challenges that tradition has posed for those seeking equity for women in athletic departments.

8. Identify moral arguments for and against Title IX.

Participation opportunities for women in sport have increased significantly since the passage of Title IX in 1972. As a result of Title IX, women are experiencing benefits of organized sport participation that were formerly unavailable to them. Not everyone is satisfied with the current landscape of athletics, however. The elimination of men's sports as a way to achieve equal participation opportunities for women has caused much concern in the sporting community. As a result of these concerns, alternative ways to achieve equity are being examined.

Is Title IX to blame for the elimination of certain men's teams from athletic programs? Should the current way that Title IX is being implemented be changed to reverse this trend? Or do the benefits accompanying Title IX stand as evidence that it should be maintained in its current form? What moral perspective might schools use to decide whether particular sports should be added to or removed from their athletic programs?

This chapter will address all of the above questions from a moral standpoint, for the purpose of clarifying the ethical issues surrounding Title IX. Furthermore, this chapter will help readers better understand how to constructively converse about these issues so that better solutions to current problems can be developed in the future.

Achieving Gender Equity Through Title IX

Title IX was created to promote gender equity in federally funded sports programs. An underlying presupposition of Title IX is that sport participation offers benefits to its participants that should be available to both sexes. Below is a brief history of Title IX and a discussion of the benefits sports participation offers to participants, along with an exploration of how women's participation in sports could result in benefits to society at large.

History of Title IX

> **Educational Amendments Act of 1972:** a comprehensive federal law that prohibits discrimination on the basis of sex in any federally funded education program or activity.

> **Title IX:** a federal law stating that no person shall, on the basis of sex, be excluded from participation in, or denied benefits of, or be subjected to discrimination under any educational program or activity receiving federal assistance.

As part of the **Educational Amendments Act of 1972, Title IX** was the first major step toward achieving equity for women in sport programs. This act prohibits gender discrimination and further affirms that, "No person in the United States shall, on the basis of sex, be excluded from participation in, be denied the benefits of, or be subjected to discrimination under any education program or activity receiving federal financial assistance."[1]

Generally, Title IX is widespread, carrying few exemptions; however, an exemption does exist for religiously affiliated colleges if a conflict exists between Title IX and their religious tenets. Equitable opportunities for male and female athletics is measured by the Department of Education[2] using one of the following three methods:

1. Participation opportunities for male and female students are provided in numbers substantially proportionate to their respective enrollments.
2. A demonstrated history and continuing practice of the expansion of programs responsive to the underrepresented sex.
3. Interests and abilities of the underrepresented sex are fully and effectively accommodated by present programs.

equal opportunities: from a Title IX athletic standpoint, providing males and females with equivalent opportunities in sport regardless of sex.

Although not actively enforced until the 1990s, Title IX mandated that **equal opportunities** and accommodations be provided for both male and female athletes. When President Richard Nixon signed Title IX on June 23, 1972, it was so broadly worded that it needed written regulations before it could be enforced. Not until 1979 did Health Education and Welfare (HEW) issue a final policy interpretation that included the three-part test that is still in use today.[3] Further hampering Title IX's effect on athletic departments was the *Grove City College v Bell*, 465 US 555 (1984) Supreme Court ruling. On February 28, 1984, the highest court ruled that Title IX only applied to programs that directly benefitted from federal funds. This ruling considerably limited the **Office of Civil Rights'** (OCR) jurisdiction in athletics programs.[4]

Office of Civil Rights (OCR): the enforcement body of Title IX.

Civil Rights Restoration Act of 1987: an act passed by Congress in 1988 that allowed the Office of Civil Rights to regain jurisdiction over athletics programs, stating that Title IX applies to all operations that receive federal funds, effectively overturning the Grove City ruling.

Not until the **Civil Rights Restoration Act of 1987** was passed by Congress in 1988, did the OCR regain jurisdiction over athletics programs. The Civil Restoration Act of 1987 effectively overturned the Grove City ruling, stating that Title IX applies to all operations of a recipient of federal funds.[5] The first case challenging sex discrimination in an entire program led to a 1988 court-ordered settlement in *Haffer v Temple University.*[3]

Before Title IX, sport opportunities for women were limited. Only about 16,000 women participated in intercollegiate varsity athletic programs in a given season just prior to its passage.[6] In educational institutions, women simply were not provided with sporting opportunities equal to those provided to men. Furthermore, women often had no input in matters concerning their athletic involvement and had no apparent choice other than to accept what was decided for them by men. French notes that women's sports at the collegiate level had little support from athletic departments because, in addition to male athletes who dominated college sport on the field, "those who sat on governing bodies and who administered intercollegiate athletics in its first century of existence were also predominantly male."[7(p63)] Title IX addressed these issues of gender inequities that persisted in intercollegiate sport. Over a period of years, Title IX has resulted in an increased number of participation opportunities for women.[8] Thus, in the 2003–2004 school year, 160,977 female athletes competed in National Collegiate Athletic Association (NCAA) championship sports.[9]

Benefits of Sport Experiences to Other Areas of Life

Sport is an arena in which boys have traditionally learned about teamwork, goal setting, the pursuit of excellence in performance, and other achievement-oriented behaviors—

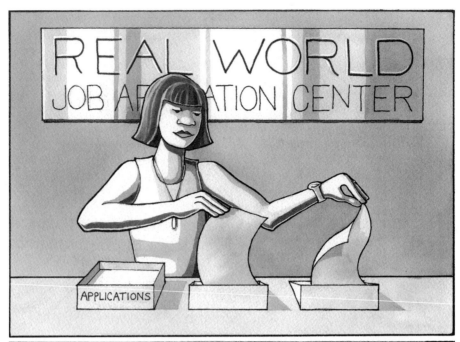

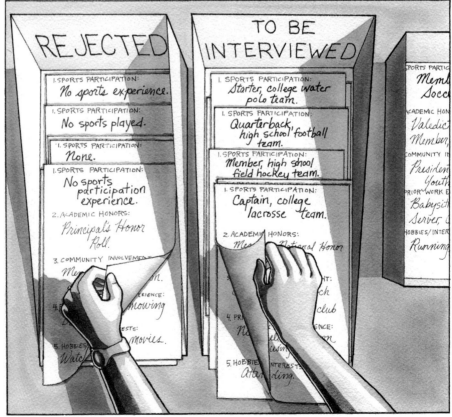

critical skills necessary for success in the workplace. It is no coincidence that 80% of the female executives at Fortune 500 companies identified themselves as former "tomboys," having played sports.[10] The Women's Sports Foundation points out the importance of equal opportunity for girls to play sports so they too can derive the psychological, physiological, and sociological benefits of sports participation. The Women's Sports Foundation also claims that sport has been one of the most important sociocultural learning experiences for boys and men for many years and those same benefits should be afforded to girls and women.[10] Deontological moral theory asserts that one should act only if those actions are based on principle and are fit to be universal to all. If boys are afforded the opportunity to gain the sociocultural learning experiences from sport, based on deontology, the same opportunities should be provided to all, including girls.

From a broader perspective, sport experiences might open one's eyes to the reality that life is not always fair. If women are denied or only have restricted access to sport participation, they may be at a disadvantage because they will not experience, through sport participation, some of the skills and values helpful to their success in society. Under teleological moral theory, one might examine fairness, justice, and beneficence. Are these three moral values applicable to equal participation opportunities in sports for females? Is it fair, just, or beneficent to females if they are denied the same participation opportunities as males?

Applying Competitive Sport Experiences to the Real World

One might argue that because sport's focus is on competition, athletes become more proficient in competing than non-athletes. If females are not provided with equal opportunities to compete in sport, they could very well be at a disadvantage when attempting to compete professionally in society against men who have had competitive sport experiences. Placing women at such a disadvantage may keep them from achieving success and becoming leaders in education, business, politics, and other areas of life. Hence, the teleologist might claim that it is unfair to deny or limit women's sport participation opportunities, because to do so amounts to **gender discrimination**.

> **gender discrimination:** actions that deny opportunities, privileges, or rewards to a person or a group because of their sex; Title IX legislation has reduced gender discrimination against women in school-based athletic departments.

Participation in athletics can take many forms and begin at early ages. Travel squads further emphasize competition and commonly provide opportunities for athletes as early as age seven in sports such as baseball and basketball. Opportunities to compete in sport continue from these early years of youth into one's middle school, high school, and college years. If these participation opportunities are gender specific—usually favoring males—males may have an advantage in professional endeavors requiring competition. There are several such professional endeavors, and because competition is a pillar of capitalism, those who learn how to successfully compete through sport might also have an advantage in a competitive society. Thus, restricting women's participation opportunities in sport is an example of gender discrimination here in the United States, because it may keep women from preparing sufficiently for life in the capitalist society in which they live. Here, the teleologist might point out the lack of fairness and respect that are directed toward women as persons and citizens when they are not provided with equal opportunities as men.

Landing jobs, being promoted, and competing against other businesses at work are three examples in which those who have experience competing, most likely will have an advantage over those who do not. The prospective job candidate may fall back on strategies that he used to "make" a sports team. Employees who strive to be promoted may very well use techniques they used to become a starter or team captain on a sports team. When competing against other businesses, the former athletes may apply social values of hard work and perseverance that helped them defeat other teams during their competitive sport years. Deontological moral theory supports the notion that if one sex receives the benefits of social values through participation, then the other sex also deserves the same opportunity.

Over the years, participation in intercollegiate athletics has benefited hundreds of thousands of women, and much of the opportunity is a direct result of Title IX. Some benefits of Title IX include the opportunity for female athletes to gain experiences of how to deal with failure and success, as well as learning about teamwork and themselves. In addition, by participating in sport, female athletes will have increased their chance of completing a college education.[8]

If women are denied opportunities to cultivate these important techniques and values through sport, they may not be able to get the jobs or promotions they desire. Hence, the disadvantages women may experience from having limited access to sport may even affect their abilities and opportunities to do what they want in life. Put another way, these disadvantages may limit their experience of freedom within their own lives.

Applying Cooperative Sport Experiences to the Real World

Team sports require a productive interaction of team members to reach a common goal, much the way a company might require the cooperation of committee members to reach a common goal. In sport, players learn how to effectively execute directives from their coach, in much the same way an employee of a company has to for their supervisor. If women are shielded from sport experiences, they do not have the chance to work with coaches and teammates and possibly develop cooperative teamwork skills under the intense conditions that sport can bring. Given the previously cited importance of developing group-related skills through sport, from a deontological perspective it seems unfair to deny women the opportunity to have the same sporting opportunities as men. To do so could prevent women from having important sport experiences that would help them develop more completely as productive citizens and human beings.

Applying Perseverance, Delayed Gratification, and Unfair Sport Experiences to the Real World

While involved in sport, sport participants often have to persevere through setbacks— something that could be helpful in achieving long-term success as an employee. Significant achievements, possibly in the form of championships, often take months or even years to achieve, as is the case with business dealings in the workplace. Experiences in sport that are not fair might be helpful in preparing sport participants for injustices that exist in the workplace and society in general. For instance, one may practice relentlessly but never achieve the success level of the naturally talented competitor.

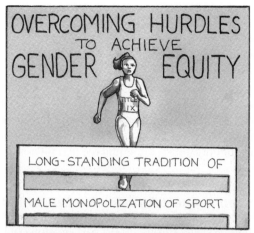

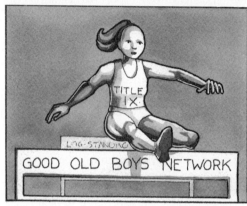

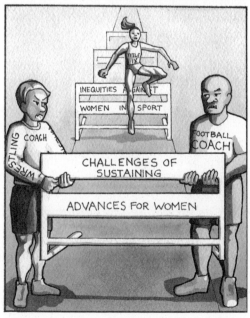

Unfair sporting experiences may prepare one for unfair work-related experiences that will inevitably take place.

Based on teleological moral theory, the deprivation of equal opportunities to participate in sport causes moral concern because it does not appear to be fair to provide opportunities to gain real world experiences through sport to one sex but not another. From a "best interests" perspective, it might be in the best interest of males to have more sporting opportunities, but is it in the best interest of females. And, is it in the best interest of society?

Equality Through Sport Participation Opportunities

The demand for equality through sport participation opportunities in educational institutions came about, in part, so women could realize the same benefits resulting from sport participation as men have realized for years. Since the inception of Title IX, there has been a real increase in sport participation opportunities for females. In 2006, there was an average of 8.45 women's teams per school. In 1970, prior to the 1972 enactment of Title IX, there were only 2.5.[8] Interesting to note, however, is the decrease of women coaches for women's teams that has taken place since the enactment of Title IX in 1972. In 1972, over 90% of women's teams were coached by females, whereas 2% of men's teams were coached by females. By 2006, the number of women's teams coached by women had decreased to less than 50%, yet still less than 2% of men's teams were coached by females.[8] From an administrative perspective, in 2006 only 18.6% of athletic directors of women's programs were female. Yet, in 1972 over 90% of women's intercollegiate athletics programs were administered by females.[8]

It is difficult to argue against the notion that sport provides its participants with myriad benefits that carry over into life dealings, including the work place. Given the overall beneficial experiences sport participation provides, it is unfair, from the teleological perspective, to provide men access to these benefits and not women. As indicated previously, such unfairness is not ethically tolerable from a consequentialist viewpoint, due to the disadvantages women might incur from unequal access to sporting opportunities. It is also, however, unethical from a deontological viewpoint, because this type of unfairness is not something one would morally wish to universally accept. If it is something that one would morally wish to accept, then men should also be willing to not gain participation opportunities, which does not at all seem to be the case. It appears, then, that the pursuit of **gender equity** in sport does indeed stand on solid moral foundations.

gender equity: the principle and practice of fair allocation of resources, programs, and decision making for both women and men.

Do Opportunities for Women to Participate in Athletics Make for a Better Society?

Making accommodations to allow females equal opportunities in sport certainly seems to contribute to the betterment of society as a whole. Although many of the benefits gained from sport might be able to be realized through other experiences, organized sport is a convenient means to do so because a large number of people have the opportunity to attend educational institutions with which sport teams are affiliated.

If women, as a result of sport experiences, are more prepared to meet the demands necessary to succeed in the work force, their professional successes will likely be an overall positive contribution to society. Additionally, as strides are made to achieve equality for all peoples, it stands to reason that as a result, people who move from a position of inequality to equality will become more satisfied and content, which makes for a more civil society. Therefore, from a utilitarian perspective, equal access to sporting opportunities is a desirable outcome that one should strive to attain in one's efforts to improve today's society. Recall, utilitarianism provides good and happiness not only to oneself but to as many others as possible.

"Unable to Work With a Corporate Team"

The year was 1971, one year before Title IX was passed into law as part of the Educational Amendments Act of 1972, which, in short, provided for equal opportunities for women in intercollegiate sport. Jan was pleased with her entire college career with one exception: not having had the opportunity to participate and compete on a women's volleyball team because one did not exist. Not one to dwell on the past, however, Jan eagerly anticipated her first professional job following graduation, a position with a major advertising firm. One of Jan's first assignments was to work with a team of seven other first-year employees to create an advertising strategy for a client. Her excitement for this task ended four days into the project, when her team members told her that she was uncooperative, unsupportive, and not working cohesively with them as part of a team. Shocked and somewhat bewildered by her team members' assessment, Jan began to question herself and even wonder if she should quit her job and seek employment elsewhere.

Questions

1. Had Jan been given the opportunity to participate in volleyball or another sport in college, do you believe her coworkers' assessment of her might have been different? Explain your answer.
2. What benefits might Jan have gained if she had had an opportunity to participate on sports teams during her college years?
3. Do you believe Jan would be considering quitting her job had she been provided with the opportunity to participate in sports throughout her college years? Explain your answer.

Unwillingness to Comply With Title IX

Unfortunately, despite positive changes brought about by Title IX, it has faced much opposition. Presented below are some examples of noncompliance, reasons for resistance, effects of legislation on attitudes, justification for noncompliance, and advocacy for changes in Title IX.

Examples of Noncompliance With Title IX

Even though enforcement exists, according to Reed, "the good ol' boys elevated foot dragging to an art form in regard to Title IX."[11(p7)] This is one reason that, more than three decades after Title IX became law, many universities and colleges still are not in compliance. In recent years, values held by those with an interest in men's sports have gained support. Reed further states that "There is no earthly reason Division I-A football programs cannot make do with 60 scholarships instead of 85 and reduce expenses for salaries as well as recruiting and travel."[11(p.7)]

Even though Title IX requires that efforts be made to make sport programs equitable between genders, many educational institutions still seem to fail to comply. For example, in 2005 it was reported that the University of Oregon agreed to pay $375,000 to settle a gender discrimination lawsuit filed by a former coach. Sally J. Harmon, who was an assistant track-and-field coach at the university for 18 years, alleged that she did not receive a fair opportunity to keep her job after Oregon merged its men's and women's track programs in 2003.[12]

Title IX mandates equity among genders in essentially all areas of athletics, including but not limited to the awarding of scholarships, practice times, facilities, equipment, and budgeting. Despite the law, for years after the inception of Title IX, women were still not being granted as many scholarships, were scheduled to practice during the least desirable times and on the least desirable fields or facilities, and were not provided equal overall dollars of support for their programs as were men. This noncompliance was unethical in that it was unjust; it created an environment of inequity in athletic departments. Athletic directors in departments that did not provide equitable opportunities for both females and males may have chosen to reason strategically and favor male athletes over female athletes as had been traditionally done in the past. In doing so, athletic directors may have failed to recognize the teleological moral values of justice, fairness, and even beneficence while arriving at decisions that pertained to participation opportunities.

In a case in Birmingham, Alabama, inequitable provision of resources, including equipment and budget, was the focus of a complaint issued by Roderick Jackson.[13] Jackson, a high school teacher and basketball coach for his girls' basketball team, complained to his supervisor in December of 2000 that the lack of adequate funding, equipment, and facilities made it difficult for him to do his job. He pointed out that the girls' team was not receiving equal treatment from the school district. Instead of responding to his complaint, the school began to give him negative evaluations and, in May 2001, took away Jackson's job as basketball coach. Supreme Court Justice Sandra Day O'Connor (as cited in Biskupic) made it clear that retaliation against a person because that person has complained of sex discrimination is another form of intentional sex discrimination.[13] O'Connor also said coaches such as Jackson are often in the best position to vindicate the rights of their students because they can see bias and bring it to the attention of administrators. In short, retaliation against someone who files a complaint of Title IX discrimination—because they file the complaint—is prohibited by Title IX.[13]

In bringing his case forward, Jackson used the moral value of fairness (inequity) as a way to obtain what he believed to be necessary funding, equipment, and facilities to do his job. One might use deontological moral theory to ask whether one would prefer to work under the same "resource-deficient" conditions under which Roderick appeared to be working.

In the past, athletic departments have chosen not to make efforts toward compliance until the threat of losing government financial support became real. Even then, efforts toward compliance often were not made willingly. For the most part, those in power made decisions that were perceived by women to be self-serving, unfair, and inequitable concerning female sporting opportunities. It was noted that many colleges and universities "slowly and grudgingly provided more equitable support for women's teams to avoid costly legal battles or negative publicity," and that "some complied under the threat of lawsuits alleging discrimination."[14(p187)] The noncompliance of male administrators created roadblocks to gender equity that allowed the traditional gender discrimination to continue within university athletic programs. Administrators often strategically reasoned to favor male athletes rather than attempting to distribute participation opportunities and available resources more equally between male and female athletes. In doing so, these male administrators chose to ignore the teleological moral values of justice and fairness and also failed to respect women's rights to quality sport experiences.

Reasons for Resistance to Title IX

Why might some men be angry about the mandates within Title IX that call for gender equity? The anger of some men might best be understood by realizing that requiring equitable opportunities for both genders in athletics has sometimes resulted in less opportunities for males in athletics than had been available in the past.[15] The perception held by many men may be that Title IX is unfair since it calls for administrative choices to be made that could result in the elimination of men's sport programs—programs such as football and wrestling that have a long standing tradition over the years. Progress toward equal opportunities for women has been met with anger by men who perceive Title IX as legislation against men's sports. The perception of some may be that Title IX is designed to unjustly punish male athletes, reducing both opportunities for male participation and the resources that had previously been available for the improvement of men's facilities and equipment. Even as recently as 2006, evidence indicates that men's programs, in fact, were being cut to meet the proportionality standard of Title IX. A decrease in men's teams and participation rates was not the idea behind Title IX. It was designed to create, not eliminate, opportunity. Since its enactment, however, more than 170 men's wrestling teams have been eliminated. Eighty men's tennis teams, 45 track teams, and 106 men's gymnastics teams have been cut.[16] From the utilitarian greatest happiness perspective, aside from gender, are a greater number of persons happy as a result of Title IX? On balance, are more persons happier with Title IX than were happy without it?

Intercollegiate wrestling has been one such sport that has suffered program eliminations as a result of Title IX. In October 2004, the court dismissed a lawsuit filed by

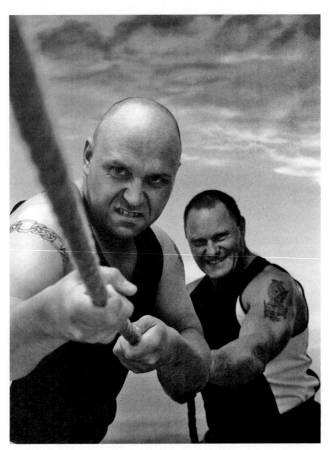

7-1 *Some males have angrily fought against universities that choose to eliminate men's sports programs to comply with Title IX.*

the wrestling coaches who had hoped to have the U.S. Department of Education's gender equity rules under Title IX declared unconstitutional. The court noted that Title IX was only one of the factors that induced colleges to drop sports, and that there was no proof that eliminating Title IX's policies would provide the relief sought by the plaintiffs. The National Women's Law Center (NWLC) filed an amicus brief in support of the Department of Education, arguing that the suit was improper because there was no guarantee that institutions would reinstate men's sports teams even if the Title IX regulations and policy were changed.[17]

Effects of Legislation on Attitudinal Changes

Can legislation change discriminatory attitudes toward a gender? Similar to racial discrimination, attitudes of gender discrimination that become part of a person at an early age seem quite difficult to overcome. As part of an effort to overcome gender discrimination, education and positive experiences may serve as two effective means of doing so. Discriminatory behaviors practiced by educational institutions (even if the behavior is subconsciously discriminatory and without malicious intent) reinforce the notion that discrimination is acceptable. Pointing out and calling for a change in such discriminatory practices may be met with strong resistance by those concerned that change will affect them negatively. Those who are faced with resistance to gender equity-related change might consider defending their position based on moral values grounded in teleology. A teleological-grounded argument might argue that the moral values of justice, respect, and fairness are lacking in athletic departments that do not offer equal opportunities for women. It is usually rare when all persons embrace change, but if more people support gender-equitable athletic departments, the change is supported from a utilitarianism perspective.

Attempting to legislate against tradition can also be met with strong resistance, which was the case when Title IX legislation was proposed to provide for equity among genders in athletic departments. If in fact, however, the legislation is equitable for both males and females, and if it is implemented fairly, then it will likely be accepted by inherently fair people. Individuals valuing fairness will recognize that certain equities may need to be mandated for a period of time in order to stifle the use of inequitable practices and improve conditions for those who have experienced discrimination. Many people in sport view Title IX's requirements as a way to provide equitable sporting opportunities for both genders.

Justifying Noncompliance

Those who might believe requirements of Title IX unfairly favor female athletes over male athletes might feel compelled to address what they perceive to be an inequity toward males. Such individuals may be inclined to simply not abide by Title IX or protest against it. Can one ethically justify not following a law?

The unwillingness to follow the law calls into question the ethics of those making the decision to not comply. Deontologically, one would have to decide if the law is able to be universalized in a fair manner to various groups—or in Title IX's case, to both genders. If a law truly does not provide the most good for the most people, a utilitarian position might support not following a law. Using teleology, an analysis of moral values might also be considered when deciding whether a law is morally sound. To this point, however, male athletes do not seem to be experiencing the difficulties female athletes faced before Title IX. Based on this analysis, not abiding by Title IX may not be morally justifiable at this time.

It might be contended that noncompliance would be an effective means to protest, especially if a large number of athletic departments share a fundamental disagreement with Title IX. But, one's personal views may conflict with those of the educational institution. If an individual is representing an educational institution and chooses to break rules—or, in this case a law—then, that college is in violation as well.

Should the individual at least consider the views of the educational institution before choosing to violate the legislation that is in place?

Furthermore, on what grounds might laws such as Title IX be questioned in that they come about through proper legislative channels? After all, the citizens' input is indirectly included through the fact that voting citizens elect officials based on their stance on issues such as gender equity. Since citizens have the ability to vote for politicians based on their stated positions on such issues, to what extent, is it ethically appropriate for citizens to question laws that were promulgated as part of a formal process? Should those who disagree with a law accept the notion that the newly developed law is best for society because it was formed by elected officials? And, should one assume a utilitarian stance by accepting that a law is in the best interests of society and will bring the most good to the most people because the law was put into place by officials who received support from the majority of voting citizens?

"The Angry Football Coach"

Coach Mann, head football coach for 27 years at Orange University, stormed into the university president's office, angry over the news that he would have to share practice times and the football field with the women's soccer team. "Are you aware that Ms. Ladi has told me that I have to share *my* football field with the women's soccer team for practice sessions as well as games, and that I have to alternate the best practice time of 3:00 to 5:00 with the women's soccer team?" The president shifted uncomfortably in his seat and replied, "Yes, I am aware of these changes. I issued this edict so that the university would be in compliance with Title IX." Coach Mann threw his hands up in the air in disgust before he turned and walked out of the president's office, muttering, "I cannot believe it. Even you have turned against me! Title IX is unfair and in protest of its unfairness to my team I am not going to abide by it."

Questions
1. List a few gender inequities that apparently have occurred at Orange University in the past.
2. In your opinion, what is at the root of Coach Mann's anger?
3. Is Coach Mann's method of protesting his perceived unfairness of Title IX appropriate? Explain your answer.

Advocating Change for a Greater Good

Others might choose to protest legislation with which they disagree by advocating changes to existing laws or new legislation that, in their view, would be more just. In other words, one might work within the existing structures of the legislative system to attempt to make changes. In doing so, one might have to convince legislators that society and athletic departments are worse with Title IX than without it—a daunting task given the perceived benefits that Title IX has provided for females. The onus of proof thus lies with Title IX's detractors; they, from a utilitarian perspective, must demonstrate that more good will come from the elimination of Title IX than from its continued implementation if it is to be justly overturned through the existing legislative process.

Three Tests of Gender Equity

To help determine whether schools were in compliance with Title IX, the United States Department of Education developed a three-pronged test for gender equity. The first and most noteworthy prong of this test is the **proportionality test.** To achieve proportionality, institutions are required to provide sporting opportunities for each gender at the respective rate of each gender's representation of undergraduate enrollment. Under the proportionality argument, the Department of Education considers the number of participation opportunities provided to athletes of both sexes. According to Feder,[17] generally, athletes who are listed on a team's squad or eligibility list at the beginning of the season are counted as participants. Next, the Department of Education determines whether these participation opportunities are substantially proportionate to the ratio of male and female students enrolled at the institution.[8] For example, if an institution has a 50% enrollment of males and a 50% enrollment of females, Title IX calls for sporting opportunities for each gender to also be at 50%. However, for reasons of flexibility, the Department of Education does not require exact proportionality.[17]

> **proportionality test:** a gender equity test within Title IX that requires athletic participation opportunities for males and females to be substantially proportionate to the undergraduate population of males and females; that is, if an undergraduate population of a college is 42% male and 58% female, to meet the proportionality test of Title IX and thus be compliant with Title IX, the athletic participation opportunities for males must be 42% and for females must be 58%.

Father of four and wrestling legend Dan Gable, who coached the University of Iowa to 15 NCAA Championships, believes Title IX should remain but that proportionality should go. Since 1990, more than 400 men's programs have been dropped.[18] Proportionality has been particularly destructive to programs at relatively low-budget NCAA D-II and D-III schools. Not opposed to the spirit of Title IX, Gable believes that if Title IX is to remain, the equity of its application should be improved to allow for fair opportunity for all participants, both male and female.[18]

Ethically, the spirit of the proportionality test of Title IX emphasizes fairness in sport offerings. It requires colleges and universities to equitably offer sports according to the male/female ratios of their student bodies. Using the moral value of fairness to argue for more equitable participation opportunities for females as compared with males has been effective.

Achieving Proportionality: Adding Women's and Dropping Men's Programs

Educational institutions have generally adopted two basic approaches to meeting the proportionality test: adding women's programs and eliminating men's programs.[16]

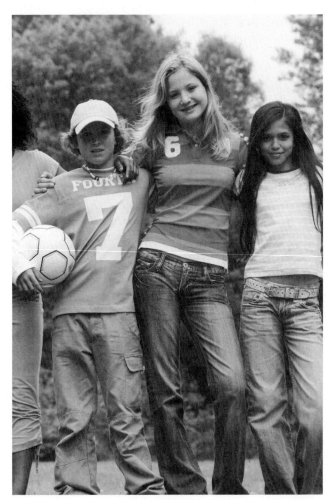

7-2 *Title IX requires schools receiving federal funds to give girls an equal chance as boys to play sports.*

Both adding women's and dropping men's sport programs are practices usually done to meet the proportionality standard of Title IX. Cutting men's sports and adding women's sports both lead to proportionality, but do both consider the short-term and long-term good of the athletes participating in intercollegiate athletics?

Whereas the overall good of adding women's programs seems apparent, the dropping of men's programs and reduction in participation opportunities for men has resulted in controversy. The elimination of non-revenue-generating men's teams is a choice that some athletic departments that chose to keep football as a sport within their departments have made. This trend has been a source of frustration among male administrators, coaches, and athletes, and has led some to blame Title IX for the elimination of men's teams. The Women's Sports Foundation contends that complying with Title IX should not result in the reduction of opportunities for male athletes to participate in varsity athletics. At most institutions, however, there is no incentive system in place to encourage maintaining sports opportunities for men.[19]

Might the approach of cutting men's sports to meet equal participation opportunities be a form of reverse gender discrimination that Title IX has brought on, because it sometimes results in a reduction of participation opportunities for men? Is the approach of cutting men's teams ethically sound, because it involves taking opportunities away from men? Is it fair and should fairness be strictly based on equal numbers, or should the history of sport offerings be considered? For example, James Madison University recently cut the most teams ever in a single episode. In July of 2007, James Madison eliminated seven men's programs and three women's programs. The men's programs included archery, cross country, gymnastics, indoor track, outdoor track, swimming, and wrestling, while the women's programs included archery, gymnastics, and fencing. In total, 144 athletes and 11 coaches were cut. According to Jim McCarthy, spokesman for the college sports council, there are 1,200 more women's teams in the NCAA than men's, yet that is not good enough as Title IX mandates the same number of athletes.[20]

Decisions to Add or Cut Driven by Money

Money could be a reason cited for cutting men's athletic teams. Schools operate under a budget appropriated for athletics; thus, administrators can be hard pressed to find funding for the offering of a new sport when it is difficult enough to continue to fund already existing lines such as equipment, travel, and recruiting. Thus, when faced with the choice of achieving guaranteed Title IX compliance by cutting non-revenue-producing men's teams, or keeping all the men's teams and adding women's teams, administrators might strategically choose to cut non-revenue men's teams because it may be in the department's financial best interest. Hence, strategic reasoning dictates that, when faced with the issue of Title IX compliance, administrators should save time, energy, and money and cut men's sports rather than investing valuable and limited resources into the task of adding new women's sports to their programs.

Meeting Title IX requirements in this manner may be legally and economically sound, but it may not be morally sound. Administrators who choose to reach proportionality by cutting men's programs are not necessarily meeting the athletic interests of women on their campus or in their region and are taking participation opportunities away from male athletes who wish to compete. In fact, in a 2005 *Congressional Research Service Report for Congress*, among the unanimous recommendations of the Commission were suggestions that the Department of Education clarify that cutting teams to achieve compliance is a disfavored practice. Furthermore, these administrators might be ignoring the fact that they could save men's programs and/or fund new women's programs by curtailing spending and not overspending on revenue-producing teams that may be using more money than needed to operate. From a teleological viewpoint, the administrators would recognize their moral responsibility to treat all teams fairly, whether they are men's or women's teams or revenue- or non-revenue-producing teams. By acting on this responsibility and by being more frugal and making a conscious effort to meet the needs of the underrepresented gender, administrators might be able to achieve Title IX compliance in a more morally responsible manner.

Moral responsibility might require administrators to commit time, energy, and money to the task of adding sports. This commitment, however, will be in the name of fairness and will demonstrate the seriousness with which the university and its administrators treat the interests of their students. The efforts on behalf of the athletes should be viewed as a show of respect for them and their interests, and as an indicator of the moral integrity of the school and its athletic program.

It is important to be aware that compliance can be achieved in other ways besides proportionality. Given the somewhat flexible approaches to achieving Title IX, athletic and school administrators are not forced to cut men's programs in order to meet Title IX requirements.

Demonstration of Progress and Meeting Underrepresented Interests

Satisfying the Department of Education's proportionality test is not the only way for programs to achieve Title IX compliance. The test provides two other possible means by which institutions can attain compliance: (a) by demonstrating that they historically have made and are continuing to make inroads toward proportionality, or (b) by providing evidence that they are meeting the athletic interests of the underrepresented sex with the current program in place.[2]

In other words, if an athletic department can demonstrate that women on a college campus do not wish to participate in sports, then the athletic department is not required to offer sports at an equitable rate for women as they have for men. By meeting one of these final two tests, the university athletic programs still demonstrate an acceptable level of commitment to gender equity and are adhering to a level of fairness while still not meeting the proportionality test.

Even though there are two additional ways in which educational institutions can achieve compliance with Title IX, athletic departments have generally relied on test #1, the proportionality prong, instead of test #2.[21] Test #2 calls for athletic departments to show a history and continuing practice of program expansion to meet the needs, interests, and abilities of a member of the underrepresented sex.[21]

In 2004, in response to a federal lawsuit filed by seven members of Baylor University's women's crew team, Baylor claimed they were Title IX compliant based on a 5-year upgrade plan to achieve gender equity. The crew team, however, contended that as a team they were victims of federal Title IX violations, saying they had no scholarships, school uniforms, or paid coaches and not enough oars and boats. The team stated that they wanted to be upgraded from club to varsity status, which would make them an intercollegiate sport. If Baylor's 5-year upgrade plan demonstrated a history and continuing practice of the expansion of programs responsive to the underrepresented sex, they would, in fact, have met the compliance criteria of test two, even though their ratio of male and female athletes participating in sport when compared with the undergraduate student body was not proportionate.

Test three of Title IX calls for the interests of the underrepresented sex to be accommodated and is illustrated in a summary of a case[17] in which female athletes at Brown University sued Brown after the school, for cost-cutting purposes, eliminated two women's sports and two men's sports. The two male teams were golf and water polo, and the two female teams were gymnastics and volleyball. The cuts made far larger reductions in the women's athletic budget than in the men's. Additionally, the cuts did not affect the ratio of male to female athletes, which remained roughly 63% male to 37% female, despite a student body that was approximately 52% male and 48% female.[17] The court focused its inquiry on whether Brown had met part three of the test, which calls for the accommodation of the interests of the underrepresented sex, which in this instance was the women. In the end, the court ruled that the existence and success of women's gymnastics and volleyball at Brown demonstrated that there was sufficient interest and expectation of competition in those sports to rule in favor of the female athletes with regard to test three of Title IX.[17]

Can one infer from this ruling that if the undergraduate population of one sex outnumbers that of the other, then any sport of the underrepresented sex cannot be eliminated? Is this fair under all circumstances, or should exceptions be made to provide for optimal fairness and participation opportunities for both sexes?

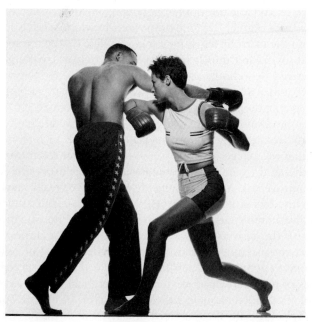

7-3 *The intent of Title IX is to provide fair participation opportunities for both males and females, not to pit one sex against the other.*

Further difficulties arise from the fact that it is difficult to gauge (a) the interest of the student body of an institution, and (b) the relevant population of individuals who should be accounted for in this process. Should school administrators and athletic directors only consider the athletic needs of current students, or should they also consider the interests of prospective students from local high schools and junior and community colleges that are major feeders of the university? From a utilitarianism perspective, are long-term best interests of both sexes taken into consideration or just the short-term interest in participating in a sport? Given the above questions and challenges, is it fair and just to place the blame for the elimination of men's teams on the spirit of Title IX legislation, or are problems related to its implementation primarily responsible for men's teams being cut?

Assessing Athletic Interests Through an Online Survey

Generally, meeting the athletic interests of women seems to be less recognized by the courts than meeting the proportionality standard. This may be changing, though. Currently, a strong push is being initiated to make acceptable a standardized online survey for the purpose of determining whether undergraduate women are interested in having additional participation opportunities in sport.

Based on recommendations from a George W. Bush-appointed Title IX Commission, the Department of Education issued new guidance in 2005 that clarified Title IX policy and the use of part three of the Title IX compliance test.[17] Again, test three calls for the interests and abilities of the underrepresented sex to be fully accommodated. The new guidance clarifies that one of the ways in which schools may demonstrate compliance with the interests test is by using an online survey to establish that the underrepresented sex has no unmet interests in athletic participation. Such a survey must be administered periodically to all students who are members of the underrepresented sex, and students must be informed that a failure to respond to the survey will be viewed as an indication of a lack of interest. Also pointed out was the fact that the survey must be administered in a way designed to generate high response rates.[17]

If the results show that women do not have an interest in additional sporting opportunities, colleges will not be required to offer them. More specifically, it should be noted that the validity and administrative procedures of this online survey are somewhat controversial. Are the results of such a survey really an accurate indicator of the athletic interests of female students? Will enough female students respond to the survey to give administrators a good understanding of the athletic interests of women on campus? If the answers to these questions are no, the fairness of using online surveys to determine the athletic needs of female students must be called into question.

From a deontological perspective, would it also be acceptable to determine the interests of male participation interests through an online survey? If so, then through deontological moral reasoning, the online survey for women could be viewed as appropriate. Teleologically, the questions of fairness in terms of how the survey is administrated and whether it is an accurate indicator of women's interests in having a sport offered must be examined. Using the utilitarianism form of consequentialism, the question as to whether the online survey will meet the best interests of not only female athletes but also male athletes, administrators, the college or university, and even the fans should be taken into account.

"Ms. Dally's Proportionality Predicament"

It has been revealed that City University is not in compliance with Title IX. The athletic director, Ms. Dally, has been aware for years that the men's sports teams outnumber the women's teams 11 to 7. As a result, when comparing male and female participation opportunities, males have a disproportionately greater opportunity. Making matters worse is the fact that the undergraduate population at City University is made up of 67% females and 33% males. The news of City University's noncompliance status has spread rapidly, eliciting phone calls from affluent alumni who are threatening to withhold any further donations to the athletic department if any men's sports are eliminated. Adding to her dilemma, City University's financial director phoned Ms. Dally to make it clear that because the university is operating at a deficit, there is no money available to fund even one new women's sports team. The unfortunate yet inevitable reality of the situation has Ms. Dally in a quandary. She is faced with the dilemma of (*a*) confronting the bitter controversy that clearly will erupt if she eliminates any of the men's sports, or (*b*) tackling the seemingly impossible challenge of adding women's sports amidst an on-going budget crisis.

Just when Ms. Dally thought she was out of options, a wrestling coach she had worked with several years ago called her and explained that she might have another option if she could prove, through an online survey, that women at City University were not interested in more sport opportunities.

Questions
1. If you were Ms. Dally, would you attempt to comply with Title IX by meeting proportionality requirements? If so, how would this provide for a more gender equitable athletic department?
2. Compare and contrast, from an equity perspective, the dropping of men's sports to the adding of women's sports as options for Ms. Dally to meet the proportionality test of Title IX.
3. If you were Ms. Dally, as a means to demonstrate that the undergraduate women were not interested in additional sporting opportunities, would you distribute the online survey to all the female students at the university?

Exemption for Revenue-Generating Sports

Part of the debate over Title IX relates to whether certain revenue-generating sports should be exempt from this law. Arguments for both sides of this issue are presented below.

Support for the Exemption of Revenue Sports Through Proportionality

After reading some of the previous points, some might ask whether sports that generate revenue should be exempt from the proportionality formula? It might be argued that revenue-generating sports such as football and men's basketball are able to finance themselves and, hence, should not be included in the proportionality formula. For example, if a college football team is financially self-sufficient, should the total number of football players be included in the proportionality formula? Football when compared with other sports is represented by a disproportionately large number of players and thus, institutions may have to decide whether to keep football and add additional women's sports, or eliminate football and not add additional women's sports. For this reason, some might argue that it is unjust that athletic programs must include football teams in their proportionality calculations, and that revenue-producing sports should be excluded from such calculations for the sake of fairness. From an altruistic perspective, revenue-producing sports might consider giving some of their money to non-revenue-producing sports to allow them to operate.

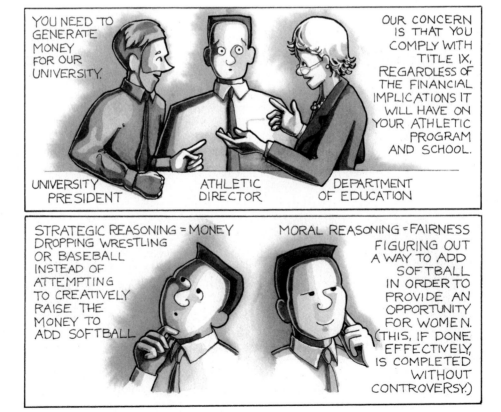

Interesting to note is that in 1975, Senator John Tower, D-Texas, reintroduced an amendment that he had introduced a year earlier that would exempt football from Title IX.[3] The amendment failed both times.

Opposition to the Exemption of Revenue Sports Through Proportionality

On the other hand, one could argue against allowing a financially self-sufficient football program to be exempt from the proportionality test of Title IX. Just because a sport generates revenue does not seem to be a valid moral reason to not provide an equal number of opportunities for women's sports programs; in fact, it appears to be a strategic reason that administrators might use to reduce or eliminate the challenges presented by Title IX. However, administrators might argue that any sport that generates revenue is helpful to the pursuit of not only equality, but also additional sporting opportunities since that revenue can be used for additional sports or to enhance the quality of the sports presently being offered. Increasing the number of sports should satisfy the utilitarian argument because more people will gain satisfaction/happiness from sport participation.

"Coach Grappler Fights to Keep Wrestling"

Balance College is in the midst of deciding how to comply with the proportionality requirement of Title IX. Coach Grappler, the head wrestling coach, is angered by the fact that his wrestling program must be included in the proportionality formula that determines the athletic department's compliance with Title IX. Coach Grappler recently pleaded his case to the athletic director by explaining that his wrestling program is financially self-sufficient through gate receipts, broadcast revenues, and fundraising efforts and, therefore, should not be required to be counted "against" the men's programs when determining proportionality, which is based on the percentage of undergraduate men and women at Balance College.

Upon learning of Coach Grappler's meeting with the athletic director, Mrs. Bennis, a physical education teacher at the college and tennis enthusiast, was outraged. Over the years, Mrs. Bennis has passionately attempted to begin a women's tennis program but has always been told that its startup and annual expenses would be too high. Mrs. Bennis scheduled her own meeting with the athletic director and explained that proportionality is fair in that it allows women the opportunity to engage in sports. She argues that proportionality is the best thing that ever happened to athletic departments because it truly provides for fair and equal participation opportunities for both women and men. Mrs. Bennis goes on to say that even though courses in higher education do not generate revenue or break even financially, they

"Coach Grappler Fights to Keep Wrestling" (*Continued*)

are not eliminated from the curriculum of academic programs. In applying this academic analogy, she states, "It makes no sense to consider exempting revenue-generating sports from the proportionality formula."

Questions
1. If you were the athletic director in a position to make a persuasive argument to the NCAA, what position would you assume concerning the exemption of revenue-generating sports from Title IX's proportionality formula? Why?
2. As the athletic director, differentiate between the issues involved in creating environments equitable to genders in athletic departments versus those in academic environments.
3. Do you agree, based on Mrs. Bennis' academic analogy, that revenue-generating sports should not be exempt from Title IX's proportionality formula? Why or why not?

Approaches and Insights in Gender Equity

Title IX legislation aside, what is the equitable approach regarding male and female sport participation opportunities? When attempting to determine what is fair and equitable, insights might be gained from examining how the needs of both females and males are met in departments other than athletics. Additional gender equity insights might be gained from examining the following three areas related to educational institutions: academics, finances, and tradition. By studying these areas and emphasizing moral rather than strategic reasoning, administrators may be able to identify and minimize or eliminate inequitable practices that maintain conditions of gender discrimination and develop improved approaches to balancing men's and women's sport participation opportunities.

Academics and Gender Equity in Other Departments

One might take an interest in how gender equity is reached in other departments or programs, such as academics and campus recreation. In academics, classes are offered equally to both males and females. Some classes may happen to draw more males than females and vice versa; however, the opportunity to enroll and attend classes is presented equally to both genders.

How is it determined whether to offer an academic course, program, or major? Certainly, market demand is an influential factor. The same is essentially true for campus recreation departments. Sports are often offered on a student demand basis. For example, if students, irrespective of gender, show an interest in participating in a particular intramural sport, campus recreation departments will usually consider offering that sport. Why should athletic departments view gender equity differently? It would seem that considering student demand as a way of meeting the needs and wants of both males and females in athletic departments would also be fair and equitable to both genders. Through the accommodation of students' athletic interests, universities demonstrate respect for the wants and needs of their students, providing them with participation opportunities that will help them better develop the skills they will need to succeed within society. In this way, universities act in accordance with utilitarianism, helping to provide for the greater good of society by preparing students more thoroughly for their lives after college.

A major and obvious difference between academic programs and sports programs is that athletic teams are separated by gender: women compete with and against women, and men compete with and against men. In most cases, academic courses, unlike sports teams, are integrated with both men and women. More women or men may enroll in a particular class, but the opportunity for each gender to enroll in the same class together is equal. If a physics class does not draw any women, that class, nevertheless, remains available for women who may choose to enroll. Using this model, and if the structure of academics is perceived to be equitable for both genders, the offering of sports for women that may not draw as well as men's sports, seems to be an equitable approach.

It would help to accommodate the interests of a greater number of female athletes and provide them with greater freedom of choice with regards to their sport participation. Thus, an academic model to sport offerings would be a fair and equitable approach for women athletes that would protect them from discriminatory practices that might accompany other approaches.

Education

When using education as the basis for athletic department decisions regarding sport offerings, educational institutions might view participation in athletics as an endeavor that provides educational outcomes for the participants. Mission statements normally focus on education for all, as opposed to education in disproportionate amounts favoring a race, sex, or group. Based on a typical mission statement, students, regardless of their sex, have equal opportunities and accommodations for education. Because the mission of educational institutions is often centered on education for all, athletics is in a convenient position to offer sport opportunities for all, which includes both females and males. An educational approach to sport offerings would be one that emphasizes the benefits that both men and women can gain from sport. It would be one that recognizes that sport has equal value for males and females and, thus, should be equally available to both groups. Thus, the educational approach might give administrators a more gender equitable way of deciding which sports to offer at their schools.

When using educational outcomes as the determining factor to decide which sports to offer, the financial feasibility of a sport and traditions within an athletic department might be considered but are not the absolute driving forces behind program offerings. Providing educational opportunities through sport for all persons, irrespective of discriminating factors such as sex, is the primary criterion when deciding which sports to offer and to whom. Using education as the premise for sport offerings should provide for equal and fair opportunities for both females and males, and supports a utilitarian mindset by bringing the most good to the greatest number of people under the circumstances.

Finances

The financial argument considers which sports programs are offered based on the cost effectiveness of each program. Programs are offered if they generate money or if they are not excessively costly and are affordable within the athletic department budget. When using finances as the factor in deciding whether to offer a particular sport, sports that are not very expensive to operate are often selected to be a part of the athletic program. Less costly sports generate revenue through tuition money from students who choose to attend a school, in part, because of the opportunity to participate in a sport. When basing sport program offerings on finances, traditions and gender equity are usually not considered. Instead, strategic reasoning is used so that the goal of making greater profits can be achieved.

When comparing academics with athletics, the fact that teams are separated by gender may have financial implications. With the previously mentioned physics class example, enough students overall, regardless of sex, may be enrolled in the class to make it financially feasible, because the class can draw from the entire student body. On the other hand, because sports teams are of the same sex, men's teams are composed of only men and women's teams are composed of only women. The probability of certain sports teams not attracting a full roster might be more likely than academic courses not filling, because the pools that sports teams can draw from are reduced, due to the fact that they are gender specific. Speaking strictly from a financial perspective, if a men's or women's athletic team does not draw enough participants, it may not be a financially prudent undertaking.

Because athletic teams are separated by sex, the notion that money being spent for a team without a full roster might better be spent to provide opportunities in other areas for that gender is one worthy of consideration. A utilitarian administrator will want to accommodate the athletic interests of the most individuals, and a teleological administrator will want to be fair to all students. However, it must be recognized that if a team does not have enough participants, it may be better for athletes to choose to participate in another sport or to transfer to a school where their sport is in greater demand. Athletes who make these choices may have better and happier sport experiences than they would have if they had been on an underrepresented team.

▸ **"The Two-Person Women's Golf Team"**

Slimborough University's athletic department has created a women's golf team as part of an effort to meet the proportionality test of Title IX, but only two females are interested in playing. Even though there are only two participants, the women's golf budget is the same as the men's golf budget, which includes money for such items as travel, equipment, coaches salaries, and the rental of golf facilities for practices and matches.

Questions
1. Is Slimborough University being unfair to another potential men's or women's sport that might draw more than two participants?
2. Even though the proportionality test is now being met by offering a women's golf team, is this offering in the best interests of males and/or females? If not, is there a better solution?

Is there a connection between sports teams that win and the generation of revenue? Teams that win usually draw more paying fans, receive donations from boosters, and, at major college levels, receive financially lucrative television contracts and revenue for post-season play. Winning, as well as quality play and heightened competition, seems to increase the popularity of the sport as well as the probability of winning and generating revenue. One might consider the years of emphasis, marketing, and overall support of men's athletics that have allowed men's sports to be the foundational stronghold of athletic departments. Is it fair, though, to use revenue generation as the sole criterion when deciding whether men's or women's sports are going to be a part of an athletic program? To what extent does it meet the greatest happiness principle of Mill's utilitarianism?

Given the historical emphasis on men's sports, it should not be surprising that some of men's sports teams are more profitable than women's programs at this point in time. If finances are the sole criterion used to determine the sport offerings of an institution, then men's programs will continue to be favored over women's to the extent that the men's programs remain more profitable than the women's. Thus, an emphasis on finances alone may lead to an unfair bias against increasing sport participation opportunities for women.

Tradition

If tradition is the criterion used to determine whether a sport should be offered, only those programs offered in the past would be offered in the future. Sports that have been a part of the athletic program in the past would continue to be part of the athletic program's present and future simply because they have historically been a part of the program. And, if tradition is the basis for the offering of intercollegiate men's or women's sports, women's sports offerings would be fewer than men's because fewer female sports have been offered in the past. Using tradition as the basis for offering programs would not allow for new programs, and hence, the offerings of women's programs would stay the same instead of increasing to the same numbers as men's.

The sole use of tradition as the determining factor in deciding which sports to offer does not allow for a genuine analysis of what is fair (teleology) and in the best interest (utilitarianism) of both female and male participants. When using tradition as the basis for deciding which sports to offer, the financial feasibility of the sport and educational benefits to the participants are not considered. Using a tradition-based approach to offering sports programs is not necessarily an approach that incorporates moral reasoning into the process and may not be the best approach when attempting to reach an equitable solution to gender issues in athletic departments. Traditionally, male athletes and administrators dominated intercollegiate athletics. If athletic programs are to move toward gender equity and away from the gender discrimination that has traditionally been a part of college sport, administrators should emphasize something other than tradition in deciding how to distribute sporting opportunities equitably.

Gender Equity

Why, prior to Title IX, did most athletic departments choose to base sports program offerings on finances or tradition and not include equality between genders? The long-standing history of what is perceived today as gender discrimination may partly speak to such previous behaviors of athletic departments. Presently, because of Title IX legislation, athletic departments must provide equal opportunities for women unless they want to risk losing federal aid.

How should schools and their athletic programs decide which sports they should offer and during what season? One case that might provide athletic directors insight regarding this matter included two fathers who brought a lawsuit on behalf of each of their daughters, who at the time were freshman athletes in the New York State Public School System. The two girls who were part of the lawsuit played on a soccer team that had its season in the spring. At the same school, the boys' soccer team played their season in the fall. The fall season allowed the boys to participate in regional and state championships, whereas the spring season did not provide the girls with the same opportunity. The girls claimed, based on Title IX, that their season should be switched from the spring to the fall so they would have the same chance to compete for regional and state championships as the boys' team.

From a consequentialist perspective, a balance of opportunities needs to be established and maintained so that the needs of the most people—both men and women— can be met. Aside from this balance, teleologists might suggest that administrators focus on fairness not only in terms of achieving equity, but in terms of providing participation opportunities that meet the interest and skill level of their student bodies. In the end, if an equitable balance is achieved and the participation needs of athletes are being met, then administrators will have acted in a good way, morally, under the given circumstances.

Looking Beyond Tradition and Revenue Generation to Achieve Equity

The solution to providing equal opportunities seems, on the surface, to be as simple as doing just that: providing equal opportunities. As discussed previously, "tradition" does not necessarily equate to fairness and equity. And, as necessary as finances can be to the successful implementation of programs, if the revenue generation of programs is the criterion driving the decisions related to sport offerings in athletic departments, the decisions are strategic gains and not moral gains.

An initial plan might be created that provides for equal opportunities for both females and males to gain educationally related benefits through sport experiences. From a moral perspective, to provide genuinely fair and equal opportunities, tradition and finance might be secondary considerations instead of the driving forces behind decisions. Once a morally sound plan is developed, based on the provision of equal educational opportunities through sport experiences, the finances obviously must be addressed but should not be the primary influencing factor behind sport offerings. Again, if equity and morality are the issues, the driving force behind the sport offerings should be the goal of providing equal educational opportunities through sport offerings for both females and males.

Given that Title IX is a law, it may be effectively used as leverage to provide for a gender equitable environment in athletic departments. Title IX has already increased participation opportunities for women in interscholastic and intercollegiate athletics. Providing opportunities for females equal to those of males has and will continue to be met with resistance on some fronts by those who have reaped benefits of past traditions that may not have been fair by standards outlined in Title IX. Given these resistances, administrators may have to choose between tradition and finances as opposed to actions they may believe to be supported through moral theory.

"Shocking Recommendations From the Title IX Consultant"

Not being completely familiar with the requirements of Title IX, the athletic director at Rounders College has hired a Title IX expert for the purpose of making recommendations helpful to Rounders College's pursuit of achieving compliance with Title IX. After a thorough review of the athletic department, the consultant recommends eliminating baseball as a way to comply with Title IX. Astonished, the athletic director replies, "I cannot believe I hired you to come up with such a drastic recommendation. With the support of our community here in Rounders, I have been running our athletic department effectively, without change, since I came here in 1963. There is no way we can eliminate baseball. Baseball provides a national visibility for our college that no other sport can replace. Our team has a long-standing reputation throughout the country as a winner, which has proven helpful for student recruitment. Eliminating baseball would cause our enrollment to drop, resulting in a financially stressed environment for the entire college. Aside from all of this, it is simply not fair to our boys

"Shocking Recommendations From the Title IX Consultant" (*Continued*)

on the baseball team. We promised them four years of baseball and you are recommending that we break that promise. I have never been one to go back on my word. Finally, I enjoy the personal recommendations I get from the community as the person who has one of the best baseball teams in the nation."

Questions

1. If you were the athletic director, would you follow the consultant's recommendation to drop baseball? Why or why not?
2. In what way would tradition influence your decision?
3. As athletic director, in what ways do you see money, ego, and national exposure affecting your decision regarding the elimination of baseball?
4. Identify basic arguments for and against Title IX implementation using this case study.

Conclusion

Title IX has played an important role in shaping the sport landscape in the United States during the last part of the 20th century and the beginning years of the 21st century. Although its future is uncertain, the increased participation opportunities resulting from Title IX are undeniable. Debate will continue over how Title IX should be implemented and the role it should play, if any, in school-based athletic departments.

As the dialogue continues regarding this important piece of legislation, those for and against it need to recognize the strengths and weaknesses of Title IX and decide what needs to be done from a moral standpoint in relation to it. Working together, the sporting community should be able to devise ways, based on moral theory, to achieve equity and offer appropriate sporting opportunities to all who want them.

References

1. U.S. Department of Labor. Title IX, Education Amendments of 1972. U.S. Department of Labor web site. Available at: http://www.dol.gov/oasam/regs/statutes/titleix.htm. Accessed May 22, 2007.
2. U.S. Department of Education. Clarification of Intercollegiate Athletics Policy Guidance: The Three-Part Test; January 16, 1996. U.S. Department of Education web site. Available at: http://www.ed.gov/about/offices/list/ocr/docs/clarific.html#two. Accessed May 22, 2007.
3. Title IX at 30: Still under fire; June 19, 2002. *USA Today* web site. Available at: http://www.usatoday.com/sports/college/stories/2002-06-19-title-ix-focus.htm#more. Accessed May 19, 2007.

4. U.S. Supreme Court. *Grove City College v Bell*, 465 US 555 (1984). *FindLaw.com* web site. Available at: http://laws.findlaw.com/us/465/555.html. Accessed May 23, 2007.

5. Gender equity/Title IX: Important facts. NCAA web site. Available at: http://www1. ncaa.org/membership/ed_outreach/gender_equity/general_info/facts.html. Accessed May 23, 2007.

6. Acosta RV, Carpenter LJ. *Women In Intercollegiate Sport: A Longitudinal, National Study: Twenty-Seven Year Update 1977–2004.* Women's Sports Foundation Web site. Available at: http://www.womenssportsfoundation.org/cgi-bin/iowa/issues/part/article.html?record= 906. Accessed April 17, 2008.

7. French PA. *Ethics and College Sports: Ethics, Sports, and the University.* Lanham, MD: Rowman & Littlefield Publishers; 2004.

8. American Alliance for Health, Physical Education, Recreation & Dance. Women in intercollegiate sport—A longitudinal, national study twenty-nine year update 1977–2006. AAHPERD web site. Available at: http://www.aahperd.org/NAGWS/pdf_files/logitudinal29.pdf. Accessed May 20, 2007.

9. National Collegiate Athletic Association. *1981–82—2003–04 Sport Sponsorship and Participation Report.* Indianapolis, IN: National Collegiate Athletic Association; December, 2004.

10. Women's Sports Foundation. Benefits—Why sports participation for girls and women: The Foundation position; August 14, 2000. Women's Sports Foundation web site. Available at: http://www.womenssportsfoundation.org/cgi-bin/iowa/issues/body/article.html?record= 577. Accessed May 19, 2007.

11. Reed B. Fault football and foot dragging, not females. *The Sporting News.* February 17, 2003;227(7):7.

12. Wolverton B. U. of Oregon settles gender-bias case. *The Chronicle of Higher Education.* July 22, 2005:A25.

13. Biskupic J. Supreme Court says Title IX protects whistleblowers. *USA Today.* March 30, 2005:A1.

14. Lumpkin A, Stoll SK, Beller JM. *Sport Ethics: Applications for Fair Play.* 3rd ed. Boston, MA: McGraw-Hill; 2003.

15. Brady E. Time fails to lessen Title IX furor; June 19, 2002. *USA Today* web site. Available at: http://www.usatoday.com/sports/college/stories/2002-06-19-title-ix-cover.htm. Accessed May 22, 2007.

16. Gender inequality: Title IX was necessary then, but now it's just unfair; October 10, 2006. *Sports Illustrated/CNN* web site. Available at: http://sportsillustrated.cnn.com/2006/writers/em_swift/10/10/title.ix/. Accessed May 22, 2007.

17. Feder J. *Title IX, Sex Discrimination, and Intercollegiate Athletics: A Legal Overview.* (Order Code RL31709). Congressional Research Service Web site. Available at: http:// www.house.gov/larson/titleix.htm. Accessed April 18, 2008.

18. Gable D. What to do with Title IX. *The Sporting News.* 2003;227(7):7.

19. Dropping men's sports—Expanding opportunities for girls and women in sport without eliminating men's sports: The Foundation position; July 23, 2000. *Women's Sports Foundation* web site. Available at: http://www.womenssportsfoundation.org/cgi-bin/iowa/issues/rights/article.html?record=84. Accessed May 19, 2007.

20. Nearman S. Title IX enforcement hits James Madison hard; October 29, 2006. *Washington Times* web site. Available at: http://washingtontimes.com/sports/20061028-115416-7089r.htm. Accessed May 22, 2007.

21. Schachter R. Title IX turns 35. *University Business.* March 2007;10(3):44–50.

Coed Wrestling

Debra, a junior at Osprey High School (OHS), wanted to try out for the men's wrestling team. Although this idea did not sit well with many of the guys on the team, Coach Roy knew he had to let her try out because OHS had no women's wrestling program. He also knew that Debra was a hard worker and a capable wrestler who could handle herself well against male opponents. At first things were very difficult for Debra. The boys on the team had never dealt with a situation of this kind before. They blamed Debra for taking a roster spot that they felt should have gone to Chris, a hard-working young man who barely made the team the previous year. None of the boys wanted to wrestle Debra in practice; they were afraid that if they lost to her, they would be ridiculed by their teammates and by the other students once word got out.

As practices continued, Coach Roy was pleased with the makeup of his team. The only problem spot appeared to be at the lightest weight class. Coach Roy decided that this was the class in which Debra might be able to win consistently. The problem with this strategy was that, for her to make weight for that class, Debra would have to lose 10 pounds. Coach Roy met with Debra and told her of his plan and that she had to drop 10 pounds as soon as possible, but gave her no further guidance. Debra had difficulty losing the weight, but managed to do so by eating and drinking very little.

The day of wrestle-offs for the first match arrived, and Debra was to wrestle her teammate Mike for the right to wrestle at the lightest class against Gull High School. To throw her off, Mike decided to grab her in inappropriate ways early in their match. Coach Roy saw this but chose not to address it to see how Debra would respond to the situation. Debra became angry and frustrated, but with increased intensity, she proceeded to win point after point against Mike and defeated him handily. After the match, Coach Roy said nothing to Mike about his unsportsmanlike behavior on the mat, but he quietly pulled him aside to let him know how disappointed he was that he "let a girl beat him." Coach Roy hoped this would make Mike more determined for the next wrestle-off the following week. Mike's teammates were not as quiet as their coach. They razzed Mike mercilessly, making him feel like a fool.

As he sat at home that night thinking about the upcoming match against Gull High, Coach Roy could not help but be concerned for Debra. Would the Gull wrestler use dirty tactics against her like Mike did? Debra was wondering the same thing. She believed Mike had harassed her on the mat that day. She was not sure if Coach Roy could see Mike's inappropriate grabs and she did not want to report Mike to the coach or anyone else for fear of being labeled a complainer or a snitch. She decided to speak to her parents about what happened that day and seek their advice on what to do.

Critical Thinking: Finding Common-Sense Solutions

1. What information should coaches provide to athletes when requesting that they lose weight? Develop a step-by-step action plan to follow in such instances.

2. Should Coach Roy have addressed Mike's unsportsmanlike behavior at the time it occurred? If so, how should he have addressed the problem?

3. Should Coach Roy have tolerated the other wrestlers razzing Mike? Explain why or why not. If not, describe in detail how you believe the coach should have handled this situation.

4. If you were Debra's parents, would you advise her to speak to Coach Roy, the athletic director, or another school official about Mike's harassing behavior? Explain your answer.

Critical Thinking: Moral Theory-Based Decision Making

5. Under what conditions should female and male wrestlers be allowed to compete against one another? Use moral values and principles to justify your reasoning.

6. Using *consequential moral theory* to guide your reasoning, determine whether it was morally good for Coach Roy to speak to Mike in the manner that he did after he lost to Debra.

7. Explain why it is important for Mike's teammates to emphasize the moral values of compassion and loyalty in dealing with him after his loss to Debra. Explain why it is important for them to emphasize these same values in regards to Debra.

Hiring Quotas at Olive University

This year, Olive University has a coaching vacancy for their National Collegiate Athletic Association's Division I women's volleyball team. They are seeking a person with 4 to 6 years of successful collegiate coaching experience, preferably at the Division I level. The successful candidate's responsibilities will include the development and implementation of a training and practice schedule; recruitment and graduation of scholar athletes; scheduling of non-conference opponents; supervision of their assistant coaching staff; and promotion of their team in a way that reflects positively on Olive University. The previous coach, Coach Sunshine, has decided to retire and move out of the state after 10 consecutive winning seasons.

Male coaches have dominated Olive University's athletic teams since Olive opened its doors in 1928. This year is no different; Olive's athletic department consists of eight women's sports and six men's sports. And, of the 14 head coaching positions, women fill only two of those positions. Even though Olive is an equal opportunity employer, their athletic department has not succeeded in hiring female head coaches at a rate equal to the hiring of men's head coaches. Dr. Jake, the athletic director at Olive University, has been instructed by the president to hire a woman for this head volleyball coaching position. Out of the 30 qualified candidates who have applied, only five were women. After a committee meeting, the pool of candidates was narrowed down to the 10 most qualified, five of whom were women. All 10 candidates were contacted for a phone interview. After the phone interviews, five candidates were invited for formal on-campus interviews; three were women and two were men.

Contradictory to the desires of Olive University's administration, the top candidate ended up being a male Caucasian, William White. Coach White met all the requirements and, after a careful and thorough review of all the candidates, emerged as the most qualified person for the position. The female candidates were qualified, but none was as qualified as Coach White. All of this puts Olive University's athletic director in a difficult position. The best female candidate is Rhonda Brown, who is also African-American. Although minimally qualified, Coach Brown is clearly less accomplished in the areas of win–loss percentages as well as overall experience when compared with Coach White. However, because of the lack of women head coaches, Coach Brown will be offered the position.

Critical Thinking: Finding Common-Sense Solutions

1. If you were Olive University's athletic director, would you have offered the head women's volleyball coaching position to Rhonda Brown? Why or why not?

2. If you were the athletic director and were required to select five persons to serve on this search committee, on what criteria would you base your selections? Would the gender or race of individuals affect your decision?

3. If you were the president of Olive University, would you have required that a woman be hired for the head women's volleyball coaching position? Why or why not?

4. If you were the athletic director and were responsible for writing the job description for the head women's volleyball coaching position, would you write it in a way that would feature strengths held by women? Why or why not?

Critical Thinking: Moral Theory-Based Decision Making

5. Using the *deontological theory* as the premise for your decision, if you were the president of Olive University, would you have required that a female be hired for the head women's volleyball coaching position? Explain your answer.

6. Using the *best interest of others* as the primary basis for arriving at your decision, as a coach on the search committee, which candidate would you support? Explain your answer.

7. Basing your decision on the moral values of *fairness* and *justice* and knowing the details surrounding the hiring process, if you were Coach White, would you accept the job when it was offered to you? Why or why not?

Gender Discrimination at the Fox Meadow Country Club

Nearly 50 years ago, Ralph and his wife, Pam, decided that they were interested in buying a country club in upstate New York. After researching the area, they decided on a country club named Fox Meadow. They purchased Fox Meadow and, along with their six children, moved to New York, where Ralph operated the club while Pam raised their three girls and three boys. When the children grew older, they all worked at Fox Meadow, usually on the golf course or in the banquet hall. The boys took on work that required physical labor and the girls completed domestic chores, including kitchen-related work. These traditional roles were quite common and accepted 50 years ago.

Fox Meadow was a financial success, which allowed Ralph to send all his children to college. When his grown children graduated from college and returned to the area, the opportunities that Fox Meadow presented to the men were quite different from those presented to the women. The men were offered ownership and management positions and the women were offered basic staff employment positions. Even if highly qualified, the women were not offered a stake in the ownership of Fox Meadow. Under no circumstances was Ralph going to allow any women to own or run his country club. Finally, Ralph decided to retire and let his sons run the club entirely, although even after his retirement, Ralph continued to oversee things and was always part of any major decisions made. Since his death 5 years ago, Fox

Meadow continued to flourish under the exclusive ownership and management of his sons.

As the next generation of the family grew older, the same gender-specific work and ownership patterns existed for the grandchildren as it had for the previous generation. Essentially, boys engaged in physical labor and girls performed domestic chores. This pattern continued until one of the granddaughters, Nancy, began to play a huge role in the club. Nancy made it a point to learn everything about the operations of Fox Meadow, especially the managerial and business aspects of the club. To supplement her practical expertise in management, Nancy attended college and earned a business degree with an emphasis in sport management. After returning home last summer with aspirations of being offered a management position at Fox Meadow, she was told that there would not be an opportunity for her there as owner or manager.

Upon hearing the news, Nancy was distraught but determined to gain a management position even if she had to sue her own family. Nancy proceeded to hire a lawyer and told her father and her uncles that she was suing them for sexual discrimination. When Nancy's sisters and female cousins learned of her lawsuit, they decided to support her at any cost. This was not only Nancy's battle, but also a battle for all the females in the family.

Critical Thinking: Finding Common-Sense Solutions

1. Ethically, should the owners (Ralph's sons) advance with the times and provide Nancy and the other qualified daughters with ownership and managerial opportunities at Fox Meadow?

2. Do the boys have an obligation to follow through on Ralph's wishes and beliefs that only the men in the family should own and manage Fox Meadow? Explain your answer.

3. Is it ethical in a family-owned business to provide family members (as opposed to non-family members) with unearned privileges, such as higher hourly wages and more lucrative working hours?

4. In your opinion, should all country clubs—both private and public—be required to allow for equal employment opportunities for all persons, irrespective of gender? Explain your reasoning.

Critical Thinking: Moral Theory-Based Decision Making

5. Are you able to identify characteristics of *strategic thinking* in Ralph's ownership and managerial philosophies? Elaborate.

6. Basing your actions on *deontological moral theory,* what actions would you take regarding the hiring practices at Fox Meadow?

7. Using *consequentialist moral theory* to guide your reasoning, how would you determine hiring criteria pertaining to gender at Fox Meadow?

Key Terms

Civil Rights Restoration Act of 1987—an act passed by Congress in 1988 that allowed the Office of Civil Rights to regain jurisdiction over athletics programs, stating that Title IX applies to all operations that receive federal funds, effectively overturning the Grove City ruling.

Educational Amendments Act of 1972—a comprehensive federal law that prohibits discrimination on the basis of sex in any federally funded education program or activity.

equal opportunities—from a Title IX athletic standpoint, providing males and females with equivalent opportunities in sport regardless of sex.

gender discrimination—actions that deny opportunities, privileges, or rewards to a person or a group because of their sex; Title IX legislation has reduced gender discrimination against women in school-based athletic departments.

gender equity—the principle and practice of fair allocation of resources, programs, and decision making for both women and men.

Office of Civil Rights (OCR)—the enforcement body of Title IX.

proportionality test—a gender equity test within Title IX that requires athletic participation opportunities for males and females to be substantially proportionate to the undergraduate population of males and females; that is, if an undergraduate population of a college is 42% male and 58% female, to meet the proportionality test of Title IX and thus be compliant with Title IX, the athletic participation opportunities for males must be 42% and for females must be 58%.

Title IX—a federal law stating that no person shall, on the basis of sex, be excluded from participation in, or denied benefits of, or be subjected to discrimination under any educational program or activity receiving federal assistance.

8 Ethical Issues in Interscholastic and Intercollegiate Sport

Learning Outcomes

After reading Chapter 8, the student will be able to:

1. Explain moral views regarding controversial National Collegiate Athletic Association issues.

2. Describe, based on moral theory, the pros and cons of compensating revenue-generating intercollegiate athletes.

3. Illustrate how the desire to attain financial benefits from college sport can affect education for athletes.

4. Distinguish between the politically correct mission of intercollegiate athletics and the actual practices that take place within intercollegiate athletics.

5. Discuss the morality of actions that often take place with regards to intercollegiate recruiting.

6. List the various ways that intercollegiate athletes can maintain athletic eligibility and the morality of those ways.

Moral issues related to interscholastic and interscholastic sport are many. Should the National Collegiate Athletic Association (NCAA) athletes be further compensated for their participation in sports that generate revenue for their colleges or universities? Is the athletic scholarship sufficient and fair compensation for their effort, or does it go too far because scholarship athletes receive complete financial remission for participation in the extracurricular activity of sports? What ethical standards should coaches adhere to when recruiting athletes to play for their schools? Should freshmen athletes be eligible to participate in intercollegiate athletics, or should their first year of college be devoted to making the academic and overall transition to university life? Should academic support services be offered to athletes and not offered to students who do not participate in athletics? Are mission statements of athletic departments transparent, politically correct statements that are in reality not followed because the pressure to win can be overwhelming? And what constraints are ethical for schools and governing bodies to place on the eligibility of athletes?

This chapter examines each of the above points in detail. Complexities that coaches and administrators need to consider when making decisions about what is right and wrong within the contexts of intercollegiate and interscholastic athletics are also discussed in this chapter. Through moral discussion, analysis, and the application of moral decision-making models, students will become better prepared to address, from a moral perspective, similar types of issues should they face them on the job in the future.

Brief History of the National Collegiate Athletic Association

Given the enormity of the NCAA as the premier sports governing body of 4-year institutions of higher education, a brief history is in order. A first step in forming what is today the NCAA took place when President Theodore Roosevelt summoned college athletics leaders to two White House conferences to encourage reforms to temper the rugged nature of football, which was resulting in numerous injuries and deaths to players. After a first meeting of 13 institutions in December of 1905, a subsequent meeting on December 28, 1905, in New York City resulted in the founding of the Intercollegiate Athletic Association of the United States (IAAUS), which included 62 members. In 1910, the IAAUS assumed its present name of the National Collegiate Athletic Association (NCAA) and was primarily a discussion group and rules-making body. In 1921, however, the National Collegiate Track and Field Championship was held, marking the first of many NCAA-hosted national championship events. After World War II, in an attempt to curb abuses involving NCAA athletes, the "Sanity Code" was adopted to establish guidelines for recruiting and financial aid. Eventually, governance has come to include the monitoring of such areas as the televising of football games, post-season bowl games, and the men's final-four basketball tournament. In 1952, with the growth of the NCAA came the need to form an executive director position to lead the organization in its newly formed national headquarters in Kansas

City, Missouri. With continued growth, the NCAA, in 1973, formed three divisions—I, II, and III. In 1980, the NCAA began administering women's athletic programs, and the following year, an extensive governance plan was adopted that included women's athletics programs, services, and representation. As of this writing, the national headquarters is located in Indianapolis, IN and consists of more than 390 office staff members.[1]

Compensation of Revenue-Generating Intercollegiate Athletes

Currently, at the Divisions I and II levels, NCAA athletes may be awarded scholarships for their athletic abilities but may not receive further compensation in the form of salaries or cash payments. Even though NCAA rules prohibit the compensation of athletes, opinions differ as to whether intercollegiate athletes deserve a stipend or salary for their athletic efforts.

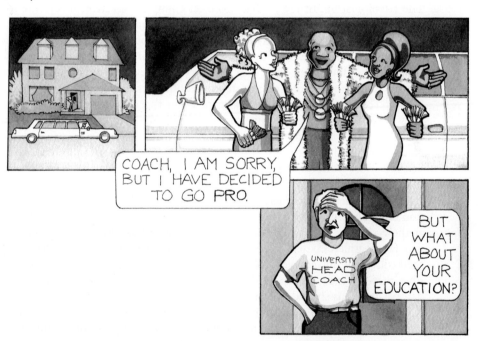

Prior, however, to beginning discussion on the compensation of intercollegiate revenue-generating athletes, it should be noted that the generation of revenue through the "so-called" revenue-generating sports is often specific to a particular college and university. In other words, not all college and university football, men's basketball, and women's basketball programs generate revenue.

How can an athletic department's existence be morally justified if it is losing money? The utilitarian might try to determine whether the benefits gained by athletic participation outweigh the amount of money lost by athletic departments. Could monies lost by athletic departments be used to benefit more persons than those gaining benefits from participating on sports teams? Recall that the utilitarian is interested in the most amount of good for the most amount of people. The teleologist might ask whether there is an element of unfairness that comes from athletic departments that lose money. Is it unfair that money might be taken from other areas to support teams that lose money? Deontologists would not want to be part of something that they would not also be willing to accept for themselves. Deontologically, the sports team that is losing money and requires financial subsidy from other programs within a university must ask themselves if they would be willing to take on an altruistic mindset and provide some of their money to others if the situation were reversed.

Many questions can stimulate discussion in relation to the compensation of revenue-generating intercollegiate athletes. Do athletes deserve more than an athletic scholarship? Is it fair to compensate only the members of revenue-generating sport teams, such as football, men's basketball, and, in some cases, women's basketball? The teleologist might argue that, from an equity perspective, if revenue-generating athletes are compensated, then non-revenue-generating athletes also deserve to be compensated. On the other hand, the teleologist could also make the argument that, in the interest of fairness, if athletes are participating in a sport that generates revenue, those athletes are deserving of part of the revenue; whereas, athletes of non-revenue-generating sports do not deserve money because they are not generating any money. Teleologists might also make the point that it is not fair and just to pay athletes of non-revenue-generating sports with money made from revenue-generating sports. A utilitarian argument, however, might support using money generated from revenue-generating sports to compensate athletes of non-revenue-generating sports because more athletes would receive a share of the wealth, thus making a greater number of people happy.

In the athletic programs that generate revenue, what effects would the compensation of revenue-generating athletes have on the vast number of non-athletes studying at these schools? Does the NCAA have a moral obligation to compensate revenue-generating athletes based on the fact that their athletic performances bring money into their college or university? Looking at this issue from the opposite viewpoint, is it possible that athletic scholarships are compensation above and beyond what athletes deserve and thus should be eliminated out of fairness for the other students not participating in athletics? Could one even go so far as to claim that, instead of receiving an athletic scholarship, all athletes should be charged a fee because sports are extracurricular activities?

If sports are truly extracurricular and are put in place to provide students who participate in athletics with sports' educational benefits, the notion of compensating athletes might be met with resistance by the teleologist. The teleologist might maintain that opportunities for as many athletes as possible to gain benefits through sport experiences might be lost because monies to operate the non-revenue-generating sports might, instead, go to the athletes of those generating revenue. If the goal is that all athletes in every sport are to be provided with the same educational benefits through the sport experience, the teleologist might argue that all athletes, regardless of sport (revenue-generating or non-revenue-generating), should be provided with the opportunity to gain educational benefits from their sport.

Further discussion below concerning whether college athletes should be compensated includes the benefits of the athletic scholarship, the view that sport participation is an extracurricular activity, the contributions of athletes to their colleges and universities, and the notion that athletes have the option to participate or not participate in sport. This discussion also sheds light on whether the scholarship is fair and just compensation for college athletes.

Benefits of the Athletic Scholarship

A full scholarship covers all of an athlete's primary school-related expenses, which include room, board, and tuition. In return, the athlete must play for the college or university's sports team that has granted him a scholarship. In addition to receiving room, board, and tuition, athletes may also apply for and, depending on their financial situation, be awarded student loans to cover additional expenses. Those same athletes who are the recipients of athletic scholarships, in some cases, may not be able to afford to attend college if it were not for the athletic scholarship.

Rare are educational institutions, such as the University of Maryland and the University of North Carolina, that offer need-based scholarships to students whose families make less than $21,000 a year. Qualified low-income students at these schools can attend debt free if they work 10 to 12 hours weekly in federal work-study programs.[2]

As previously discussed, teleology attempts to determine moral correctness through a moral values approach. Justice and fairness are moral values of teleology that are often applied to real scenarios to make moral assessments. One way to examine whether athletic scholarships are fair and just compensation for the efforts made by the athlete is to compare the benefits athletes receive from athletic scholarships with the benefits that non-athletes receive. Both students who participate in sports and those who do not are confronted with financial challenges while attending college. Often, after completing college, students are saddled with significant debt due to student loans. However, athletes who are under full scholarship and choose not to borrow and spend can graduate without huge debt. Overall, it is apparent that full scholarship athletes benefit more financially when compared with non-athletes who are not on comparable academic scholarships.

Education as a Priority and Sport Participation as an Extracurricular Activity

If education is the primary purpose of institutions of higher education, then it might be argued that the focus of education should be equal educational opportunities for all. This could weaken the argument for compensating athletes, because such compensation could reduce the amount of financial support colleges and universities have available for educational initiatives. On the other hand, even though all athletically related revenue does not go toward education, one could certainly argue that if a school's athletic program is turning a profit, then its academic programs should be receiving a significant portion of the monies available. Utilitarian ethical theorists would be quick to point out here that more good can be done for more of the student body if profits from athletic programs are shared with academic programs and other programs that enhance the educational experiences of students. Given this point, the argument against compensation does gain strength when one considers the educational welfare of all students rather than the economic welfare of athletes.

If one holds that athletics are extracurricular activities, then *any* form of compensation for athletes might be considered above and beyond what is fair. Is it fair that athletes receive money to gain educational experiences through sport participation when other students are paying for educational experiences gained from academic programs? In fact, one might argue further that if higher education is providing athletes with learning experiences above and beyond those available to other students, the recipients (the participating athletes) of those experiences should be charged a fee instead of receiving money. Participating in sports might be considered experiential learning, much like an internship within an academic curriculum. Athletes on college sports teams receive expert instruction from superb coaches in much the same way other students pay for and receive expert instruction from professors. On the other hand, is it fair that athletes are not paid when the revenue-generating sports in which they participate generate money?

Contribution of Athletes to Their Colleges

The fairness of athletic scholarships may also be analyzed from the perspective that athletes' contributions in many cases generate money for their college. For example, in the 2005 to 2006 season, the football programs at Ohio State, Texas, Florida, and Michigan made $28.5, $42.5, $32.4, and $37.6 million, respectively.[3] Because some major Division I men's basketball and football teams generate large amounts of revenue, it could be argued that the athletes playing for these teams deserve some of that revenue.

One might argue that athletic scholarships are adequate compensation, because athletes receive a free education, meals, housing, and increased earning potential on completion of their degrees. Are scholarships fair and just compensation for college athletes who, through their athletic skills, help generate revenue for their college or university? Or, do the NCAA and athletic departments have a moral obligation to compensate athletes commensurate with their abilities and earning power that ultimately generate revenue? Concerning both the athlete and the college or university, what is fair?

Outstanding athletic performances help create winning teams that generate greater revenue through post-season competitions such as football bowl games and basketball tournament games. In fact, for the rights to televise the 2003 March Madness Division I NCAA men's basketball tournament, CBS paid the NCAA $370 million dollars. Televising of games, football bowl independently negotiated by the large conferences, is also lucrative for colleges and universities. During the 2002 to 2003 season, the Southeastern Conference earned $22 million from bowl games, with the league getting $15 million from its football championship game. Overall, the Southeastern Conference reported earning $122,488,264 during the 2002 to 2003 fiscal year.[4]

Without athletes, this money would not come to colleges and universities; thus, one might argue, from a teleological standpoint, that it would be fair and just to compensate the athletes for their hard work and successful performances. The deontologist might call for consistency in behaviors or actions. In other words, paying all athletes in all sports might be a consideration from the deontologist's viewpoint. Paying all athletes who are part of teams that generate money is another decision that might be supported by the deontologist, because there are consistent criteria as part of deciding which athletes to pay. Or, not paying any athletes might be another option considered by the deontologist because the decision is being applied to all athletes without exception.

Is it, however, presumptuous to assume that particular athletes on teams are responsible for generating revenue? One could also argue that when an athlete opts *not* to participate, there is always another talented athlete interested *in* participating. The earning power of individual athletes can certainly be questioned, especially if there is a steady line of capable athletes, who can effectively perform, ready to fill empty roster spots. In terms of earning power, it could be argued that no one or two athletes are responsible for the revenue generated by men's basketball and football teams. Generally, when a superstar athlete chooses to bypass college and play professionally, the college game as a whole does not seem to suffer financially. Another talented athlete simply steps in and takes the previous athlete's place. As teams compete to advance in post-season tournaments, the superstar athlete who bypassed college is all but forgotten. For example, when Kobe Bryant, and more recently LeBron James, bypassed college to go directly to the National Basketball Association (NBA), the NCAA men's basketball season and post-season tournament experienced the same general popularity and revenue generation as always.

Similarly, but to a much lesser degree in terms of revenue generation for a university, when tennis players Jennifer Capriati, Anna Kournikova, and Maria Sharapova turned professional as teenagers, universities did not miss the potential revenue that these young tennis stars may have produced for their universities. The decision of whether to bypass college for professional play is one that pits education against money. Tennis, in general, will not generate money for either player or educational institution at the interscholastic or intercollegiate level, but will generate money for the player and tournament at the professional level. According to Clarke, the lure of money from endorsements, sponsorships, and international fame is the attraction that causes athletes to bypass the remainder of formal high school and enrollment in a college or university.[5]

In actuality, individual athletes may not be as responsible for generating revenue for the NCAA and its member institutions as many believe. Other athletes seem to emerge as fan favorites and box office attractions. And, regardless of which players make up a team, long-standing team rivalries within the sport and the excitement surrounding amateur competition seem to continue to draw large numbers of paying fans and lucrative television contracts.

Choosing to Participate

The question of whether a scholarship is fair and just compensation may not be as important as it first appears, because athletes may exercise their option not to participate in intercollegiate athletics at any time. An argument against compensation of **revenue-generating athletes** can be made based on the fact that athletes are not forced to participate in intercollegiate sports, and when they make the choice to participate, they are also making the choice to abide by the rules of the governing organization of the sport. In essence, athletes are not bound by any rules until they choose to attend and play for an NCAA college or university. If a player strongly disagrees with NCAA rules and regulations regarding compensation, he or she can simply choose not to participate and, thus, avoid having to follow rules with which they disagree.

> **revenue-generating athletes:** intercollegiate players on sports teams that make money, primarily through gate receipts and television contracts, for their athletic department and college or university; football, men's basketball, and sometimes women's basketball at major universities are normally the sports in which revenue-generating athletes participate.

Many college football and men's basketball players exercise this option each year when they bypass or leave college and enter professional drafts. The lure of an exorbitant salary at the professional level has been too strong for many young athletes to ignore, influencing them to play professionally instead of intercollegiately because it is against NCAA rules for them to receive a salary as collegiate players. If athletes are not talented enough to play professionally, they can also choose to play in semi-professional leagues, in recreational leagues, or not at all. In any case, an athlete can choose not to participate in NCAA sports and thus not be required to abide by NCAA rules that disallow compensation for participants.

There is, however, an age restriction that prevents high school athletes from going straight to the NBA. With the implementation of the NBA collective bargaining agreement in June of 2005, the issue of high school players bypassing college to go straight to the NBA has become nearly nonexistent. Both the National Basketball Player's Association (NBPA), under the leadership of Billy Hunter, and the NBA, under Commissioner David Stern's leadership, agreed in contract to a minimum age requirement of 19 (plus one year removed from high school) for NBA players.[6] This means the days of high school phenoms like LeBron James and Kobe Bryant jumping from high school to the NBA are over. No longer will high school players have the opportunity to earn exorbitant NBA salaries immediately after finishing high school. In all cases they will have to wait until they are 19 years old before entering the NBA.

A Legal Perspective

From a legal perspective, it is possible that initiating the compensation of revenue-generating athletes would establish the legal grounds for an overall compensatory model for intercollegiate athletics. Legally, compensating the members of one team might open the door for the compensation of all university athletes—non-revenue-generating athletes included. Although there would seemingly be sufficient funds to provide compensation for athletes in revenue-generating sports, the funds might deplete quickly if all athletes, including the non-revenue-generating athletes, in athletic departments were to be paid. If this were to take place, the risk of jeopardizing the offerings and quality of non-revenue-generating sports might become real. Thus, more persons might be negatively affected, which would go against the utilitarian model, which calls for the most amount of people being happy.

Somewhat unusual was the donation of $10 million for scholarships to Indiana University for non-revenue-generating sports for the 2005 to 2006 season. If donations such as this one were commonplace in sport, athletic departments might be able to afford to pay all athletes, revenue-generating as well as non-revenue-generating, a sizeable stipend to complement their athletic scholarships, which are used for room, board, and tuition. Rupp (2005) claims, however, that without such additional donations, athletic departments would run the risk of falling short of operating funds if they were to open the door for athlete compensation across the athletic departments.[7] From a consequentialist point of view, the question would then be whether compensating revenue-generating athletes would be worth risking the benefits that non-revenue-generating teams provide for participants if those programs would not be able to exist financially. Given the emphasis that the NCAA and its member institutions have placed on the educational value of intercollegiate athletics, such a risk would seemingly be unacceptable.

The process involved in creating NCAA rules can provide a perspective on the views related to compensating intercollegiate athletes. Colleges and universities have an influence over NCAA legislation. Delegates from institutions in Divisions II and III hold mass votes at the association's annual convention, and, even though Division I colleges do not vote directly on their own rules changes, campus executives as well as smaller committees of athletic administrators meet throughout the year to consider NCAA policies and rules changes.[8] Input from NCAA member institutions, as part of the process, does seem to add a component of validity to legislation that is passed or rejected through it.

Winning and Reaping the Financial Benefits at the Cost of Quality Education

Is intercollegiate athletics an extracurricular activity that serves a valid educational function, or has its primary purpose become winning and the generation of as much money as possible for those who manage the sports? Teams that consistently win games usually generate large sums of money through such means as gate receipts, television contracts, and increased alumni donations. Furthermore, conferences make money based on how well men's basketball teams have done in the championship tournament. The more games that members of conferences play in the tournament, the more lucrative the payday is for conferences.[4]

"Ridiculed for Putting Class Ahead of Soccer"

Coach Opaque was irate when she learned that her top soccer player scheduled a class that conflicted with the 3:00 p.m. Monday, Wednesday, and Friday soccer practices. Coach Opaque screamed at Julia, "How on earth could you compromise the potential success of this team by allowing a class to get in the way of practice? You owe a responsibility to your teammates and I and should be ashamed of yourself." Julia was nearly in tears and whimpered the following to her coach, "But coach, this is the final class that I need for graduation and it is the only time it is offered. If I do not take it, I will have to stay an extra semester." The coach would hear nothing of it and screamed at Julia again, this time saying, "You should be completely ashamed of yourself for putting yourself in front of the team. The only way you can redeem yourself at this point is by dropping the class."

Questions
1. If you were Julia, would you drop the class? Explain why or why not.
2. What are the conflicting values in this case? What values appear to be held by Coach Opaque? What values appear to be held by Julia?
3. Discuss the social value of leadership as it relates to Coach Opaque as a head coach and Julia as the top soccer player on her team.
4. Under the consequentialist theory, supported by utilitarianism, how might this dilemma best be resolved?

Major college sports have become money-focused endeavors, with many parties reaping some form of benefits. Athletic administrators who manage and control sports teams may be the ones reaping the most significant benefits from the revenue generated from sports teams. Benefits that coaches receive include bonuses received for signing their contracts, and additional bonuses and perks for such things as winning a specific number of games, defeating rivals, participating in post-season tournaments, and having high team graduation rates—accomplishments that all carry some form of monetary reward.

One benefit of major college coaches is their lucrative coaching contracts. The most lucrative of all coaching contracts might be the one held by Duke University head men's basketball coach Mike Krzyzewski. Leveraging the interest expressed in him as a candidate for the Los Angeles Laker's head coaching position, Krzyzewski was granted a lifetime contract by those in power at Duke. With such tenure normally being reserved for the likes of college professors and Supreme Court justices, Duke has set the bar even higher for other colleges and universities in their pursuit to attract the best coaches for the purpose of winning and revenue generation.[9]

On the other hand, could one argue that players are gaining, through sport participation, an education above and beyond the education received by other college students? Are the experiences athletes have as members of sports teams educational in nature? As alluded to previously, sport participation might be considered similar to an internship or apprenticeship. Certainly, players are exposed to the skills of coaching and managing on a day-to-day basis. As members of a sports team, players have the opportunity to learn, through observation, educational principles of business and marketing, because major college sports do seem to be based and operated on business principles. In some cases, while participating on sports teams, players might even serve as the ones who implement such principles.

Largely due to mass media attention, interscholastic sport is highly focussed on winning. In many cases, schools take the measures necessary to have the best sports programs in their local community, state, or nation. For example, in 2003, the Valdosta High School football team in Valdosta, Georgia raised close to $500,000 in total revenue. On Friday nights they play in a newly renovated $7.5 million stadium. In high school basketball, some teams in Indiana and other basketball frenzied states will reap money as the result of their teams being televised nationally. The height of interscholastic media attention may have taken place in Ohio with Akron's St. Vincent-St. Mary's LeBron James, who was featured on the cover of Sports Illustrated as a sophomore.[10]

Has money corrupted college sports to the point that fundamental educational values are being lost? If such values as respect, honesty, and compassion are overridden by money, the sport is not operating from a strong teleological foundation. Has the strong emphasis placed on winning and making profits in college sports compromised the quality of the education athletes receive, thus not leaving athletes as well prepared for a non-athletic professional future as their fellow college students who do not participate in athletics? If so, sports that overemphasize money are not operating from a strong utilitarian foundation.

The Mission Statement of Intercollegiate Athletics as a Facade

Are **mission statements** of intercollegiate athletics that speak of focusing on the education and well-being of athletes being followed, or are they facades covering the hidden agendas of administrators of higher education? Are genuine efforts being made to meet the objectives of mission statements? An analysis of college and university mission statements and athletic department mission statements is of interest. Such an analysis might help in determining whether missions, in fact, are being carried out as stated. Mission statements that are created to cover hidden agendas and that generally are not intended to be put into practice do not adhere to the moral value of honesty and are teleologically unsound.

mission statements: statements drafted by organizations (i.e., a university or sport department) to define their core purpose: why they exist, their reason for being; the declaration of values, goals, and aspirations that authoritative groups agree upon as describing the central unique mission of the organization.

Athletes' perceptions as to the benefits of athletic participation might also be of interest, as the student/athlete is usually a centerpiece of the mission statement. Do athletes perceive that their schools are actively implementing measures on their behalf to meet mission statements? Or, are the mission statements simply empty catch phrases, summarizing politically correct goals that serve as a public relations strategy on behalf of colleges and athletic departments? If mission statements of colleges and intercollegiate athletic departments are created with the intent to genuinely and comprehensively carry out what is stated, the efforts of those creating the mission statement are honest and therefore gain teleological credibility.

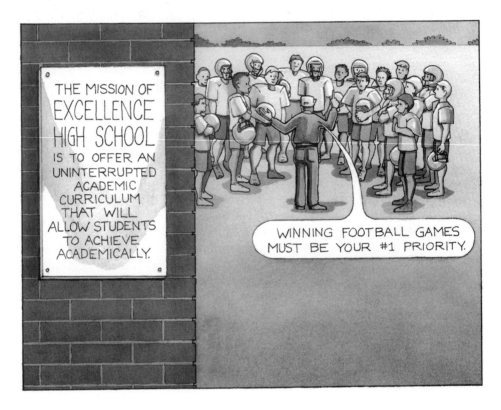

Of concern is that athletes are not gaining the educational benefits outlined in mission statements. An analysis of school and athletic department mission statements is helpful in determining whether (a) mission statements are in alignment with acceptable standards in higher education, and (b) the objectives stated within those mission statements are being met. If it is found that colleges and athletic departments are meeting the objectives of their mission statements, they deserve praise and, again, should be recognized as meeting the moral value of honesty. If, on the other hand, the objectives of mission statements are not being met, the teleologist would likely criticize the university for being dishonest and would suggest that they implement the necessary measures to align what is being stated in the mission statement with what is actually being practiced. Morally good athletic directors and university administrators will recognize their responsibility to athletes and make sure that they have a fair chance to gain the educational benefits that universities have to offer them as well as the benefits associated with their athletic participation.

Recruiting

Recruiting is the process by which coaches seek out and persuade players to play for their teams. Sports programs rely on effective recruiting to win games. With the focus on winning, coaches and administrators are fully aware that they must recruit the most talented players and players who fit within a program's system to win consistently. A case in point is Harry Statham, a coach who has won 903 men's basketball games at McKendree College in Illinois. Statham understands full well the importance of recruiting good players who fit within a system to win games. Over his 40-year coaching career, Statham has recruited players who are academically sound and also love basketball. According to Statham, when he has not been able to get this type of player, his teams have not been as good.[11]

Adding to the pressure to recruit well in major college revenue-generating and/or popular sports is the head coach's awareness that he or she may be fired if not successful. Coaches know that having more talented players than the opposition is one of the primary factors that will allow them to have winning seasons.

The pressure to win and the accompanying temptations to break recruiting rules to acquire players is an issue worthy of moral analysis. Deontologically, if a coach believes the rules of recruiting should apply to other coaches, he too should follow those same rules. If a coach looks at the consequences of breaking the rules and believes that recruiting players illegally is not immediately hurtful to others, he may rationalize breaking recruiting rules through consequentialism, but only if he can show that it results in a greater good. Recall, however, that the consequentialist attempts to look at what appears to elicit good consequences, or a positive outcome, without regard for moral values. Teleological moral theory, on the other hand, bases decisions on moral values such as honesty, fairness, and trust. Honest, fair, or trustworthy coaches will choose not to break recruiting rules.

Recruiting to Meet the Unrealistic Demands of Winning

The pressure to win is present in many intercollegiate athletic programs. The simple understanding of the fact that 50% of all teams will win and 50% will lose demonstrates, however, that expectations for coaches to win will often not be realistic ones. For example, if all high school and college coaches' jobs depended on their teams winning 60% to 70% of their games, as many as two-thirds of coaches could lose their jobs based on the mathematical impossibility for all teams to win at that rate. Even though the odds to win games are stacked against coaches, the demands to win remain. In efforts to meet these demands, coaches aggressively recruit the most talented players available.

The need to recruit highly talented players to meet the demands placed on coaches to win sometimes causes coaches to recruit players who are less academically qualified than a college or university would prefer. It was reported in 2006 that the athletic director of Dixie State College in St. George, Utah fired his head football coach for not maintaining necessary academic standards on the part of his football players. The team grade point average was 1.96. The firing was somewhat surprising in that the head coach, Greg Croshaw, over the course of 24 seasons had compiled a record of 214-56-1, with 17 Western State Football League wins and two runner-up finishes. In this case, it appears that the emphasis on academics overrode an emphasis on winning.[12] This decision appears to be more morally based rather than strategically based, because strategic reasoning would have supported keeping a coach who makes money for the athletic department. Instead, the long-term best interest of future athletes appears to have been considered because poor academics will no longer be allowed.

Reasons Cheating Takes Place in Recruiting

Many sport governing bodies have rules in place to govern recruiting. For example, the NCAA has specific rules and regulations pertaining to actions that are acceptable and unacceptable in the recruiting process. Many coaches abide by these rules and many do not.

Even though NCAA intercollegiate athletic programs that are caught breaking recruiting rules receive widespread media attention, it is possible that a larger problem exists in the Amateur Athletic Union (AAU) ranks. In 2006, the Knight Commission heard testimony from Bishop O'Connell High School's head boy's basketball coach Joey Wootten, who spoke of summer league coaches who offer players up to $15,000 or seedy trips to Las Vegas to join their teams. Both are violations of NCAA rules. Wootten also said that summer league AAU coaches probably recruit 10 times more than college coaches. Furthermore, according to Wootten, travel teams are employing full-time coaches to field star-studded summer league teams that can play in top tournaments that will grab the attention of college recruiters.[13]

Unscrupulous recruiting might be linked to a strong desire of coaches to win, rewards that accompany winning, and negative repercussions coaches wish to avoid from losing. As players and coaches become immersed in competitive situations, the desire to win sometimes becomes even stronger, drawing out the competitive instincts of both players and coaches. Knowing that to compete successfully, talented players are needed, coaches are aware of the need to acquire the best players possible, which might cause some coaches to disregard rules put in place to govern recruiting.

"New Cheerleading Expectations"

When Coach Triumph began her coaching career, her purpose was to help and develop young people as individuals. As her high school administration placed more and more emphasis on the exposure that national cheerleading competitions brought to her

"New Cheerleading Expectations" (*Continued*)

school, the pressures to acquire the most talented athletes and perform at the highest levels increased. Coach Triumph was told that her cheerleading teams must finish in the top 10 over any 5-year period or she would be fired. These winning expectations, according to Coach Triumph, have completely changed her coaching approach. Now, instead of focusing exclusively on the well-being of her athletes, Coach Triumph focuses on winning and its rewards. Primarily, though, she focuses on doing whatever it takes to make sure her cheerleading teams finish in the top 10 at the national cheerleading competition at the end of each season. Coach Triumph is frustrated with herself because she now places all of her coaching emphasis on winning instead of the well-being of her athletes.

Questions

1. Describe the ethical dilemma that the administration has created for Coach Triumph.
2. In this case, describe how the newly established expectations of winning have changed Coach Triumph's approach to coaching.
3. How would you have responded to the newly established expectations for winning? Would you have changed your coaching style? Explain.

The rewards—both intangible and tangible—provided to coaches who win are other influencing factors that may move coaches to recruit in ways that violate established guidelines. Intangible rewards include the praise and adulation that can make coaches stars within their sport and are not related to money. On the other hand, tangible rewards coaches receive for winning come in the form of cash bonuses, multi-year contracts and extensions, apparel contracts, and increases in their program's budget. Awards might tempt those involved in sport to participate not for the good of the sport but for hedonistic reasons, to make themselves happy. After winning the national championship with a 41-38 Rose Bowl victory over the University of Southern California, Texas head football coach Mack Brown was promptly rewarded with more than a $300,000 salary increase, for a package worth $2.5 million per year.[14] In 2006, Ohio State football head coach Jim Tressel, who coached the Buckeyes to a 2002 national championship, renegotiated his contract, which was set to expire after the 2008 season, and received a $500,000 signing bonus as part of his new contract through 2013.[15] In 2005, the University of Kansas head football coach Mark Mangino received a new contract that raised his annual salary from $128,438 to $220,000. Mangino's professional services monies, which are compensation for public relations and promotional duties, increased from $475,000 to $1.28 million per year. Mangino's increases were based on the fact that he led Kansas to two bowl game appearances in the past 3 years.[16] Keep in mind that just because coaches makes exorbitant sums of money does not mean that they are being driven by strategic reasoning or various forms of consequentialism. Persons, including coaches, can make lots of money and still be driven by and base their actions on moral theory.

Finally, negative repercussions from losing may also factor into coaches' decisions to cheat during the recruiting process. From a coaches' perspective, a severe negative repercussion from losing games is getting fired. To keep their jobs, some coaches might go to extreme measures to win by recruiting the best players, even if that means breaking established recruiting rules.

Coaches who break recruiting rules to protect their own interests are not acting from a utilitarian mindset because they are not considering the best interests of all. The same coaches are also not basing their actions on teleological reasoning, because they are not adhering to the moral values of honesty, fairness, trustworthiness, and respect. Coaches who break recruiting rules are being disrespectful to the process that was established to create the rules.

Improper Inducements

> **recruiting violations:** breaking rules (usually NCAA) that are put into place to provide coaches fair and equal opportunities to attract and persuade prospective athletes to enroll in their colleges and play on their sports teams.

> **improper inducements** (to players): inappropriate recruiting efforts that are against the rules; attempts by college athletic personnel—including but not limited to coaches, administrators, staff, or boosters—to improperly persuade prospects/players to attend a college or university and play on one of its sports teams by offering prospects such appealing items as cars, cash, and luxurious off-campus living accommodations.

Despite NCAA regulations that clearly outline improper recruiting behavior, many coaches choose to use illegal recruiting practices. **Recruiting violations** commonly take place in the form of providing **improper inducements** to players. In an effort to persuade prospects to sign with their college or university, coaches, administrators, staff, or boosters may improperly offer prospects such appealing items as cars, cash, and luxurious off-campus living accommodations. During on-campus visits, it has not been uncommon for recruits to be induced through parties that feature the availability of alcohol and sex.[17]

Although offering the above inducements is against NCAA recruiting rules, they have proven to be effective in attracting prospective athletes to sign with colleges and universities, and, hence, continue to be used during the recruiting process. In this case, strategic reasoning seems to be dominating the decision-making process.

The Dilemma of Committing Recruiting Violations and Punishing Cheaters

Are the punishments sanctioned by the NCAA effective in deterring recruiting violations by colleges and universities? A brief analysis of major college sports can provide insight into the question of whether, from a strategic perspective, it "pays" to cheat. Having the ability to separate strategic reasoning from moral reasoning and to base one's actions on moral rather than strategic reasoning has an important role to play in helping to "clean up" the recruiting process in intercollegiate athletics.

As discussed previously, because major college sports such as football and men's basketball can be tremendous revenue generators, colleges and universities aggressively compete for their share of revenues by doing what is necessary to win. Generally, the more a team wins, the more money it will make from the NCAA.

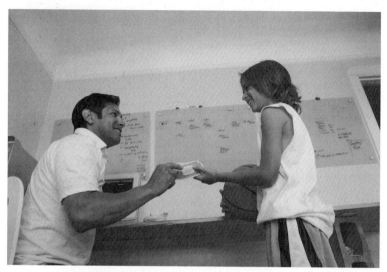

8-1 *Improper recruiting inducements in the form of cash are against many amateur sport organization recruiting rules.*

Football bowl payouts, television contracts, and multiple appearances in the men's basketball tournament may result in millions of dollars in revenue for schools.[18] It is the responsibility of the head coach to attain these financial rewards by leading the team to victory.

Coaches' moral values may be challenged as they try to win and in doing so give in to the temptations of recruiting dishonestly to attain players. Coaches often must decide whether they want to recruit honestly, abiding by the NCAA's rules and possibly risking being less successful, or engage in dishonest recruiting practices that could result in winning more games. No matter how coaches choose to act, some coaches will probably cheat in recruiting and might very well sign some of the best players when doing so. The possibility realistically exists that some honest coaches are fired for losing, whereas some dishonest coaches are applauded and rewarded for winning. Thus, the pressure to win truly does test coaches' moral values when making choices about how to recruit.

If "everyone" is breaking rules of recruiting, is it then appropriate for others to also break recruiting rules? Deontology calls for one to act only on the principle of which, then and there, you would be willing to make general law. Thus, if one is willing to live under the same rule-breaking conditions that they themselves are creating, they are accepting of the same actions from others, which is a component of deontology. Keep in mind, however, that deontology is based on principles worthy of being acted on and not merely willingness to live under the same conditions that you are imposing on others. The teleological moral value of honesty, however, is being disregarded by the coach who decides to break recruiting rules—even if all the other coaches are doing it. If a situation exists where all coaches are in agreement to break particular recruiting rules, eliminating the rules might be considered.

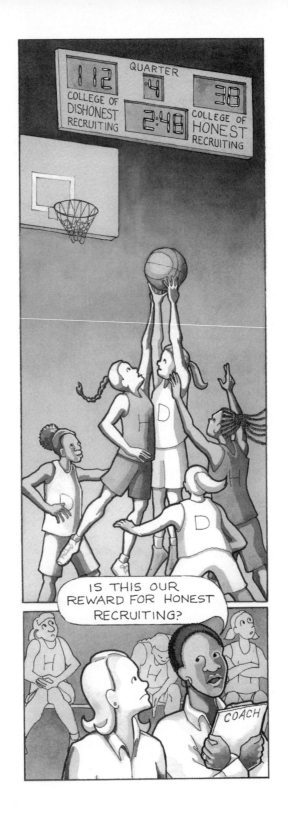

The financial rewards for winning are clear and without dispute, but are the punishments for recruiting violations severe enough to deter cheating? When allegations of recruiting violations surface with regard to a program, the athletic department of the college or university in question is often given the opportunity to self-impose sanctions against the accused team. The NCAA may also conduct its own investigations and, if conclusive evidence is found that supports the allegations, may also impose sanctions against the accused team and/or the athletic department.

Punishments are typically more severe if they are levied by the NCAA. These generally include such things as loss of scholarships, exclusion from post-season competition (a penalty that can be quite costly), or even the firing of the head coach. In the most severe cases, teams may receive the "**death penalty**," which bans them from all NCAA competition indefinitely.

> **death penalty**: in NCAA athletics, a ban on a member institution's entire sports program for gross rules violations within the program. In 1987, Southern Methodist University's football program was issued the "death penalty" as their entire season was cancelled for violating NCAA rules.

Should athletic departments impose sanctions on their own teams because they fear that, if they do not do so, the NCAA will? Or should athletic directors and departments take it upon themselves to impose sanctions against their teams because they acted dishonestly in breaking recruiting rules? For a consequentialist, the end result here would be the same because, in either case, the school would receive the same self-imposed sanctions and penalties from the NCAA regardless of whether they were acting from strategic or moral reasoning. Teleologists, on the other hand, would hope that athletic directors and departments would sanction themselves out of a commitment to the moral value of honesty, whereas deontologists might adhere to the principle that one should always tell the truth. Again, it seems that even though the latter situation is more ethically desirable, athletic directors and their departments often tend to do what they think will be in their own best interests rather than doing what they believe to be morally correct.

Given that the aforementioned sanctions are some of the most severe, coaches might be tempted to ask whether it is worth the risk of being caught violating recruiting rules. When approaching decisions in this manner, they are essentially dismissing moral reasoning and adopting a strategic approach that helps them assess what might be gained or lost from cheating. Those who knowingly violate rules may or may not consider the possibility of getting caught. Nevertheless, athletic department personnel are aware of the punishments that are generally associated with recruiting infractions.

What *do* coaches and athletic administrators have to lose from cheating? What do athletic directors and universities have to lose from not punishing cheaters? A not-so uncommon form of punishment imposed against coaches who have committed recruiting violations or allowed such violations to occur under their watch is job termination. It is usually the coach's college or university that does the firing. Depending on how coaches' contracts are structured and the number of years remaining on them, coaches may or may not receive a salary after termination.

Many major college coaches who are fired for rules violations end up unemployed for a year or two and then are hired by a new college or university seeking to improve its program. The list of coaches fired for cheating and rehired by another college or university is somewhat extensive. Kelvin Sampson, after being fired by Oklahoma in 2006, was just as quickly hired by Indiana. Even though Bob Huggins was found guilty of lack of institutional control at the University of Cincinnati in 1998, it did not stop Kansas State from hiring him as their men's basketball coach in March of 2006. Dennis Erickson was hired to coach Idaho's football program after leaving Miami in 1994 just before Miami was put on probation for multiple infractions. Todd Bozeman was formerly the head men's basketball coach at California until he was fired for NCAA recruiting violations in 1996 and then eventually rehired by Morgan State.[19]

This trend of being rehired after being fired for cheating indicates that coaches do not have much to lose from committing recruiting violations, even if they do get caught. In 2006, Cannella stated, "One thing to remember if you are planning to cheat in college sports: be a coach. Otherwise you will have to pay the price."[19(p16)] It seems that strategic reasoning sometimes prevails over moral reasoning within the context of major intercollegiate athletics. If this situation is to improve, moral values and principles must be practiced instead of just talked about by coaches and administrators.

"Coach Mobile's Cheating Methods"

Coach Mobile was in the second year of a 5-year contract at his university. Much like his previous seven head coaching positions, Coach Mobile was expected to win in a big way. At each of his previous positions he turned programs around from "no-name" losing teams to "household name" winning teams. Coach Mobile had accumulated three national championships and had a reputation of being one of the most successful recruiters in the history of college coaching. With this new season came some new additions, including a new assistant coach, Coach Upright, who was fresh out of college and who was hired to recruit. On coach Upright's first recruiting trip, Coach Mobile handed him a briefcase with $20,000 dollars in it and said that it was to be delivered to the parents of the most sought-after recruit. Coach Upright told Coach Mobile that he was *scared* to hand over the money because it was against the rules. Coach Mobile replied saying, "Listen coach, I did not win three national championships by waiting around for players to come to our team because they like me, the university, or a silly academic program. When we get fired, we will take a year off, and then someone else will hire us to build their program into a winner. My method of recruiting is proven; now go and give this money to our number one recruit's parents.

Questions
1. If you were Coach Upright would you follow Coach Mobile's directive and give the $20,000 to your number one recruit's parents? Why or why not?
2. Identify at least two conflicting values that Coach Upright may have to reason through before choosing to act.
3. Based on moral reasoning, if you were Coach Upright how would you (a) act, and (b) justify your actions?
4. Knowing Coach Mobile's past history of recruiting violations, would you hire him as your coach? Explain.

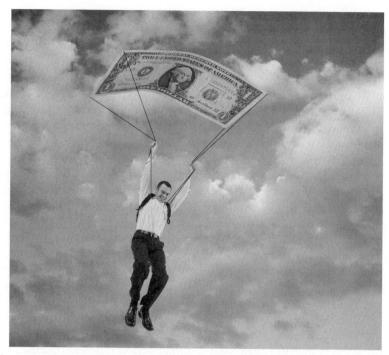

8-2 *The over-reliance on money by athletic departments can affect moral judgment.*

What about athletic directors? Does it pay for them to cheat? Again, examining this issue from a strategic perspective, the temptations to dismiss moral reasoning as a foundation for decision making are many. Athletic directors are largely responsible for the athletic department budgets and must make sure that enough revenue is generated to operate effective sport programs within the department. Winning is the primary measure of success, and, as such, is a primary means of revenue generation. Although athletic directors are often not culprits actively committing rules violations, they ultimately will be held responsible for all rules compliance and may also be held accountable for the actions of their employees.

The situation of the athletic director is not dissimilar to that of the coach. After rules violations have been identified within a program, athletic directors may be forced to resign. As with many coaches, athletic directors, unless fired, may have little to lose from rules violations, whereas the benefits they stand to gain from winning are quite substantial.

If the aforementioned strategic analysis is accurate, it might be worth the risk for athletic directors to hire coaches who have reputations of committing the type of recruiting violations that can attract extraordinarily talented players. If those same coaches have a proven track record of winning games, selling out arenas, and attracting lucrative television contracts, the desire to hire them might be even further enhanced.

The question begs as to how could such a hiring be justified morally? Could athletic directors make a case that hiring a coach with a past record of cheating provides a greater good? Could coaches, from the standpoint of consequentialist moral theory, perhaps argue that the aforementioned goods that might accompany their hiring outweigh the fact that they are rule violators? It is hard to see how such a claim could be made in favor of hiring coaches who have acted unscrupulously in the past. The athletic directors must then consider the past of coaches when hiring them. There is a serious question as to whether a head coaching candidate with past success but also a record of unethical transgressions should be considered "the best person for the job" in any job search.

The position of athletes should also be considered when examining recruiting violations. If boosters provide prospective players with illegal inducements, it is largely the college or university that is held accountable for the transgressions. When analyzing the situation strategically, cheating boosters, much like cheating coaches and athletic directors, might have more to gain by cheating than to lose by being caught cheating. Given the lack of financial security of many players, they might believe that the risk of getting caught accepting improper gifts is worth taking.

Usually, if and when players are provided with improper cash payments, boosters and coaches make sure no one other than themselves is present to witness the transgression. As a result, players normally remain free from blame unless they come forward and incriminate themselves. If they are found to have taken money illegally, players may be suspended for a specified period but often escape more serious punishment. Teleologically, regardless of whether players are caught, these acts are still morally wrong due to the dishonesty of the behavior of the players and the boosters paying them. Furthermore, these individuals are likely not acting in an honest manner. Hence, from a deontological perspective, they are also acting unethically in accepting and offering illegal payments.

Negative Recruiting

positive recruiting: the use of honest and positive comments by a recruiter regarding his own program to persuade the prospect to join this program.

negative recruiting: the use of negative and dishonest comments by a recruiter regarding other programs that a prospect is considering to persuade the prospect to join the recruiter's program.

There are many recruiting strategies: some are positive and some are negative. **Positive recruiting** is best described as speaking honestly and positively about one's own program and the programs of others. **Negative recruiting,** on the other hand, is a concerted effort to convince players *not* to join another program by emphasizing and/or exaggerating the negative aspects of that program.

When recruiting athletes, it is ethical for coaches to honestly feature the strengths of their schools in trying to convince prospects to sign letters of intent. Strengths that may be featured include the academic reputation and social atmosphere of the school, credentials of the coaching staff, and past successes of the sport program, including the frequency at which players continue on to the professional ranks. The ethical coach will "sell" by highlighting the school and community in a persuasive yet honest manner. Additionally, to recruit in an overly persuasive manner, albeit positive, to the point where one is being dishonest is morally irresponsible and unethical behavior on the part of the coach.

What, specifically, constitutes negative recruiting, and under what conditions might it be unethical? Providing negative information about another school's program might very well be perceived as unethical. But is it ethical or unethical to provide one's honest opinion, even if it is perceived to be negative, in response to questions a recruit may ask about another program? A case can be made in support of providing any and all factual information, whether positive or negative, about any program. The teleological moral value of honesty is not being abridged, and one might argue that the best interest of the athlete is being addressed when a coach provides honest information about sports programs other than his own to prospective athletes. This question is of particular concern because the prospective recruit is attempting to make an important career choice and needs all relevant information to select a college or university that most effectively meets his or her career needs.

Although some of the questions as to what constitutes negative recruiting are debatable, others are clearly identifiable as negative. Providing false information about another college or university to persuade a recruit to attend one's school is dishonest in that it is nothing less than lying; thus, teleology is not being followed because the moral value of honesty is being disregarded. From a teleological standpoint, all information presented to recruits must be presented honestly. Furthermore, recruiters who lie in such a way are violating the moral value of trust in betraying the trust of the prospective recruit. They are choosing to lie to recruits in a manner that they would not want to be lied to, and to lie about rival schools and programs in a way they would not want to be lied about; therefore, the behavior is not supported deontologically. Hence, a coach who provides a prospective recruit with untrue information is acting unethically from both teleological and deontological perspectives.

Eligibility Issues

The NCAA, under the guidance of athletics professionals, creates academic requirements within the intercollegiate sporting environment that have implications within member institutions' academic culture. Minimum academic requirements for eligibility on admission, NCAA high school course requirements, and standards for satisfactory academic progress are academic requirements created by the NCAA that affect the lives of students who participate in athletics on college campuses.[20]

Of moral concern is when personnel within college and university athletic departments are allowed to influence academic policies. The educational institution may run the risk of compromising its academic integrity if athletic personnel influence policy in a way that serves their athletic interests. If academic policy developers take a utilitarian approach, the needs of the student body at large would, likely, be the primary focus, with concern also being taken into account for students who participate in athletics. Further inconsistencies within policy creation take place when structures developed for major universities are also applied across the board for all colleges, despite being less applicable to the missions of smaller colleges.[21]

Freshman Eligibility Advantages and Disadvantages

Should intercollegiate athletes be eligible to compete on sports teams as freshmen, or should eligibility rules be passed that require freshmen to wait until their sophomore year in college to compete? Because this issue directly relates to the welfare of athletes, their best interests should be considered throughout the decision-making process. Utilitarianism, the universal form of hedonism, calls for the best interests of athletes to be taken into account when considering the most amount of good for the most amount of people.

Making a successful transition from high school to college can be equally challenging in athletics and academics. As a result, athletes might be better off if they did not have to take on both academic and athletic challenges as new students and were allowed, instead, to spend their first year making the academic and overall transition to college life. Freshman ineligibility might provide athletes with a better foundation that would help them succeed as students as well as athletes.

In 2004, for the first time since 1972, the NCAA considered a ban on freshman eligibility. A 27-member panel examined the pros and cons of returning to the days when freshmen athletes would not be allowed to participate on the varsity team. In the end, the panel decided to continue to allow freshmen to participate in athletics on their initial entry into college. Low graduation rates of male basketball players were the focus of the discussion. The concern was that athletes are isolated from the rest of the campus and have a hard time adjusting to the general college life. A goal behind a freshman eligibility plan would be to provide athletes with a better opportunity to concentrate on their studies and integrate themselves more easily with teachers and other students who do not participate in athletics.[22]

Adjusting to such things as moving to a new town, living with a roommate, developing study skills for the rigors of college courses, and being active in university clubs and other activities are just a few of the experiences freshmen face in their first year of college. Would these and other challenges be more effectively met by freshmen if they did not also have to make the adjustment to athletics?

Former North Carolina basketball coach Dean Smith has been a longtime advocate of freshman ineligibility. Smith prefers to call an athlete's freshman year "a year in residence" and claims that it would boost graduation rates. According to Smith, freshmen athletes should be students, first and foremost, and then have the privilege to play varsity basketball.[23]

Certainly, students who do not compete in athletics have more time to adjust to their new climate and lives, but does this extra time actually help them make a smooth and successful transition from high school to college? In addition to their college-related responsibilities, students frequently must work full- or part-time jobs to help pay for their education. Are the demands of such jobs comparable to the responsibilities of athletic participation? Are working students able to adjust to having both job and additional college responsibilities? If so, then it could be argued that freshmen are also capable of making the adjustment to athletic competition while adapting to their new college responsibilities.

It might also be argued that as students become more engaged in college life, the high school-to-college transition becomes easier. One might also note that if athletes are not required to make the adjustment to athletics during their freshman year, they could establish a non-athletic lifestyle that would make their adjustments to athletic life the following year even more difficult. Thus, it could be in the best interest of athletes to make the athletic adjustment early in their careers as a freshman, because that is the lifestyle in which they will be involved throughout their college careers.

If, however, freshman participation in college sports is simply too daunting for athletes when combined with their other new responsibilities, the demands that college athletics places on them may need to be re-examined. Perhaps the overall demands on freshmen have become too overwhelming and need to be scaled down somewhat.

From a moral consequentialist's perspective, a middle-of-the-road approach might serve athletes best in this instance. By allowing athletes to practice or train during their freshman year but not compete until their sophomore seasons, administrators would allow athletes to maintain an active athletic lifestyle, yet at the same time allow them more time to adjust to being college students. Athletes might even be granted permission to travel to away games that do not conflict with their academic responsibilities, so they could experience the rigors of travel before their sophomore seasons. This middle-of-the-road approach could help freshmen adjust to college life while, to some extent, preparing them for their future lives as athletes.

Again, the best interest of the athletes is one way to decide legislation pertaining to freshman eligibility. Recall, if a decision such as freshman eligibility is made on the basis of strategic reasoning, the self-serving interest of those in the position to create academic legislation might be the driving force behind the legislation.

Graduation Rates

Moreover, in addition to the issue of freshman eligibility, the NCAA administrators might also consider re-examining the overall academic abilities of athletes. If the academic abilities of athletes are not reflective of the average abilities of students who do not participate in athletics, this may be an issue that deserves attention.

The NCAA has, in fact, developed a way to measure the academic capabilities of intercollegiate athletes, most notably those recruited for the sports of football and men's basketball. This approach involves measuring the graduation rates of athletes, especially of football and men's basketball players at the Division I level, because their rates are lower than those of athletes in other sports. The progress rate of athletes is measured on an annual basis. Athletes are expected to have completed 40% of the school's graduation requirements after 2 years, 60% after 3 years, and 80% after 4 years.[24] If a program's progress rates are subpar, they will face penalties that begin with a warning letter and can progress to reductions in scholarships, recruiting, and playing seasons.

If improvements are still not made, a post-season tournament ban may be imposed on teams, and ultimately, the NCAA may take away the school's share of conference tournament money. In certain instances, the NCAA may consider granting waivers to teams that perform below the academic standards but have a graduation rate above that of their overall student body.[25]

In the past, administrators and coaches have often only paid "lip service" to the academic interests and goals of athletes. However, with the ever-increasing emphasis that the NCAA has placed on graduation rates, athletes must take real matriculating classes that will lead to a degree. Instead of filling an athlete's schedule with fluff courses and just dropping the athlete after his or her eligibility expires, athletic programs must demonstrate legitimate academic progress on an annual basis that will, after 5 years, result in an undergraduate degree.[26]

Often, athletes at more academically select universities are poorer "academic fits," creating an incongruent relationship between academic profiles and graduation rates of athletes, which may be perceived as exploitation of athletes on the part of the university.[27] The prevailing assumption is that universities make an academic tradeoff by accepting athletes with lower academic credentials than the general student body in hopes of producing winning sports teams. This is not a new concept, as universities have used the visibility of successful athletic programs to enhance their reputations since the late 1800s.[28]

The upgraded expectations of academics in NCAA intercollegiate athletics have resulted in increased efforts by athletic programs and teams to meet those expectations. The goal is to increase graduation rates of athletes. To accomplish this and maintain eligibility through academic progress, colleges and universities have taken approaches that include investing money in academic services programs that feature team study halls and one-on-one tutoring for athletes. From an incentive perspective, coaches are being provided with "perks" if the graduation rate of athletes on their team reaches predetermined levels. For example, the University of Iowa offered their head coach a $75,000 bonus to increase graduation rates of football players at the school. The head coaches of Ohio State, Florida, Florida State, and Auburn were also offered several thousand dollars to maintain respectable graduation rates of their programs.[29]

Providing money to coaches as incentive to assure high athlete graduation rates is an extrinsic form of motivation that may lead to the best interest of athletes, thus supporting utilitarianism.

Gaining Eligibility Through Preparatory High Schools

To meet NCAA eligibility standards, some high school athletes have elected to attend preparatory schools that often operate with little or no oversight from accreditation agencies, state departments of education, or school districts. Also referred to as nontraditional high schools, some preparatory schools are primarily attended by athletes for the sole purpose of receiving the necessary grades to meet NCAA eligibility standards. A most extreme example is an unaccredited correspondence program based in Miami that reportedly had no classes or teachers, yet awarded high grades to high school athletes who enrolled in the program as seniors and went on to play college sports. The school shut down after *The New York Times* publicly examined it.[30]

Given the fact that many of the preparatory high schools in question are not regulated by an educational body, the NCAA has decided to scrutinize unusual student situations linked to such programs. Among the red flags that now draw increased scrutiny from the NCAA are schools that allow students to complete an abnormally large number of classes, allow students to take courses simultaneously that normally require an ordered sequence, and offer a disproportionate number of courses compared with the size of their faculties. In more extreme cases, a school may simply offer a diploma for a flat fee.[30] Strategic reasoning seems to be the predominate form of reasoning taking place in the previously mentioned examples. Most, if not all, of the moral values that are the foundation of teleology do not support providing courses and degrees without education.

Also found guilty by the NCAA of providing athletic eligibility through inappropriate means was Cal State Northridge. They were placed on probation by the NCAA when a NCAA panel ruled that a coach tried to arrange for a player to receive credit for a course he never took. The unscrupulous activity took place when Northridge's basketball coach persuaded assistant coaches of the baseball and volleyball teams, who taught kinesiology courses, to inappropriately give credit to an athlete. The volleyball coach agreed to the scheme and followed through by providing a copy of the final examination and an answer key to the basketball coach. The basketball coach then persuaded the volleyball coach to give the athlete an "A" to keep him eligible, according to the report of the committee.[31]

In the case of giving the athlete an "A" to keep the athlete eligible, the teleological moral value of honesty was violated because grades were fabricated and not earned. Respect for the educational system was violated, as well as respect for the student's right to gain a valid education. Fairness was also violated because it was unfair to the students who actually had to work to earn their grades.

Tutoring Athletes

In most colleges or universities, tutoring is available to the general student body, which includes athletes. At many schools, however, additional tutoring programs are provided exclusively for athletes. And, as indicated previously, many athletics departments are devoting increasing sums of money to academic-support programs. For example, the University of Texas at Austin has its own academic advisors specifically for the football team.[32]

Should academic support services be offered that are exclusive to athletes, or do such offerings constitute an unethical form of preferential treatment for athletes? Of further concern is the fact that some athletic tutoring programs have been used to keep athletes eligible rather than to assist them with their learning needs. Some sports programs might even go so far as to *require* athletes to take part in tutoring programs. Should ensuring athlete eligibility be the primary focus of tutoring programs

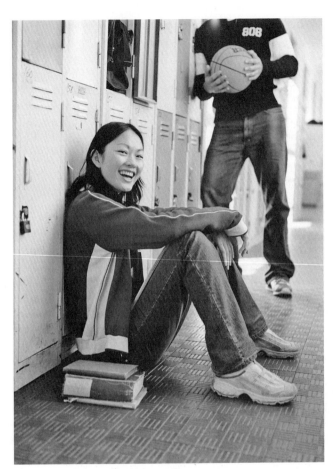

8-3 *Academic support services exclusive to athletes have been scrutinized on the basis that it is unfair not to offer the same services to non-athletes.*

for athletes? Is it unfair that college athletes are the beneficiaries of special tutoring services developed and provided exclusively for them?

The teleological moral values of fairness might be examined through several approaches. Are special tutoring services fair to the athletes and students who are not athletes? It could be argued that the provision of tutoring services is unfair to students who are not afforded the same services. On the other hand, it could also be argued that athletes are deserving of special athletic tutoring services because an athletic contest is a college-related function that often requires them to miss classes to compete.

Furthermore, although it may be easy to decry the existence of special support programs for athletes, it may be that the offering of such services is warranted. Again, one could argue that athletes are providing a service for their college by participating

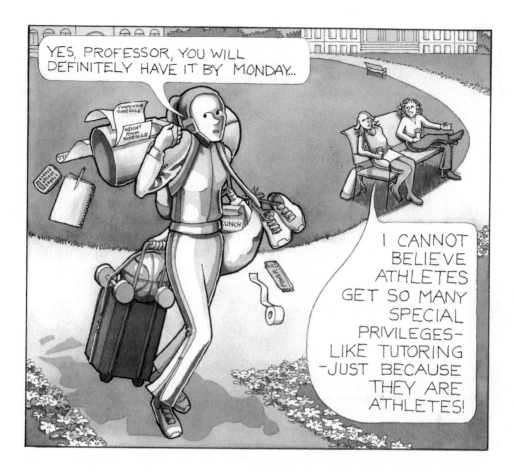

in intercollegiate athletics. Colleges may choose a strategic approach for the purpose of reaping financial benefits from their athletes' efforts but also may gain positive public relations and, arguably, increased enrollments. To serve their schools and help them garner these benefits, however, athletes must remain eligible.

The athletic demands placed on athletes hamper their efforts toward academic achievement by taking away from the amount of time they have to study. The time that athletes must use to train, practice, and participate is extensive. In a study that compared intercollegiate athletes with non-athletes, it was suggested that highly selective schools that choose to admit athletes with lower academic credentials and whose athletic programs make great time demands on these athletes need to provide the support and assistance they need once on campus. It was also found that the difficulties athletes often encounter have to do with finding time to study and achieve. Interestingly, no evidence was discovered to support what might be referred to as athlete stereotypes. Athletes were not found to be less academically ambitious, grade conscious, or interested in devoting time to study.[33] Often, athletes are unable to attend courses when traveling to and from away games, and many have trouble keeping up in their courses as a result. Because of some of the factors mentioned, it seems fair to offer athletes academic support services that may not be as readily available to the college student who is a non-athlete.

The tutoring issue is further complicated by the potential for cheating within programs. Tutoring programs that are nothing more than systematic efforts on the part of universities, coaches, and administrators to keep players eligible at all costs fly in the face of the spirit of higher education. The completion of papers, homework assignments, and take-home tests by tutors are just a few ways in which cheating can take place within tutoring programs. Carelessly monitored tutoring programs could thus become "eligibility machines" that jeopardize the integrity of athletic programs as well as colleges and universities. Under the above conditions, the moral value of respect for the academic integrity of the institution could be lost.

But should all tutoring programs for athletes be banned because cheating has been traced to a few unscrupulous tutoring programs? This action seems a bit extreme. If tutoring programs for athletes serve a worthy purpose, such as helping athletes improve necessary academic skills, it might make more sense to put measures in place to prevent cheating instead of eliminating tutoring programs entirely. If tutoring is causing the most amount of good for the most amount of people, the utilitarian would recommend keeping athletic tutoring programs yet at the same time implementing measures in an attempt to prevent morally corrupt activity. If tutoring programs are known to be allowing athletes to cheat and not meet academic competencies, consideration should be given to correcting these wrong behaviors instead of eliminating the entire tutoring program. This question of whether to ban tutoring programs because they may be calculated efforts to cheat is quite different from the question of whether tutoring programs are fair and equitable provisions for athletes. Seemingly, checks and balances to prevent cheating within such programs could be implemented in such a way that athletes would be able to gain academic benefits from them, while at the same time helping athletes to honestly maintain their eligibility.

No Pass No Play

To what extent should academic achievement be emphasized in determining the eligibility of interscholastic athletes? Requiring that athletes meet rigorous academic standards to be eligible to participate in sport might reinforce the notion that athletics are extracurricular activities. In addition, allowing athletic participation only after such academic standards have been met may be in the long-term best interest of athletes.

What role does athletics play in the pursuit of a high school education? In a 2003 study conducted by Ryska in which 235 members of high school starting teams were surveyed, it was found that the athletes, both male and female, had greater-than-average scholastic competence.[34] The strong interest athletes have in participating in sport may be used to motivate them to achieve academically. If athletes are required to reach established academic standards in the classroom to be eligible to participate in sport, they may be motivated to achieve those academic standards. In the long run, academic achievement of athletes is good for the athletes as well as society.

Eligibility Based on Residence

Is it ethical for a high school athlete to live in one location yet establish official residency in another so he or she can be eligible for athletic competition in that school district? Residents living in the zone of a particular high school are restricted to attending that particular public high school, unless they choose to pay for and attend a private school. An athlete, however, might prefer to play for a school's athletic program different from the one in his or her district. Residency rules normally allow only those living in the district to play for the school in that district.

> **residency rules:** regulations in place that provide geographical boundaries outlining the residences that are affiliated with particular school systems as well as their athletic programs; residency rules allow interscholastic athletes to only play for the athletic program in their district.

To circumvent **residency rules** that allow athletes to only play for the program in their district, athletes have established official residency with a relative in the desired district while continuing to live with their parents in their original district. This *official* but fictitious change of residence allows students to attend and play sports at the public high school of their choice even though they are not legitimately a resident of that district.

"Attracting Players by Providing Parents With Jobs"

The baseball coaches at Eastside High School had just finished a dismal season, and no one was looking forward to their annual end of the year meeting among the coaching staff. The head coach, Coach Weary, assured his assistants that he would not spend more than 30 minutes meeting because his message and future plans were short and simple. At the beginning of the meeting, Coach Weary started by saying that he was so sick and tired of losing that he was ready to implement a plan that would never allow for another losing season. Now having gained his staff's full attention, Coach Weary said, "Thank goodness for the new automobile plant that will be part of our community next year. As a staff, beginning today, we will track the top 50 players in the area and contact their parents to offer them a job at the new automobile plant. If they are skilled laborers, managers, or willing to put in some time, we can find them work and make sure they are paid handsomely. Of course, their son will have to move into our school system and play baseball for us. Finally, our losing days will be over."

Questions

1. Is it ethical on the part of Coach Weary to persuade/recruit players outside of Eastside High's district lines to relocate by providing their parents with jobs?
2. Is Coach Weary's plan in the best interest of the players? parents? opposing teams? coaches? Eastside High School?
3. Is Coach Weary's plan to acquire players a fair one?

Athletes might be influenced to establish residency outside their district for many reasons. A winning tradition of a sports program, the opportunity for increased media exposure for the purpose of gaining a college scholarship, and the opportunity to play for a renown coach all might be reasons that draw an athlete to a school. Sometimes, coaches might even persuade a player to officially change residency by offering him or her cash.

Such actions violate the spirit of public interscholastic athletics' residency rules. In theory, the zoning of districts might have an overall effect on the level of competition within areas. If zones encompass populations similar in number, the talent pool of athletes within zones should be somewhat equal over time. If, however, players circumvent the residency rule and the zoning process, a system of haves and have-nots might result that would make for a disproportionate distribution of talent among teams. Such unequal distributions of talent might make for less competitive environments and take away from the interest in particular sports.

Is it fair that athletes are restricted from participating on sports teams other than the ones located in their home district? If athletes are talented enough, why should they be prevented from participating on strong sports teams in districts other than the one in which they live?

From a teleological perspective, breaking or circumventing residency rules violates the moral value of honesty. Unless a person is actually living within the boundaries assigned to the district in which she is participating in athletics, she is violating the moral value of honesty. The moral values of fairness and respect are also being violated. Intentionally breaking the residency rule is a display of disrespect for the rule and the process under which the rules were established. Breaking residency rules is often done for self-serving purposes and is unfair to those who are following the rules. If all persons involved in a league broke the rules, leagues might experience instability, with players moving from one team to another by changing their address at a moment's notice. From a stability perspective, it seems to not be in the best interest of the league to allow players to live in a district yet play in another district of their choosing. Thus, deontology does not support the circumvention of residency rules because it is unfair and not something that coaches and players would be willing to apply universally to each team.

One should keep in mind that athletics differs from academics in that it operates under a competitively based performance structure, which, in essence, means that no matter the circumstances, one team will win and another will lose. In academics, usually specific standards are established for achievement that allow all students the opportunity to score at the highest levels on such academic measures as standardized tests and homework assignments. Although standards exist in athletics, teams that consist of highly talented players usually achieve success in the form of winning. Given the impact of talented players on winning, special guidelines such as residency rules are necessary to help keep the playing field level in public high school sports.

Homeschooling and Sport

In 2003, there were more than 1.1 million youths homeschooled in the United States, up from 850,000 in 1999.[35] One report estimated that 2.5 million people were being homeschooled in 2005.[36] With this growth in popularity, the practice of homeschooling, in itself controversial, has also raised new ethical questions related to sport.[35] Should students be allowed to participate on the local high school sports teams if they are being homeschooled? For athletes to be eligible to play for a particular public high school, they must not only reside within the boundaries established for that particular school, but they must also be enrolled in and perform at acceptable levels within a formal academic curriculum at that school. Should these reasons prevent homeschooled students from participating on school-based sports teams?

To answer these questions, the broader question of the academic legitimacy of homeschooling must also be answered. If a goal of interscholastic education is to attain state learning outcomes, does the process by which one achieves those learning outcomes matter? Public school education might be looked on not only as a state mandate, but as a service provided by the state through tax payer dollars. If parents prefer to assume the finances and burden of **homeschooling** and if the homeschooled students demonstrate acceptable learning outcomes, then homeschooling might appear to be an acceptable educational teaching practice.

> **homeschooling:** educating a student from his or her home instead of from a traditional classroom in a school building.

However, whereas students might be able to effectively gain the benefits and achieve learning outcomes related to academic content areas such as math or science through homeschooling, it is not possible to gain the benefits of organized sport competition within the home. Students must join teams in organized competitive leagues to reap benefits that come from learning to compete and to cooperate with teammates in pursuit of a common goal. Some fitness and recreation-related centers have recognized the homeschooled population as a target market for fitness-related activities. Centers have designed programs with a focus on socialization that include making new friends and having fun.[36]

However, despite these fitness and sport alternatives, the question arises as to whether homeschooled students residing in a particular school zone should be eligible to participate on a sport teams at that school. It has been pointed out that participation in sports provides a necessary socialization aspect for some homeschoolers.[37] If the participation in sport does provide a necessary component of socialization, should districts allow homeschooled students to gain such socialization through sport? And, should all students residing in the district be eligible to participate on the school's sports teams, even those receiving their education at home?

In addition to these issues, the potential for exploitation in the area of athletic eligibility is also a concern. Might homeschooling be a convenient way to circumvent interscholastic eligibility rules? Can parents be trusted to record valid grades for their own children? More specifically, is the homeschooling environment more conducive to academic fraud? Does homeschooling provide the type of structured learning environment necessary to prevent cheating?

When establishing eligibility standards for those enrolled in public schools, how should the homeschooled student be evaluated? As of this writing, the NCAA has given homeschoolers equal status with traditional students and streamlined their access to its academic eligibility clearinghouse. In other words, courses taught at home by parents are acceptable, much in the same way as courses taught in traditional high schools by certified teachers.[35] However, increased academic oversight of homeschooling is being proposed in the form of curriculum approval, instructor credentials standards, academic progress review, and/or standardized testing.[36]

On the other hand, nothing is in place in traditional schools to completely prevent teachers from dismissing standards by doing the same things that may take place in homeschooling. For example, teachers in traditional classroom environments can also give inflated grades to undeserving students; not teach the curriculum that, in part, is necessary to receive program accreditation; and inadequately teach the course materials, despite having outstanding credentials in the form of multiple degrees, while still allowing students to reach learning outcomes.

Arguments, however, can be made against homeschooling as a legitimate means of educating and reaching equal learning outcomes as traditional schools. If marking period grade point averages are included as part of the assessment criteria used to determine academic eligibility, can the same measures be used to determine the eligibility of a homeschooled high school athlete? What if parents elect to use non-traditional methods of evaluation that do not facilitate the calculation of grade point averages? How could homeschooled students be evaluated under such circumstances?

"Achieving Eligibility the Nontraditional Way"

Sam is an outstanding player with aspirations to play sports in college but is worried that his grades will not be good enough. The athletic director of his high school encouraged Sam by telling him that if he completes all of his homework assignments and studies hard for his tests, he should make the necessary grades to be eligible to play college sports. Sam's athletic director also assured him that if studying hard and completing his homework does not work, he can improve his grades by going to a nontraditional preparatory school. Furthermore, Sam's athletic director told him that if preparatory school does not work, arrangements can be made for his own parents to homeschool him. Sam's athletic director finally said: "All I know for sure, Sam, is that we will make sure you are eligible to play sports in college next year." Sam, not being familiar with the nontraditional preparatory school or the concept of homeschooling, is more confused now than before he began the conversation with his athletic director. Sam cannot understand why there are ways outside of the traditional high school to gain eligibility to play sports in college.

"Achieving Eligibility the Nontraditional Way" (*Continued*)

Questions

1. Do you agree with preparatory schools, correspondence courses, and home-schooling as ways to achieve and maintain eligibility for athletes? Explain.
2. Was the athletic director or "the system" exploiting Sam in that he was provided with various opportunities to become eligible for college athletics? Explain.
3. In this case, were those who developed and participated in preparatory schools and homeschooling betraying the integrity of education by doing so? Explain.

If the integrity of homeschooling as an effective method of teaching is to be maintained, then serious efforts should be made to answer these and other questions concerning the athletic eligibility of homeschooled students. Strategies must be examined to structure homeschooling in a way that does not permit exploitation, such as padded grades or unmet learning objectives.

Exploitation can also take place in a different context. Athletes who are being homeschooled for the purpose of taking a route of less resistance to gain eligibility are exploited in that they do not gain a legitimate education because they do not have to meet the same criteria as those in the public school. Furthermore, there are many criticisms concerning the legitimacy of the athletic eligibility standards currently in place within public school systems. Instead of dismissing homeschooling because of the *potential* for wrongdoing, administrators should consider weighing potential negatives against the overall benefits of allowing homeschooling students to participate on public school sport teams. If, for eligibility purposes, homeschooling is exploited, measures should be taken to correct it.

Discussion should ensue as to whether moral values of teleology such as fairness, honesty, respect, and compassion are enmeshed in homeschooling and athletic eligibility issues associated with homeschooling. After teleological moral theory is addressed and necessary moral values are found to be a part of homeschooling and athletic eligibility, deontological moral theory might also be addressed. If homeschooling is grounded in teleology, it might be more readily universalized to all students and athletic programs; hence, it would be supported by deontological moral theory.

Conclusion

Many ethical issues have arisen in intercollegiate and interscholastic athletics over the years. Several of these are complex in that their resolution requires that educational, ethical, and strategic concerns all be considered as parts of the decision-making process. Coaches and administrators, thus, must decide which of these elements will take precedence over others. Although academic concerns seem to generally take moral precedence over athletic interests, the strategic temptation is strong to reverse these priorities when wins and profits are on the line. Coaches and administrators must figure out how to balance their ethical responsibilities to their athletes and schools with the expectations that they will produce winning teams. This difficult task warrants special attention if the contexts of intercollegiate and interscholastic sport are to demonstrate moral as well as athletic excellence.

References

1. History of the NCAA. NCAA Web site. Available at: http://www.ncaa.org/about/history.html. Accessed May 29, 2007.
2. Making college affordable. *University Business.* June 2004;7(6):58.
3. Wieberg S, Whiteside K. Why bigger is better at Ohio State; January 23, 2007. *USA Today* Web site. Available at: http://www.usatoday.com/sports/college/2007-01-04-ohiostate-finances-cover_x.htm. Accessed May 29, 2007.
4. Suggs W. Big money in college sports flows to the few. *Chronicle of Higher Education.* 2004;51(10):A46–A47.
5. Clarke CV. Too young to go pro? *Black Enterprise.* 2005;36(2):142–146.
6. NBA, NBPA reach agreement in principle on new collective bargaining agreement; June 22, 2005. Available at: http://www.nba.com/news/cba_050621.html. Accessed May 17, 2008.
7. Rupp A. $10M donation to Indiana big boost for non-revenue sports. *USA Today* Web site. July 13, 2005. Available at: http://www.usatoday.com/sports/college/other/2005-07-13-indiana-donation_x.htm?csp=34. Accessed September 6, 2006.
8. Suggs W. NCAA creates panel to review its governance structure. *Chronicle of Higher Education.* 2001;47(25):A44.
9. Ratto R. Paperwork a formality for Coach K. ESPN Web site. November 15, 2001. Available at: http://sports.espn.go.com/columns/ratto_ray/1278554.html. Accessed September 6, 2006.
10. Gehring J. H.S. Athletics out of bounds, report warns. *Education Week.* 2004;24(9): 1,18,19.
11. Cherner R. College hoops' biggest winner. December 26, 2005. *USA Today* Web site. Available at: http://www.usatoday.com/sports/college/mensbasketball/2005-12-26-statham-record_x.htm. Accessed September 5, 2006.
12. Associated Press. Dixie State football coach fired. *Community College Week.* February 27, 2006:11.
13. Associated Press. Reform panel hears reports of widespread corruption. ESPN Web site. January 30, 2006. Available at: http://sports.espn.go.com/espn/news/story?id=2312683&campaign=rss&surce=NCBHeadlines. Accessed September 5, 2006.
14. Associated Press. Brown gets salary boost after leading Texas to national title. *USA Today* Web site. January 29, 2006. Available at: http://www.usatoday.com/sports/college/football/big12/2006-01-29-texas-brown-raise_x.htm?POE=SPOISVA. Accessed September 5, 2006.

15. Associated Press. Ohio State's Tressel to make almost $2.4 million this season. *USA Today* Web site. May 18, 2006. Available at: http://www.usatoday.com/sports/college/foot-ball/bigten/2006-05-18-ohiost-tressel_x.htm. Accessed September 5, 2006.

16. Moore CJ. Mangino's contract increases expectations. *Kansan* Web site. September 5, 2006. Available at: http://www.kansan.com/stories/2006/sep/05/contract/?print. Accessed September 5, 2006.

17. College town grapples with recruiting scandal. February 18, 2004. CNN Web site. Available at: http://www.cnn.com/2004/US/Central/02/18/university.assault.case.ap/index.html. Accessed May 29, 2007.

18. 2006–07 NCAA postseason football finances. NCAA Web site. Available at: http://www1.ncaa.org/membership/postseason_football/finances. Accessed May 31, 2007.

19. Cannella S. Slime and punishment. *Sports Illustrated*. 2006;105(6):16–17.

20. Academics and athletics. NCAA Web site. Available at: http://www.ncaa.org/wps/por-tal. Accessed May 31, 2007.

21. ASHE Higher Education Report. *The Athletics System in Higher Education*. 2005;30(5): 15–35.

22. Conrad M. NCAA to consider ban on freshman basketball eligibility. WRAL Web site. June 10, 1999. Available at: http://sportslawnews.com/archive/articles%201999/NCAAban.html. Accessed September 5, 2006.

23. Carlson K. Former UNC basketball coach calls for freshman ineligibility. WRAL Web site. 2004. Available at: http://www.wral.com/news/2815738/detail.html. Accessed September 5, 2006.

24. Beland J. NCAA board approves athletics reform. *Academe*. 2004;90(5):13.

25. Associated Press. NCAA says bad grades could cost schools plenty. ESPN Web site. August 2, 2006. Available at: http://sports.espn.go.com/ncaa/news/story?id=2537617. Accessed September 5, 2006.

26. Holsendolph E. When academics and athletics collide. *Diverse: Issues in Higher Education*. 2006;23(4):22–23.

27. Ferris E, Finster M, McDonald D. Academic fit of student-athletes: an analysis of NCAA division I-A graduation rates. *Research in Higher Education*. 2004;45(6):555–575.

28. The rise of intercollegiate football and its portrayal in American popular literature. The University of Georgia Web site. Available at: http://www.uga.edu/honors/curo/juro/2001_10_13/Turano6.html. Accessed May 31, 2007.

29. Fish M. College football coaching contracts filled with lucrative incentives. *Sports Illustrated* Web site. December 23, 2005. Available at: http://sportsillustrated.cnn.com/2003/writers/mike_fish/12/19/coaching.contracts/index.html. Accessed September 5, 2006.

30. Trotter A. NCAA boosts scrutiny of 'nontraditional' high school. *Education Week*. 2006;25(36):5.

31. Suggs W. NCAA penalizes Cal State at Northridge for academic fraud. *Chronicle of Higher Education*. 2004;50(32):A37.

32. Wolverton B. Making the grade. *Chronicle of Higher Education*. 2006;52(27):A36.

33. Aries E, McCarthy D, Salovey P, Banaji MR. A comparison of athletes and non-athletes at highly selective colleges: academic performance and personal development. *Research in Higher Education*. 2004;45(6):577–602.

34. Ryska TA. Sport involvement and perceived scholastic competence in student-athletes: a multivariate analysis. *International Sports Journal.* 2003;7(1):155–171.

35. Ruibal S. Elite take home-school route. *USA Today* Web site. June 7, 2005. Available at: http://www.usatoday.com/sports/preps/2005-06-07-home-school-cover_x.htm. Accessed September 8, 2006.

36. Roberts L. How to develop a recreation activity program for homeschoolers. *Parks and Recreation.* September 2005;40(9):112–115.

37. Romanowski MH. Revisiting the common myths about homeschooling. *The Clearinghouse.* 2006;79(3):125–129.

Tragedy at the Post-Game Party

Alcohol use among high school athletes is a problem that has existed for a long time at the small, rural Farmtown High School. Although eligibility policies exist and students are required to sign a contract at the beginning of each season acknowledging their understanding of them, the policies do not always deter students from drinking.

Substance abuse policies vary from school to school in the area, but are basically quite similar, with game suspensions as well as alcohol and substance abuse counseling being the primary consequences. Coaches at Farmtown High School are responsible for the enforcement of these policies and, at their discretion, have the option of making the penalties stricter.

For the first time in many years, Farmtown High School's substance abuse policies had to be enforced when students were found to be drinking at a post-prom party last year. This drinking incident resulted in the suspension of several student-athletes, which adversely affected the seasons of the baseball and softball teams.

Before the next year's girls' basketball season began, the varsity coach, Coach Needer, spent a considerable amount of time and effort making sure that his players would not drink during the sport season again. At a pre-season meeting with the girls, Coach Needer emphasized his zero-tolerance policy that included doubling any school-imposed penalty for violators.

Coach Needer has been a guidance counselor at Farmtown High School for over 30 years and has coached the girls' varsity basketball team for the past 15 years without having a losing season. Additionally, during this time, his teams have won league, sectional, district, regional, and state championships. This year, Coach Needer was expecting nothing less than an undefeated season ending in a state championship.

At the end of the first week of games, the team won their annual Tip-Off Tournament in a thrilling, hard-fought contest. After the game, the coaches went out for their usual post-game drinks and appetizers and talked about the game and the team. The coaches always drink responsibly at these post-game gatherings.

The players also decided to celebrate the victory with drinks, but not responsibly. One of the boy's basketball players, Tom, threw a party at his house because his parents were out of town. After a couple of other boys obtained and stocked Tom's house with alcohol, the stage was set for an evening that ultimately ended in tragedy.

Four players from the girls' team, six players from the boys' team, and many other Farmtown High School students were at the party. It did not take long for most of the persons at the party to become quite intoxicated. In an effort to behave responsibly, Ray, one of the boys' team members at the party, called his friend Jill, who was a member of the girls' team and was at home rather than at the party. Ray explained to Jill that he was too drunk to drive and needed a ride home. Jill, wanting to help, arrived at the party with her friend Kerry, who would be the designated driver. After "hanging out" at the party for a few minutes, without drinking, Kerry prepared to drive Ray home.

As Kerry began to slowly back out of the driveaway, Warren, a friend of Ray's, was leaning, from the outside, in the passenger window trying to convince Ray to stay. As Warren was talking, he slipped and his entire body fell underneath the car. Kerry continued to back down the driveway and unknowingly drove over Warren's abdomen. Warren later died at a local hospital as a result of internal injuries.

Coach Needer, the school's only guidance counselor, was extremely involved with the situation that followed. Needer spent significant time counseling his players, family members and friends of the players, and the entire student body. Nothing, however, could heal the severe pain felt throughout the community and the school as a result of Warren's death.

Following several days of counseling, the school administration decided it was time to discuss eligibility issues related to this tragedy. As a first step, a committee was formed to review and discuss the eligibility consequences established by the written policy, which could be modified at the committee's discretion.

Coach Needer believed he should have been part of the committee, but was not included. The decision from the committee was to suspend the first-time offenders for four games and to require them to attend alcohol counseling. Any athletes who had attended the party—drinking or not—were considered at least first-time offenders. Second-time offenders—a group that included almost everyone caught drinking after the prom last year—were suspended for eight games.

Coach Needer now stood to lose six of his 13 players, three of whom were starters, for a significant number of games. In addition, if Coach Needer enforced his own penalty of doubling the school's punishment, the team's chance of winning any championships would be highly unlikely. In the end, Coach Needer decided not to double the suspension, because the students were suffering enough with the loss of a close friend. Coach Needer also believed that the penalty was too harsh for the two girls who only came to pick up their drunk friend.

Coach Needer stated that he has always told students, in his role as guidance counselor, that friends do not let friends drive drunk, and he believed they should not have been punished as severely as those who were at the party and drinking. Some saw this decision, however, as controversial, because these girls also happened to be the two best players on his team.

Critical Thinking: Finding Common-Sense Solutions

1. If you were a teacher that was a member of the committee formed to determine appropriate consequences for those involved in the party and the accident, would you have banned Coach/Guidance Counselor Needer from being a member of the committee? Why or why not?

2. If you were Coach Needer, would you have enforced the double penalty rule that you created? Why or why not?

3. Given the role that alcohol played in this tragedy, if you were one of the coaches, would you continue to celebrate victories over a couple of drinks at local establishments where parents and athletes may also be present? Why or why not?

4. If you were the athletic director, would you consider making changes to the current substance abuse policies because they did not prove to be effective in this instance? Why or why not? If so, what changes would you make?

Critical Thinking: Moral Theory-Based Decision Making

5. Using the *deontological theory* to guide your reasoning, what decisions regarding the eligibility of Jill and Kerry would you make as the leader of the eligibility committee? What decisions would you make concerning the other girls' basketball team players at the party? Explain how your decisions are grounded in the *deontological theory*.

6. Using *teleological moral* theory to guide your reasoning as a coach, which moral values would you emphasize in making decisions regarding penalties for Jill, Kerry, and the other girls' basketball team players at the party?

Tom's Dilemma Over Wrestling Injured

The College Athletic Association (CAA) has grown into a powerful organization that has over 1200 members, consisting of nearly every college and university across the country. Major football and men's basketball teams bring in millions of dollars each year to many of the high-profile intercollegiate athletic programs throughout the nation. Although football and men's basketball are the two primary revenue-generating sports for major intercollegiate athletic departments, wrestling is the breadwinner of the athletic department at Fracas University.

For nearly 30 years, the head wrestling coach at Fracas University, Chuck Champeen, has enjoyed overwhelming success. Coach Champeen has coached 12 Eastern Seaboard Conference (ESC) Championship teams, nine national champion wrestlers, and 31 All-American wrestlers. Entering this season, Fracas University was the two-time defending ESC wrestling champion and was expected to challenge for a third consecutive championship.

As the season progressed through January, Coach Champeen's team was winning with ease and everything was going as planned until Fracas University's best wrestler, Tom Tussle, went down with an injury. Tom suffered a tear of the ulnar collateral ligament (UCL) in his right thumb, a condition in athletic training known as "gamekeeper's thumb." Although Tom was able to withstand the pain and finish his match, his participation in the remaining 4 weeks of the regular season, the ESC Championship, and the national tournament was in serious jeopardy.

The next day, the team physician explained to Tom that the UCL injury was a clean and complete tear and was in need of a special surgical procedure to repair the ligament. The physician explained further that if Tom was willing to put off surgery for a 4- to 6-week period, he would be able to continue his wrestling season with the assistance of a custom-made Orthoplast splint. In putting off surgery, however, the ligament would only return to 75% of its original strength. Alternatively, if Tom chose to end his wrestling season and have surgery on the thumb immediately, his thumb would regain 100% of its original strength and effectiveness. As one can see, Tom has numerous things to consider when deciding whether to continue his wrestling season.

Others close to the situation have their views and opinions as well. Coach Champeen, desperately wanting to win another national championship, wants Tom to wrestle. Concerned for Tom's health and welfare, Tom's parents want him to immediately undergo the surgery and forget about the rest of the season. Tom's teammates want him to wrestle because they believe the risk and sacrifice are a small price to pay for another championship. Instead of telling Tom what to do, the athletic trainer has outlined the pros and cons associated with the injury and is leaving Tom with the final decision.

Throughout his wrestling career, Tom has always placed the highest priority on meeting his personal goals. Despite only being a sophomore at the time of this injury, Tom barely missed being an All-American his freshman year. He really wanted to attain All-American status this year, and perhaps challenge to be a national champion. Tom knows that if he succumbs to this injury, he will have only two remaining years of eligibility to reach his goals.

Critical Thinking: Finding Common-Sense Solutions

1. If you were Tom's teammate and he chose not to wrestle, how would you respond to him and why?

2. If you were Coach Champeen, how would you respond to Tom if he chose to participate? If he chose not to participate? Explain your reasoning.

3. If you were the team physician, would you take a stance regarding whether Tom should continue to wrestle? Why or why not?

4. If you were the athletic director at Fracas University, would you assume the position that Tom has a responsibility to continue to wrestle for Fracus because he is on a full scholarship? Why or why not?

Critical Thinking: Moral Theory-Based Decision Making

5. Using the *consequentialist theory* as the foundation for your reasoning, would you continue to wrestle if you were Tom? Why or why not?

6. If you were Coach Champeen and were reasoning *egoistically*, could you make a case to support winning over Tom's welfare? Why or why not? Could you make the same case as the athletic trainer, team physician, Tom, and Tom's parents? Why or why not?

7. From the following moral values, select and describe the ones that you would emphasize as Tom's parents in deciding whether he should wrestle: *fairness, compassion, responsibility, beneficence,* and *loyalty*.

Academic Support Services Investigation at Hoops University

Hoops University is a Division I school that is the home of a very successful men's basketball program, currently coached by Coach Winner. Coach Winner's teams have advanced to the *Sweet 16* each of the past two years despite losing some star players to academic ineligibility. This year's team returns every starter from the previous two seasons, which makes the goal of winning a national championship realistic.

The athletic director of Hoops University and Coach Winner have a long-standing relationship, going back to the time they played on the same national championship college basketball team. Both realize the strong potential of this year's team. In fact, Coach Winner has gone so far as to postpone his planned retirement, because he believes this team is capable of winning a national championship.

Also instrumental in Coach Winner's commitment of at least one more year is the fact that a new academic support system has been formed and implemented for the athletic department.

In the past, Coach Winner blamed poor academic performance of his players on the lack of qualified tutors that were available at the student support center on campus. Winner has said that, "The lack of competent tutors at Hoops University has cost me at least two final four appearances and maybe even a national championship."

Because the athletic department operates the new academic support system, it is that department who is responsible for hiring the tutors. Mrs. Tutor, the office assistant, is the director of the tutoring program and takes on the responsibilities of scheduling tutoring times, monitoring the progress of the players, and keeping Coach Winner informed as to the academic status of his basketball players. Mrs. Tutor also makes sure that the players' take-home tests and papers are completed and submitted to their professors on time. A very bright, organized, and helpful person, Mrs. Tutor happens to be the daughter of the athletic director.

As a result of the new academic program, the basketball players' academic performance improved dramatically. The most noticeable indicator of this improvement is the significant increase in the men's basketball team grade point average.

This unusually strong academic performance has also caught the attention of the president of Hoops University. Although the president is excited about the team's performance on the court, he has heard anonymous reports that the academic support team has committed academically fraudulent acts favoring the men's basketball team. Adding credence to the rumors is the fact that the football team did not experience the same level of academic improvement as the basketball team. In fact, the football team had several academically ineligible players, whereas the basketball team had none.

The president's suspicions were now to the point where he felt compelled to find out more about the "overnight" academic improvement of the men's basketball team. Because of the inconsistent academic performances of the football and men's basketball teams and the accusations of academic fraud against the latter, the president decided to conduct an internal investigation of Mrs. Tutor and her academic support system. Fearing the worst from this internal investigation, Mrs. Tutor submitted her resignation as head tutor for athletics.

Critical Thinking: Finding Common-Sense Solutions

1. As the athletic director, would you have responded in any way after noticing the "overnight" increase in the men's basketball grade point average? If so, how?

2. Given the available evidence, would you have called for an internal investigation if you were the president? Why or why not?

3. If you were one of the tutors at Hoops University, what level of help would you believe to be appropriate from a tutor? For example, where would you "draw the line" between assisting an athlete with a paper and writing the paper for the athlete?

4. If you were Mrs. Tutor, what measures would you have taken to prevent academic fraud from taking place within the academic support services program?

Critical Thinking: Moral Theory-Based Decision Making

5. Do you believe it was *fair* for Coach Winner to blame past poor academic performances of his basketball players on Hoops University's academic support services? Why or why not?

6. Is it in everyone's *best interest* that the president called for and is conducting an internal investigation? Explain why or why not.

7. Using *deontological theory* as a basis, what actions would you have taken as athletic director, if any, based on the rumors of fraudulent activity favoring the men's basketball team?

The Back-Stabbing Assistant Coach

As a member of Competition College's (CC) women's lacrosse coaching staff this past season, Coach Victim found herself the victim of lies and untrue rumors. The stress she felt as a result of this experience was magnified because she was a first-year assistant coach attempting to keep up with her many responsibilities during the beginning of the conditioning phase of the season.

In an effort to reduce the workload for her and the other assistant, the head coach, Coach Delegator, hired a third assistant coach, Coach Sneaky. Coach Delegator carefully created and outlined responsibilities for his three assistant coaches to perform. These duties included such things as running drills in practices, meeting with players to discuss their concerns, and monitoring their grades.

During the conditioning season, the coaching staff met several times to make sure duties were being fulfilled in the most efficient and effective ways possible. Practice plans were designed daily and were based on specific goals to be met by specific deadlines. During these meetings, Coach Victim often got the feeling that Coach Sneaky may not have been thinking along the same lines as the rest of the coaching staff.

Coach Sneaky seemed to frequently misrepresent what was said in meetings. For example, once when Coach Victim stated in a meeting that the team did not have the speed to run an up-tempo offense, Coach Sneaky told several players that Coach Victim referred to them as lazy and that she did not believe in them. As a result of such misrepresentations, a growing environment of distrust was building against Coach Victim, but was also present, to a lesser degree, among all the coaches and the team. Coach Sneaky seemed to be pitting coaches against coaches, players against coaches, and even players against players.

As the first week of actual practice began, athletes were continually approaching Coach Victim about negative rumors they heard concerning her, them, and the team. It was evident that even though the regular season had just begun, they were not together as a team. As a result of this poor team cohesion, Coach Victim became very upset.

According to Coach Delegator, there had been no problems related to the spreading of false rumors and lies or cohesion on his teams over the past 2 or 3 years. In fact, Coach Delegator's teams had a reputation of getting along well, working well together, and having strong team unity.

Finally, about five practice days into the season, team morale hit rock bottom as their mistrust and inability to function as a team increased. Players were upset to the point of apathy and began to disclose information from any and all conversations in which they had been involved. As more and more information was brought forward, it became clear that Coach Sneaky was the person fully responsible for creating the dissent that had overtaken the team. After a players-only team meeting, the captains delivered the news back to Coach Delegator, telling him the details of Coach Sneaky's lies and false rumors and how he communicated them (phone, e-mail, or in person). The number of lies told by Coach Sneaky that surfaced was astounding. One of the most disrupting things that came to be known was that Coach Sneaky manipulated the youngest kids on the team into believing that Coach Victim and the other assistant were "out to get them."

Critical Thinking: Finding Common-Sense Solutions

1. If you were the head coach, what would you do with Coach Sneaky on learning the facts? Would you fire him? Why or why not?

2. In deciding whether to fire Coach Sneaky, to what extent would you consider the additional workload that would be placed on the other assistants?

3. What factors would you consider when deciding what actions to take as you try and bring the team "back together?"

4. Should the hiring and firing of assistant coaches lie solely in the hands of head coaches, or should the administration be involved in the process as well? Explain.

Critical Thinking: Moral Theory-Based Decision Making

5. What preventative measures should be put in place so a similar situation does not occur again? Using *consequentialist moral theory*, describe how you would resolve the above situation. How would you include the "best interest of others" in your reasoning when arriving at a decision concerning whether Coach Sneaky should be fired?

6. From the list of moral values below, choose one and discuss how it would help you resolve the issue of how to deal with Coach Sneaky: *justice, honesty, respect,* and *compassion.*

Revoking of Max's College Basketball Scholarship

Max, a senior at Diamond High School, is an All-American high school basketball player being recruited by major Division I colleges and universities. At 41.3 points per game, 9.2 rebounds, and 8.3 assists per game, Max is one of the most sought-after players in the country. Max's future has all the makings of fortune and fame as a basketball phenom.

Since childhood, Max has dreamed of playing at Northern Avon University, which is one of the top programs in the country, coached by one of the top coaches in the country, Luther Legend. Last week, when Coach Legend and members of the Northern Avon University basketball team arrived at Diamond High School to watch Max play, Max was "up" for the occasion and scored a school record 67 points. Impressed with the performance, Coach Legend made Max's lifetime dream a reality the next day, when he offered him a scholarship and Max accepted, agreeing to play for Northern Avon University for the next 4 years.

Unfortunately, as quickly as Max's dream of playing for Northern Avon University seemed to be coming true, it turned into a nightmare. Three days after signing the letter of intent, Max was one of 24 area students arrested during a major drug raid by local authorities. Max was charged with four drug-related felonies: two counts of possession with intent to sell and deliver marijuana; one count of sale and delivery of marijuana; and one count of sale, possession, and delivery of a controlled substance on school grounds. The raid took place after weeks of gathering evidence by undercover officers at Diamond High School.

The "fall out" from Max's arrest was significant. The administration at Diamond High School immediately suspended Max from the team for the rest of the season, and the local judge placed Max on probation while at the same time sentencing him to community service. But, most hurtful was the action that Coach Legend took. After thinking long and hard, Coach Legend decided to revoke Max's scholarship to play for Northern Avon University.

Heartbroken and worried that his basketball career might be over, Max was determined to "make good" on any second chance that might come his way. However, the only major college coach that expressed an interest in Max, after his arrest, was Santana State University's Eric Yearning. Before offering Max a scholarship though, Coach Yearning decided to take it upon himself to learn first hand, from persons close to Max, more about Max's character and the charges filed against Max. Through lengthy and thorough discussions, Max's coaches, teachers, and high school administrators, as well as his family and friends, portrayed Max as a respectful and decent person who had made some bad choices.

Coach Yearning was pleased to hear the many positive comments regarding Max. But, given the very serious charges against Max, Coach Yearning is still undecided as to whether he will offer Max a scholarship.

Critical Thinking: Finding Common-Sense Solutions

1. If you were Coach Legend, would you have revoked Max's scholarship? Why or why not?

2. If you were Coach Yearning, when deciding whether to offer Max a scholarship to Santanta State University, would Max's extraordinary basketball abilities be reason enough to overlook his criminal charges? Why or why not?

3. If you were Max, would you have approved of Coach Yearning researching your personal life? Why or why not?

Critical Thinking: Moral Theory-Based Decision Making

4. Having learned of Max's criminal charges, if you were the athletic director at Diamond High School, when applying the *teleological theory*, which of the following moral values would you emphasize when deciding what to do with Max: *justice, fairness, honesty,* and *respect*? How so?

5. If you were Coach Yearning, when deciding what is *good for Max* versus what is *good for others*—including the fans at Santana State University, the team at Santana State University, and Max's friends and family—would you have offered Max a scholarship? Explain your reasoning.

6. If you were Coach Yearning, do you believe you would be *betraying the integrity of the sport* of basketball by offering Max a scholarship? Why or why not?

Key Terms

death penalty—in NCAA athletics, a ban on a member institution's entire sports program for gross rules violations within the program. In 1987, Southern Methodist University's football program was issued the "death penalty" as their entire season was cancelled for violating NCAA rules.

homeschooling—educating a student from his or her home instead of from a traditional classroom in a school building.

improper inducements (to players)—inappropriate recruiting efforts that are against the rules; attempts by college athletic personnel—including but not limited to coaches, administrators, staff, or boosters—to improperly persuade prospects/players to attend a college or university and play on one of its sports teams by offering prospects such appealing items as cars, cash, and luxurious off-campus living accommodations.

mission statements—statements drafted by organizations (i.e., a university or sport department) to define their core purpose: why they exist, their reason for being; the declaration of values, goals, and aspirations that authoritative groups agree upon as describing the central unique mission of the organization.

negative recruiting—the use of negative and dishonest comments by a recruiter regarding other programs that a prospect is considering to persuade the prospect to join the recruiter's program.

positive recruiting—the use of honest and positive comments by a recruiter regarding his own program to persuade the prospect to join this program.

recruiting violations—breaking rules (usually NCAA) that are put into place to provide coaches fair and equal opportunities to attract and persuade prospective athletes to enroll in their colleges and play on their sports teams.

residency rules—regulations in place that provide geographical boundaries outlining the residences that are affiliated with particular school systems as well as their athletic programs; residency rules allow interscholastic athletes to only play for the athletic program in their district.

revenue-generating athletes—intercollegiate players on sports teams that make money, primarily through gate receipts and television contracts, for their athletic department and college or university; football, men's basketball, and sometimes women's basketball at major universities are normally the sports in which revenue-generating athletes participate.

9 Ethical Decision Making of Sport Managers

Learning Outcomes

After reading Chapter 9, the student will be able to:

1. Express ways that sport managers can emphasize ethics in sport organizations.

2. Describe how sport managers can ethically manage incompetent employees.

3. Discuss different ways to ethically obtain accurate information for the purpose of decision making in sport organizations.

4. List various ways that ethics drive decisions made by sport managers.

5. Cite steps to establish an ethical workplace in sport organizations.

6. Explain the role of athletic directors in the professional advancement of their coaches.

Today's sport managers face the difficult task of operating departments and organizations in a business climate in which winning and profits are often valued above all else. At times, moral values and standards are de-emphasized or even ignored within sporting contexts because of the immense importance placed on winning. When controversies arise, sport managers must decide how strongly they value ethics and to what extent they want ethics to influence the direction and reputation of the organization. In expecting a level of ethics within their sport organizations, leaders must determine the level of moral excellence they will require of their employees.

In athletic departments, the athletic director is the employee who normally has the responsibility of understanding, interpreting, and communicating the value system of the sport program. Therefore, those who are in positions of sport leadership must possess a strong sense of priorities, purpose, and ethics for themselves and their programs in an attempt to effectively reduce harm to sport.[1] Athletic directors with a sense of ethical purpose have the prerequisites necessary to develop a sport program from a firm ethical foundation.

This chapter will examine some of the challenges faced by sport managers today and the elements and reasoning they might use in making difficult decisions. It begins with a look at the ways in which ethics are stressed within sport organizations and goes on to examine how sport managers might deal with incompetent employees and how they should go about collecting and verifying information they will use in their decision making. Throughout the discussions within this chapter, several references are made to the many types of sport managers and administrators, including athletic administrators, general managers, leaders in sport, and athletic directors. In some cases, when discussing general management issues that are germane to most athletic-related entities, the various sport management–related titles are used interchangeably. The many management stances sport administrators might adopt toward ethics and ethical standards will also be examined. Finally, the chapter will conclude with a look at the role that athletic directors should play in the advancement of coaches under their employment.

Emphasizing Ethics in Sport Organizations

Sport managers must arrive at decisions while factoring in not only the best interest of athletes, coaches, and fans, but also society as a whole because sport and athletics pervade and affect, even if just in a small way, today's culture. How can sport managers best meet both the ethical and performance expectations placed on them in the "win first" culture of American sport?

Frequently, athletic directors will be called on to make decisions that have both strategic and ethical implications. In a study in which 354 Divisions I, II, and III National Collegiate Athletic Association (NCAA) coaches were surveyed, 90% agreed that athletic administrators should be responsible for the conduct of athletes, coaches, and fans. It was also believed by 79% of the coaches that institutional administrators should be held accountable for enforcing a conference code of ethics. In other words, a large share of the responsibility for emphasizing and ensuring good moral behavior within athletics falls on the shoulders of sport managers.[2]

Recruiting Ethical Employees as a Priority

Employing persons who are guided by strong internal moral values and standards is essential to the development and maintenance of ethical sport organizations. To this end, although educational endeavors such as workshops and seminars are necessary and helpful, the recruiting and hiring of employees with sound moral character should be the primary focus. Even with the help of educational offerings, it is not easy to change the mindset of persons who have practiced unethical behavior over time.

Based on the belief of some sport philosophers, ethical behavior is instilled in children by adults who model and have them repeat proper behavior.[3] In other words, it is difficult to instill ethical behavior in someone if he or she did not practice ethical behavior as a child. Given the previously cited knowledge, the screening of prospective candidates and the gaining of an understanding of their past behavior prior to hiring is critical to hiring morally upstanding employees. With the help of letters of recommendation and the interview process, sport managers should be able to ensure that prospective hires have a history of doing the "right thing" and the moral constitution to continue doing so in the future.

Hiring those in athletic departments who will "do the right thing" is, on occasion, explicitly recommended by groups or commissions that have an influence on sport organizations. For example, the Knight Commission—which is made up, in part, of leaders from higher education, business, and athletics—issued its first report on college sports reform in 1991. That report, "Keeping the Faith With the Student-Athlete," focused on the primary responsibility of college and university presidents to ensure the appropriate educational and ethical operation of their institutions' athletic programs.[4] Presidents might begin meeting this challenge by demanding that athletic directors hire employees, including coaches, in their athletic departments who are ethically sound.

If sport managers wish to develop ethical sport organizations, they must place a priority on hiring employees who have high ethical standards. Without morally upstanding employees, organizations will, at best, run the risk of being marred with unethical behavior. The adage "an ounce of prevention is worth a pound of cure" can be applied to the process of hiring employees in athletic departments. When interviewing and hiring, if a sport manager does not consider the moral character of employees, a rash of problems is likely to occur over time throughout the organization.

"Who Should I Hire?"

Mr. Smith is the athletic director of a medium-sized university that has 21 men's and 21 women's sports teams. The athletic activity seems to be unending; seasons of different sports overlap, and players as well as coaches hardly have a chance to recover from the past game or season before the next one begins. However, nothing compares to the intensely demanding job of the sports information director (SID). Unable to cope with the pressures of the job, the fourth sports information director in less than 4 years just quit. Job stress related to deadlines and ferociously demanding coaches was, once again, cited in the letter of resignation. Mr. Smith is now confronted with the unenviable task of hiring another SID and feels fortunate that two candidates have applied. One candidate, Stewart, is easy-going, considerate, and grounded in an

"Who Should I Hire?" (*Continued*)

unshakable value system. The other candidate, Ken, is a bit rough around the edges, can be aggressive and even abrasive at times, and has a slight reputation of not being completely moralistic. Normally, Mr. Smith would not even consider hiring a person with less than a pristine moral past and a congenial personality. For the first time, though, given the revolving door of SIDs and the overall difficulty of the job, Mr. Smith is considering hiring someone such as Ken.

Questions

1. Who would you hire? Why?
2. Would you consider compromising values for competency?
3. Would it be worth it to you to consider hiring Ken over Stewart if you believed Ken might be able to withstand the pressures of the SID job and stay longer than a year?
4. In your opinion, in whose best interest would it be to hire Ken? Stewart? Explain.

Overall, the process of recruiting ethical employees begins with the inclusion of ethical criteria in job descriptions. Prospective job candidates should have an understanding and record of adhering to organizational rules. Job descriptions should also be created in a way that requires candidates to be of good moral character.

> **job description:** a written statement describing an occupation and listing its required and preferred qualifications.

A **job description** created to attract candidates of high moral character should require prospective candidates to demonstrate evidence of moral character traits and values such as honesty, responsibility, fairness, and beneficence. Those hiring athletic department employees should include in the job description a requirement to demonstrate evidence of having successfully completed formal education related to ethical behavior. Results of a survey in which 400 high school principals were studied showed that over 41% of the principals believed that it was essential or very important to be educated in the area of ethics to succeed as a high school athletic director.[5]

Being an athletic administrator who expects, practices, and makes ethical behavior a priority can be demonstrated in several forms. One such form is the addition of sport ethics programs to one's sport organization. For example, athletic administrators at six major institutions—Arizona State University, Iowa State University, the University of Alabama at Tuscaloosa, the University of Georgia, the University of Maryland at College Park, and Virginia Tech—have included an external sport ethics curriculum into their football programs.[3] These athletic administrators are demonstrating their personal interest in teaching athletes how to practice good moral behavior by exposing them to ethical programs.

Manipulation of Affirmative Action Policies in Hiring Coaches

The importance of hiring morally strong employees who understand the difference between ethically acceptable and unacceptable behavior is apparent. But how far should sport managers go to hire such persons? When attempting to hire ethical employees, the temptation to **circumvent hiring policies** might present itself. Can sport managers justify circumventing such regulations if they believe it is in the best interest of their organizations?

> **circumvent hiring policies:** to not follow the established guidelines when hiring an employee.

If sport managers have confidence in their abilities to identify the best candidate for the job, are they justified in ignoring affirmative action policies? As was established in a previous chapter, if sport managers disregard affirmative action procedures, they run the risk of creating inequitable hiring practices that are unfair to minorities and may cause harm to the organization over the long term. From a teleological perspective, the morally good sport manager who focuses on the values of justice and responsibility will adhere to affirmative action policies out of commitment to these values. Even if the teleological sport manager may see merit in circumventing hiring procedures, in the interest of not compromising moral values, he or she will not do so. From a deontological perspective, if a sport manager decides to circumvent affirmative action policies and believes it is also acceptable for all other sport managers to do the same, the deontological component of not acting in a way that one would deem unacceptable for all others to act is being met. However, if all others believe it is acceptable to circumvent affirmative action procedures, based on a generally agreed-upon principle, affirmative action policies should be revisited and possibly modified in a way that is generally supported by sport managers. If the policies gain universal support and by and large are perceived to be grounded in strong teleological moral values, the policies, likely, will be more effective.

Although the ability to make effective independent decisions is essential for sport managers, they should be cautious when acting beyond the parameters of policy. As a general rule, sport managers should put aside their personal feelings and adhere to and enforce previously established hiring policies. Employees in sport organizations, other than the sport manager, may attempt to manipulate or circumvent search procedures as well. Employees who circumvent search procedures are not showing respect for the policies that are currently in place and are also not showing respect for the process under which the rules were developed. In such cases, sport managers should consider assuming the responsibility of enforcing regulations and maintaining ethical conduct within their organizations. Sport managers who turn a blind eye to employees in the sport organization who blatantly disregard search procedures of the sport organization are reinforcing unethical behavior within the organization. Thus, sport managers may have to put aside their personal impressions and desires, and instead consider the long-term moral good of the sport organization as they focus on maintaining ethical hiring procedures. The sport manager might choose to adhere to the consequentialist approach of considering the best interests of all—or, in this case, the best interests of the sport organization as a whole.

Instilling a Sense of High Ethical Standards Into Employees Through Education

Rudd emphasized the need for sport administrators to consider character from a moral perspective, and suggested education as a first step in developing moral character in sport.[6] A more balanced emphasis—one that does not favor social character over moral character—needs to be encouraged as part of the actual competitive-sport experience. Such an approach includes the development of honesty, fairness, responsibility, and respect for opponents.[6] Even if sport organizations recruit employees who have a strong foundation of moral values, the sport managers should continue to emphasize the importance of ethical behavior by offering a variety of educational training programs for their employees.

Ethical training programs could consist of case scenarios that call for moral decision making. A discussion of the various moral theories and the theories most appropriate for areas such as policy development, conflict resolution, and organizational vision might also be practiced through ethical training. Requiring ethics training for employees at the workplace of a sport organization will demonstrate to its employees that good ethical behavior is a point of emphasis in the athletic department.

Employees often follow the behavioral patterns established by their managers. If a sport manager consistently offers and encourages or mandates employee participation in ethical training programs, sound ethical conduct will likely be enhanced and sustained. On the other hand, even though 80% of employees behave ethically, most persons will violate their personal ethics if they think their job requires them to do so.[7] An ethics committee might even be established to help sport managers implement and oversee some of their strategies for maintaining high ethical standards. Regardless of the process through which ethical standards are implemented, sport managers should be vigilant in their efforts to protect their organizations from corruptive forces that may arise within sport organizations.

There are several ways to establish a culture of positive ethical behavior in athletic departments. Establishing an overall goal of becoming a lifelong learner of ethics will assist sport managers in instilling positive ethical behavior into their organizations on a daily basis. To that end, as previously indicated, coaches may be required to attend one or more ethical training seminars or workshops. Also, clear and readable ethics guidelines can be distributed to all employees. Ethical guidelines can be grounded in teleology along with an understanding and working knowledge of deontology.

It has been suggested that employees attend ethical lectures and that managers should create an environment in which employees learn about ethics in the workplace and feel comfortable discussing ethics.[7] In-service workshops related to ethics may be brought to sport organizations or may be sought out at local, regional, national, or international professional conferences. And, requiring employees to collect continuing education credits in this manner might be an effective way for sport managers to encourage and foster ethical behavior in their organizations.

One sport organization taking a lead in emphasizing the importance of ethics is the National Association of Basketball Coaches (NABC). Division I head coaches of the NABC have collectively accepted the responsibility of organizing a plan of action to further enhance the overall integrity of the game. One goal is to continue to enhance the ethical and moral expectations of all college basketball coaches. The NABC has committed to reviewing and providing recommendations on stiffer penalties for secondary recruiting violations. Additionally, the association's Board of Directors has authorized the Ethics Committee to institute a plan to formally respond to unacceptable behavior, including penalties that could include suspending membership rights. Also included in the ethics plan of action was a five-session professional development program mandated for all Division I assistant coaches at the Final Four in San Antonio. The professional development program was organized for the purpose of developing workshops covering recruiting rules, diversity, coaching character, ethics, and morals.[8]

It should be stated, however, that the encouragement of ethical behavior is only a beginning step in the creation of an ethical sport organization. In sport organizations, good ethical behavior must be reinforced and unethical behavior must be corrected or punished. Also, remember that ethical sport organizations often result from the individuals within the organization who consistently practice moral values.

If sport managers truly want their sports programs to exhibit good moral behavior, they must be proactive in their quest to do so. As is often done with winning, sport managers must reinforce good ethical behavior with worthy rewards. Sport managers could require coaches to implement reward systems for team members who exhibit or promote sportsmanlike behavior. From a team perspective, sport managers, including athletic directors, could select coaches and teams who display ethical conduct throughout their seasons to receive awards for their positive actions. If good ethical behavior is positively reinforced, it likely will occur more frequently.

Balancing Ethics With Competency

Sport managers may find it challenging to identify employees who have high moral standards and are also highly competent. Obviously, for sport organizations to achieve goals and objectives, organizational leaders must emphasize employee competency, but at what cost to ethics? Sport managers must decide what should be expected of their employees and what constitutes minimal levels of job competency as well as ethical conduct. They must make these determinations on the basis of the goals and objectives of the sport organization.

If sport managers prefer organizations that operate under the highest ethical standards, they should hire employees who have extraordinary records of ethical conduct or provide evidence of their potential to be ethically strong employees. On the other hand, if sport managers place a strict emphasis on productivity-related outcomes instead of ethics, then employees who can "produce" should be hired over less productive employees who have demonstrated a stronger moral background. However, if a morally questionable employee is hired, sport managers may have to monitor employee behavior more closely to make sure that it at least meets minimal standards of ethics expected by the sport organization.

In addition, sport managers should ensure that their employees understand the moral values of fairness and honesty and how a disregard for these can detrimentally affect the organization. A positive and productive work environment might also depend on the practice of moral values such as beneficence, altruism, compassion, and respect for others in the organization. Employees who are primarily focused on strategic reasoning might benefit by understanding how moral values affect the productivity of the organization. The sport manager might also benefit from a utilitarian mindset that seeks the greatest amount of good for the greatest number of employees in the sport organization.

Decisions Related to Incompetent and Unwanted Employees

Unfortunately, even the best efforts to hire employees who are competent as well as ethical are not always successful. More specifically, interscholastic administrators are not always in a position in which they can select the highest quality coaches.[9] Despite the best efforts of sport managers, incompetent coaches and other employees are hired from time to time.

Competencies expected of interscholastic coaches include the teaching of rules, skills, and tactics. In addition to these expectations, coaches are usually also expected to win games. State standards sometimes are weak—probably because of the high demand for coaches—in terms of what is expected of coaches. Less than one-third of the states specify that coaches must have a teaching certificate, and often coaches learn how to coach "on the fly," with no formal training. Interscholastically, coaches lack training in coaching principles, basic first aid, and how to teach basic sport skills. Lack of training in these areas can result in the incompetence that may be displayed in the following ways: incompetent teaching of players, use of improper physical training techniques, disorganized practices, psychological abuse, and malpractice in injury treatment.[10]

Incompetent coaches in school districts can not only result in an increase in parent-related problems, but also in legal problems. Despite what might be perceived to be low coaching standards by certifying boards in some states, sport managers should maintain their own high levels of coaching competencies when seeking out prospective coaches for their organizations.

There are factors that adversely affect the supply of competent coaches. Since the increase of salaries in the mid-1980s due to the Teachers Enhancement Act, many teachers no longer need to supplement their income through coaching. Other factors causing teachers, who are also competent coaches, to elect not to coach include the pressures of winning, beginning families, time demands of gaining teaching certifications, and the difficulties of balancing teaching and coaching.[9]

As can be seen, the attempt to find coaches who are qualified, competent, and also of strong moral character is a challenge. Again, sport managers are often forced to hire coaches who barely meet minimum qualifications. If athletic directors choose to hire coaches who have no formal education or coaching experience, they must be prepared to deal with incompetence.[10]

When such incompetence surfaces, the organizational leader must take action. Sport managers have three options when dealing with incompetent employees: (a) dismiss the employee; (b) retain the employee and provide them with improvement programs; or (c) dismiss the employee and assist them in obtaining employment within sport organizations that better match their talents. What factors should sport managers consider when deciding which option is best under any one set of circumstances? To what extent should the well-being of the coach or other employee be considered in such situations?

Dismissing or Providing Improvement Programs for the Employee

Is it ethical for sport managers to dismiss employees because of incompetence, even though the incompetence was not revealed during the interview process? To what extent, if any, are sport managers justified in firing and replacing incompetent employees as expeditiously as possible to improve or preserve the quality of their sport organization? Improving the quality of the organization would likely provide the most amount of good for the most amount of people in the organization and might meet the needs of the organization as a whole—both of which are supported by the utilitarian component of consequentialism. Sport managers might model termination procedures after those used for faculty, which are more formally established than those for coaches and other sport personnel. The termination of incompetent faculty centers on the needs of the students. If a faculty member's level of instruction or pedagogical skills are far below the professional standards of the university, it is a disservice to students to permit him or her to continue to teach.[11]

These same standards might be used to fire incompetent coaches. When the standard of skill instruction, player-personnel decisions, human relations dealings, training methods, and game strategies are judged to be far below professional standards, then it is a disservice to the players to allow the coach to continue to coach.

In firing incompetent workers, sport managers may choose to protect the overall reputation and interests of all the employees in the organization above the perceived well-being of the incompetent employee. To ensure that the greatest amount of good comes from an unfortunate situation, sport managers may assume this utilitarian stance out of a sense of loyalty and responsibility to their organization and employees.

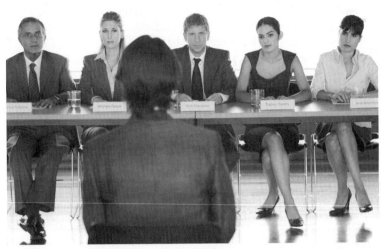

9-1 *Terminating incompetent employees may be in the best long-term interest of a sport organization.*

"What to Do With the Incompetent Employee"

The athletic director and assistant athletic director of Mosey College disagree as to whether to fire a coach for being incompetent. Coach Incompetent was hired 6 months ago and is one of the nicest coaches in the department. She is, however, completely incompetent. With every new day comes a new problem for the athletic director, caused by Coach Incompetent. Today, Coach Incompetent did not meet the deadline to turn in her squad list, yesterday a parent called complaining that her daughter—a member of Coach Incompetent's team—was upset with the coach, the previous day she held her practice in the wrong location and upset two coaches, and three days ago a coach in the league called complaining that she had, inappropriately, invited a player on another team in the league to join her team. It just never ends. Unfortunately, Coach Incompetent does not understand the NCAA rules and could jeopardize the department by violating the rules. The assistant athletic director argues that Coach Incompetent should not be fired, but instead be given the opportunity to improve through training. The athletic director argues that Coach Incompetent should be fired immediately so that the athletic department can stop worrying about her inadequacies. In other words, according to the athletic director, the sooner Coach Incompetent is fired, the sooner the athletic department can get back to business as usual.

> ## "What to Do With the Incompetent Employee" (*Continued*)
>
> ### Questions
> 1. If you were the assistant athletic director, would you try to persuade the athletic director to (a) fire Coach Incompetent, or (b) provide Coach Incompetent with training? Explain.
> 2. Regarding what to do with Coach Incompetent, describe the considerations involved in arriving at a decision based on utilitarianism.
> 3. Using teleology, what moral values would you consider in arriving at your decision?
> 4. In whose best interest would it be to fire Coach Incompetent? To provide Coach Incompetent with training?

On the other hand, sport managers might base their actions on the teleological moral value of compassion in this instance and provide the incompetent employee with opportunities to improve, instead of firing him or her. One could argue that because the screening process that was designed to determine qualified and competent employees was ineffective, employees with difficulties should be allowed to participate in improvement programs. The improvement programs should be designed to help employees overcome their problems and become productive and valued members of the organization. If sport managers have doubts about their organizations' recruiting and hiring processes, they may have an obligation to provide incompetent employees with such opportunities for success.

A third option, which some sport managers have used successfully in the past, might be to help the incompetent employee find employment in a more suitable position within another sport organization, taking advantage of well-established networks of professional relationships. This option is one that might be considered good and fair for both the employee and the organization at which they were originally hired. From the employee's standpoint, the sport manager has acted beneficently and compassionately in helping the employee gain new employment. From an organizational standpoint, the sport manager has acted responsibly in removing an incompetent employee who had been negatively affecting the organization and helped to maintain the reputation and integrity of the organization and its employees.

Circumvention of Termination Procedures to Remove Unwanted Employees

If a manager of a sport organization becomes aware of an unacceptable act committed by an employee but does not have the needed documentation to fire her, is it ethical to "build a case" against her in other areas for the sole purpose of terminating her employment? Policies are developed, in part, to prevent situations from being resolved inconsistently and independently. Is there a point, however, at which it is acceptable for a sport manager to take it upon himself to override policies if he believes it is in the best interests of the organization? This type of activity probably happens more frequently than one would expect. Are there cases in which it would be considered ethical? Or, are manipulative strategies of this kind always unethical?

For example, informally, it may be widely known that a coach is sexually harassing his players. However, players may be afraid to come forward because the coach controls such things as scholarships, starting positions, and playing time. Hence, the athletic director may not have enough direct evidence to justify firing the coach. Knowing this, should the athletic director attempt to "build a case" against the coach in other areas? Would it be ethical for the athletic director, for example, to manipulate subjective evaluation criteria of performance evaluations and annual reviews in a way that reads negatively against the coach to provide the necessary documentation to dismiss the coach? Here, from a teleological perspective, a sport manager could experience a clash of moral values. Should the athletic director attempt to build a case for firing the coach out of compassion for and responsibility to the athletes? Or should he focus on being fair and honest in assessing the coach's performance?

When sport managers manipulate established policies, they are implying through their actions that they believe the current procedures are ineffective and that they know, from an independent perspective, what is best under the circumstances. The circumvention of established procedures becomes risky if those procedures were established based on input from the various persons affiliated with the sport organization. In a specific case, even if the majority of persons in the organization agree with the circumvention and the manipulation of evidence to terminate an unwanted employee, this act is risky because it may open the door for the athletic director or others to break additional organizational rules with which they disagree. If it should become apparent, however, that the procedures currently in place are not effective, those procedures should be re-examined through a formal process established for that specific purpose.

The long-term results of circumventing agreed-upon procedures and rules could cause more harm than good in situations such as the one previously mentioned. On the other hand, the long-term results of keeping an employee known to have committed an unacceptable act might also not be in the long-term best interest of the employee. A more thorough moral analysis may be in order. Examining the situation from a deontological perspective might also be helpful. If the situation were reversed, would the sport manager accept being fired for an act that could not be proven? In other words, using deontology as a basis, what is acceptable for one person must also be acceptable for all persons.

Obtaining Accurate Information for the Purpose of Decision Making

An essential component of sound decision making in sport organizations is accurate information. Ethical parameters, however, should restrict the means by which sport managers obtain such information. Should information be collected only through gossip: either fact-based idle talk or rumor, especially about the private affairs of others.

formal processes such as meetings, or is informal **gossip** an acceptable means through which to gain information? And, prior to basing decisions on obtained information, are there ways that sport managers should verify the accuracy of the information?

Formal Meetings

Obtaining information through formal meetings, where information exchanges take place in an open forum, is perceived to be ethically acceptable. However, sport managers must consider that formal meetings will not necessarily disclose all of the activity—including deviant actions of some employees—that is taking place in their organizations. The acquisition of extensive information is necessary for sport managers to make the best possible decisions in many situations. Hence, it is important to assess what informal means of gathering information are ethically acceptable or unacceptable for sport managers to use.

Informal Meetings

One way that information is exchanged is through informal, unscheduled meetings. Informal meetings may help sport managers supplement information obtained through formal meetings. Such meetings can take place anywhere but often come about when employees visit with leaders of an organization in their offices. Leaders should not act too quickly on information obtained during informal meetings, especially when persons being discussed are not present. When obtaining information through informal meetings, the accuracy of the information should be verified before acting on it. By doing so, administrators of sport are acting fairly and responsibly toward the employees who have been informally discussed and, by basing actions on the moral values of justice and responsibility, are acting in accordance with teleological moral theory in this case.

Is it ethical to have informal discussions concerning people who are not present? The extent to which the information in question benefits the sport organization and those within it might help to determine whether discussing individuals when they are not present is ethical. The way that information will be used might also be taken into consideration in such instances. Whether the information will be used in support of or against the person being talked about is also something that should be considered.

When verifying the authenticity of information being articulated, the sport manager must consider the credibility of the source. Unless the person delivering the information is willing to do so formally, his credibility might be called into question because he is shirking accountability by not disclosing the information publicly. For example, if, during an informal meeting with an athletic director, a player or coach mentions the name of another coach who is physically abusing his or her players, the athletic director should not rush to judgment. In fairness to and with respect for the coach being accused, the sport manager should not prejudge him or her. Using teleology as a basis,

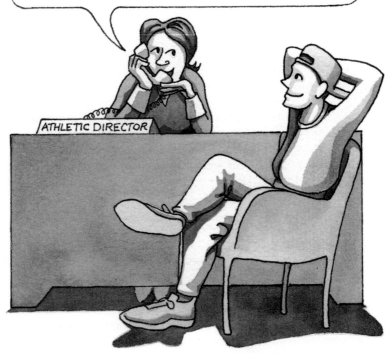

any information stated about another person should be verified to ensure that it is accurate and honest information.

Gossip and Rumors

The passing of information through gossip and rumors is similar to, but even less formal than, the exchange of information through informal meetings. One would be naïve to believe that gossip is not a common form of obtaining information in sport organizations. Furthermore, at least anecdotally, gossip seems to be an effective means of disseminating and obtaining information.

> **rumors:** a statement or opinion widely circulated from person to person, though unconfirmed by facts or evidence.

Rumors arise when the demand for information exceeds the amount offered through institutional channels. Gossip, on the other hand, is not an opinion and not a story but a special mixture of the stories and opinions about the stories, and it has a special role in opinion spreading. Gossiping is a transport network of information—a small news network.[12]

Should sport managers use gossip as part of their decision-making process? To better understand the position of the sport manager, one should first examine whether it is unethical to gossip. To answer this question, utilitarians would weigh out whether gossiping would bring the most good to the most people in the organization. Deontologists, however, would likely find gossiping to be ethically unacceptable because it is disrespectful to those who are the subject of the gossip. They might claim that because people would not want to be the subject of gossip, it is not a universally acceptable behavior.

Is it ethical for sport managers to acknowledge or entertain rumors or gossip? Should they turn a deaf ear to all forms of gossip or selectively entertain certain forms of it? If sport managers will accept only certain types of gossip, what are those types and how will they be identified as being ethical? Finally, is it necessary to ask whether gossip may be harmful or hurtful to the person being gossiped about?

"Gossip in the Athletic Department"

Gary Gossip was insecure with his position as the head boys' ice hockey coach at Victory High School. The boys' ice hockey team has a long-standing reputation of being a powerhouse that wins games. For the past two years, however, for the first time in the history of the school, the girls' ice hockey team has won more games than the boys' team. The athletic director has taken notice and has rewarded the girls' team by providing them with more money while not increasing the budget of the boys' team. Deeply disturbed by the overall situation throughout the past two years, Coach Gossip was prepared to do anything to win more games than the girls and, once again, be recognized as one of the best hockey teams in the state or, at least, the best hockey team at the high school. Coach Gossip decided to damage the credibility of the girls' program by spreading a rumor. Coach Gossip began by telling his assistant coaches that the girls' head hockey coach was providing her players with performance-enhancing drugs. Before long, the rumor had reached the athletic director as well as the girls' head hockey coach. When the girls' coach first heard the rumor, she laughed at its outrageousness, then she became angry, and finally, when she realized how damaging it could be to her and her program, she began to cry. When the athletic director heard the rumor, he was not quite sure what actions to take, if any. The only thing he knew for sure was that the athletic department was in a state of disarray; many of its members held distrust for one another because of what had taken place.

"Gossip in the Athletic Department" (*Continued*)

Questions

1. If you were the athletic director, what actions would you take, if any?
2. If you were the head girls' coach, what actions would you take, if any?
3. If you were the athletic director, what precautionary measures would you take to prevent the spreading of future rumors?

It is not uncommon for sport managers to learn information for the first time through gossip. This in itself may be harmless enough, but acting on this information may be harmful. Basing decisions exclusively on gossip stands a reasonable chance of resulting in a detrimental or hurtful outcome for the individual being gossiped about, the sport manager, and the organization.

half-truths: a partially true statement intended to deceive or mislead.

Acting in a way that hurts others infringes on the moral values of compassion and beneficence. Sometimes gossip includes **half-truths** and inaccurate information, which infringe on the moral values of honesty and fairness. Given gossip's potential for breaching several moral values, acting or making decisions impulsively based on gossip is ill-advised. To make sound decisions, as many facts as possible should be gathered, and, as with informal meetings, the reliability of the sources must be considered.

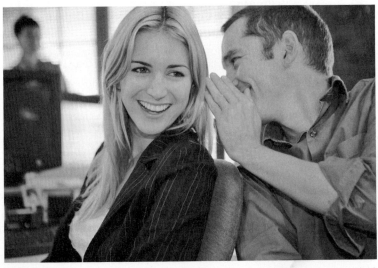

9-2 *Gossip in sport organizations that includes half-truths and inaccurate information infringes on the moral values of honesty and fairness.*

Gossip has been described as the primary mechanism for communicating negativity and causes missed communication that can lead to conflict, deadlines not being met, strained relationships, and the disruption of teamwork. Gossip is destructive, hurtful, and a divisive form of communication that permeates the workplace and can sabotage a team's ability to work together.[13] A decrease in productivity can result from gossip and is one example of the destructive effect gossip can have on a workplace. As a manager, keeping communication vacuums filled with positive, accurate, and timely information can help prevent it from being filled with negative or incorrect information.[14]

Given the negativity and harm that can result from gossip, when determining whether the information should be used, the benefits of the information to the sport organization might be weighed against the potential harm to the person who is the subject of the gossip. The sport manager who manages as a utilitarian would attempt to estimate the overall amount of good that would come from acting on gossip and whether the actions would be in the best interest of the sport organization. If information is obtained that could be helpful to the organization or individuals within it, then a case might be made from the sport manager's perspective to confirm the accuracy of the information and then act on it.

Validation of Information

Rather than acting or passing on information heard through the grapevine, the information should first be verified by asking the person who communicated it.[14] Sport managers should have an effective process to validate information upon receiving it. The process of substantiating facts might include directly asking persons whether specific rumors about them are true. Discussing information with others close to a particular situation might also be helpful when attempting to distinguish true statements from false ones. The credibility of the person who is gossiping should also be considered. A process to validate rumors will help the sport manager make decisions that are fair and in the best overall interest of the sport organization.

Categories of Ethical Management

In a time when winning is in high demand, can sport organizations meet the wants of their fans and sponsors in an ethical manner? To what extent must sport managers operate from a sound ethical foundation? Sport managers can be divided into three categories of ethical management. Some resist temptations to cheat and are able to win and generate revenue ethically. Others, however, focus on expectations of winning with only partial concern for ethics. Still others concentrate exclusively on winning at all costs, acting with complete disregard for ethical values and standards.

Decisions Driven Exclusively by Ethics

Ethical behavior in sport oftentimes requires moral courage, which means having the resolve to stay with one's values in unsavory times and to resist pressures for short-term actions that are not in the team's or institution's long-term best interests.[1] Sport managers who consistently manage in accordance with generally accepted standards of ethical conduct allow ethical standards to direct their actions rather than the persuasions of others.

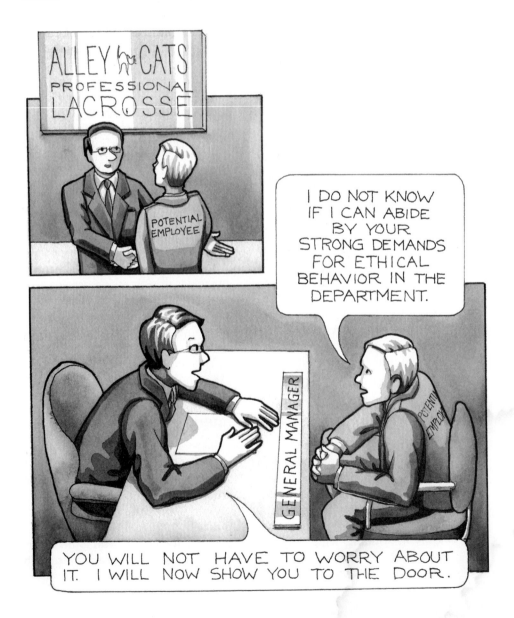

A part of being a professional is adhering to the highest organizational and personal ethical standards. Sport managers should make it clear from the outset, i.e., during the interview process, that unethical behavior will not be tolerated in their organization. Leaders as well as followers in any group must establish the ethical tone for the organization. If leaders at all levels of an organization choose to act beyond reproach, reward correct behavior, and refuse to tolerate wrong doing, there is a much greater chance that members of the organization will behave ethically.[1]

Serving as an example is the NCAA's Division III Empire 8 Commissioner, Chuck Mitrano. Mr. Mitrano is the chair of the Division III Commissioner's Association (DIIICA), which is responsible for creating the Sportsmanship and Ethical Conduct Committee. A goal of the committee is to dedicate a portion of the DIIICA Web site (www.diiicomm.org) to sportsmanship and sports ethics policies. Additionally, programming is available to serve as a resource to other member institutions and conferences who are seeking such information when creating their own programs.[15]

Carrying out decisions based exclusively on ethical guidelines will bring moments of controversy in which individuals with greater power may question sport managers' decisions. If a sport manager's **ethically grounded management philosophy** is to be carried out, she must adhere to her moral values even in times of controversy. However, support from the sport manager's supervisor is necessary if this is to be accomplished. Without support from high-level administrative personnel, the effectiveness of sport managers' decisions may be compromised or the decisions themselves overridden. For example, if an athletic director decides to punish a coach for breaking a rule and the principal of the high school overrides the athletic director's decision, the athletic director's ability to consistently carry out the ethical expectations of his employees may be undermined. When the athletic director's efforts to foster ethical behavior in a sport organization are not upheld by his superiors, the athletic department might be in jeopardy of being overrun by unethical behavior.

> **ethically grounded management philosophy:** an approach in which sport management is based on a foundation of moral values.

Persons of power not directly related to sport organizations may also attempt to manipulate and control the management of sports teams. For example, if a booster is donating extraordinarily large sums of money to a specific sport team, he or she may want to control player personnel decisions, including deciding who "makes" the team, who "starts," and how much playing time particular players may receive. In such a case, the sport manager must decide whether this generous booster's continuous interference in team affairs is worth the money he or she is giving. If a booster is continually meddling in the day-to-day affairs of the athletic department or a particular sports team, the sport manager may decide it is not worth receiving the booster's money for the amount of trouble being caused by the booster. The sport manager may decide to risk losing the booster's donations if their input is negatively affecting the team or its performance.

One of the most generous boosters to an athletic department is T. Boone Pickens, who was ranked by Forbes Magazine as the 207th richest person in the United States. In January of 2006, Pickens gave his alma mater, Oklahoma State University, $165 million, which was the single largest donation ever to a college athletic program.

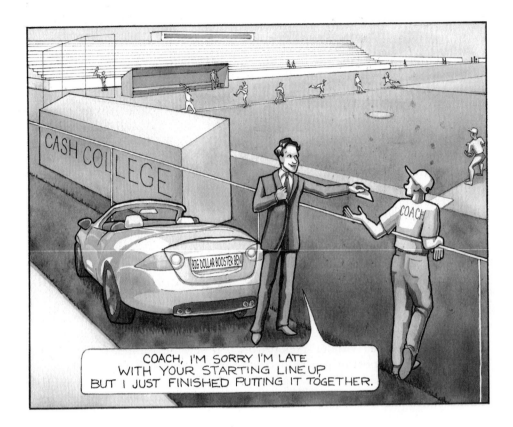

The football stadium, Boone Pickens Stadium, is named after him. Few boosters, if any, write checks as sizeable as Pickens', and, thus, few boosters have as much direct or indirect influence over an athletic department as Pickens. Although Pickens claims that he does not directly call plays or voice concerns about strategy, he has been known to make general comments regarding the preparedness of the team. Pickens has also made it clear that he wants to know what is going on and wants to have an influence on who might come in to replace a coach who is leaving.[16]

If money being given to a program provides good to a large amount of people, utilitarianism might support compromising some power to the donor in order that benefits continue for coaches, players, fans, and the community. If, however, moral values are being compromised or rules broken, teleology would not support giving the donor team-related power to continue receiving money. On the other hand, if good results from receiving money and no moral values are violated, the decision to continue to accept money from boosters gains moral support from a teleological and consequentialist viewpoint.

Leaders of high school athletic programs have also been confronted with controversy related to boosters giving money to athletic programs. In 2006, it was learned that boosters affiliated with the Bellevue football program in the state of Washington had paid coach Butch Goncharoff $55,000, annually, above and beyond his $5,600 coaching stipend. As a result, the Washington Interscholastic Activities Association conducted a survey around the state to find out about how much money their athletic coaches earn and where it comes from. The concern of the Bellevue school district is the fairness, or lack thereof, of allowing schools to pay one coach so much.[17] If a particular school is gaining an unfair advantage because of a booster who supplements a coach's salary, sport managers and athletic directors throughout the league may have to address the situation. Sport managers may consider legislating against the subsidization of coaching salaries through private donations. Moral theory should be considered when creating such legislation.

At some point, when a sport manager's decision-making philosophy of adhering to ethical standards is challenged, as previously indicated, he or she will need the support of higher administrators. It is helpful if coaches, athletic directors, and presidents of universities are all on the same page regarding controversial ethical issues in athletic departments. For example, a president of a university may pressure a coach and athletic director to allow a high-paying donor control over a sports team in return for giving money to the university. Given the power of upper-level administrators and the fact that boosters are willing to give money, the ethical decisions of the athletic director and coach may be compromised. In this case, the athletic director may have to be prepared to assume a management position in another sport organization where upper administration is more supportive of strong ethical standards. In the most extreme of cases, one may choose to resign from one's job in the interest of ethics. Or, in other cases, it may be the upper-level administrators who adhere to sound ethics but the coach and athletic director who might prefer to behave unethically for the purpose of personal gain.

Decisions Driven by Ethics With Convenient Exceptions

A somewhat less controversial and seemingly more common approach is one in which sport administrators manage according to widely accepted ethical standards, but make exceptions if in the best interest of the sport organization. In certain situations, sport managers might follow the "path of least resistance." In doing so, their organizations will appear to operate smoothly and with minimal conflict because they compromise their ethical standards now and then to prevent conflict. This type of ethical management style is likely to be less controversial than the previous mode of management, because when a controversy does arise, sport managers will act in a way that eliminates the controversy—even if their actions are not completely ethical.

Employees used to working in environments where ethical standards are valued may initially experience frustration when their managers make exceptions to these standards in times of controversy. Over time, however, employees will likely adjust to this "exception-based" style and anticipate when exceptions will be made.

Using the example in which the booster is donating large sums of money to an athletic program to gain control over a particular sports team, an athletic director might attempt to persuade the coach to allow the booster to make certain player personnel decisions. In granting the booster this control, the athletic director hopes to avert the controversy that will inevitably follow when upper administrative personnel find out that the wealthy booster has stopped donating. If the booster were to cease donating money, the president of the university might begin to apply pressure on the coach to allow the booster input to ensure that the booster reconsiders and begins donating once again.

"The $25,000 Offer"

The athletic director at Small College is feeling tremendous levels of stress over the fact that the football program's operating expenses are unsustainable. Game attendance has decreased, causing gate receipts to drop. For the first time in his 10-year career, the athletic director will have to cut the budgets of the other sports in the athletic department by 3% in order to allow football to survive. Interestingly, the athletic director has been presented with one other option. Knowing of football's dire financial state, Mr. Booster has approached and offered the athletic director a $25,000 gift to the program, which would easily solve all of the program's financial problems. Mr. Booster's only request is that his son, who is currently a third team linebacker, be a starter for the entire season.

Questions
1. If you were the athletic director, would you attempt to persuade the head football coach to start Mr. Booster's son so the program could receive the $25,000?
2. From a utilitarian perspective, how might one form an argument that supports accepting the $25,000 from Mr. Booster in return for inserting his son as a starter?
3. In whose best interest is it to start Mr. Booster's son in return for the $25,000? Explain.
4. In whose best interest is it to decline the $25,000 offer from Mr. Booster and continue to make unforced football-related personnel decisions? Explain.

Although seemingly effective in the short term, it is likely that a management approach that permits exceptions to be made regarding ethical standards will cause long-term problems. Teleologists would argue that such an approach would be unacceptable because it would permit sport managers to ignore ethical values and principles when they believe circumstances warrant exceptions. Deontological moral theory would support making exceptions to prevent problems if the members of the athletic department approved an exception-based management model. The utilitarian perspective of consequentialism would approve of such a model if it provided the most amount of good for the most people in the department or overall. However, when sport managers acquire a reputation of compromising their ethical standards in the face of controversy, others might perceive this behavior as a weakness and attempt to exploit it for self-serving purposes.

Moreover, if an athletic director has a reputation of avoiding controversy at all costs, some coaches may choose to break recruiting rules because they know the athletic director is unlikely to confront them about unethical behavior. The athletic director must then decide whether to overlook the illegal recruiting behaviors of the coaches, or uncharacteristically confront the perpetrators. Situations such as this could escalate to the point at which unethical behavior becomes epidemic within the organization. Therefore, sport managers should be selective in making exceptions for unethical behavior so that immoral behavior by athletic department employees does not go unchecked.

Decisions Made Without Consideration for Ethics

Some leaders of sport organizations disregard ethics when making decisions. Their decisions may be driven by money or politics but are not influenced by ethical values, principles, or standards. Why might sport administrators manage their organizations without regard for ethical standards? The high demand to win placed on coaches by their schools is one factor. Winning games generates revenue, and some programs are willing to break rules to increase their leverage to win and fill the seats at football stadiums.[18]

When winning is the absolute focus of a sport organization and commercialization takes over, sport managers may lose sight of ethics as an important aspect of their decision-making process. To address the unethical behaviors that sometimes take place in order to win, the Coalition on Intercollegiate Athletics has been formed from members of six athletic conference faculty senates, governing boards of universities and colleges, and the NCAA.[18] In February of 2004, this coalition met with athletic directors of various schools and found that the athletic directors believed that there was a strong disconnect between the values that govern athletics policy and the problems encountered related to highly commercialized, large-stakes athletics programs. Sport managers who allow or support this disconnect are taking a shortsighted approach to winning and fame, which often results in serious long-term problems for sport managers and organizations alike. When sport managers fail to reprimand coaches or other employees for rules violations or other unethical behaviors, the organization runs the risk of being enmeshed in scandal.

Steps to Establish an Ethical Workplace in Sport Organizations

Conn and Gerdes[1] recommend five steps professionals can follow to establish an ethical workplace. The steps logically begin with the leader of the organization:

1. Clearly define and articulate the organization's values in no more than three sentences. Act according to published values.
2. Conduct ethics-awareness training for members of the workplace community.

3. Outline specific responsibilities for decision making to ensure accountability.
4. Encourage open discussions about controversial issues, ethical questions, and anything that might fall into gray areas.
5. Weigh all decisions against published values.

Conn and Gerdes also offer some questions that might be helpful for leaders such as sport managers as they engage in the decision-making process. To effectively weigh a decision, individuals must identify and understand the facts and the options available to them. Indeed, professionals must recognize that even though a decision can be made without considering outside factors, the effects of the decision may be far reaching and will reflect their integrity and that of their organizations. In addition to the decision-making models presented in Chapter 1, the following are some general questions offered by Conn and Gerdes[1] that may help professionals (i.e., sport managers) as they consider a values-centered approach to decisions in athletic departments.

- Do I have all the information needed? Do I need to speak to someone else, such as the legal staff, to obtain what is needed?
- What are the options? Are they legal? Do they violate any federal, state, district, or league organizational policy or standard?
- Do the options support my values and personal ethics? Can I justify them in the light of my values and business ethics? If not, the option probably is not ethical.
- What are the short-term and long-term consequences of each option? Who or what does each option benefit? Who or what does each option harm?
- Am I still comfortable with the options? How will they be perceived by others? Could they embarrass any party involved?[1]

After leaders weigh the options against their ethical standards, they are ready to make their decision and share it with those involved. The leader must make sure he conceptualizes and articulates the decision so that subordinates view it as consistent with the stated values and ethics of the sport organization. The leader cannot completely protect himself and his programs from the unethical behaviors of associates and other related parties, but he can build into his programs a strong ethical foundation that will keep him and his organization strong in both good times and bad.[1]

In 1932, businessman Herb Taylor developed the Four-Way Test of moral character, and in 1942, gave the right to use this famous test to the prestigious business and community service organization, Rotary International.[19] **Taylor's Four-Way Test** requires responses to four basic questions when attempting to make decisions and certainly could assist sport managers in arriving at decisions. The four basic questions are as follows:

> **Taylor's Four-Way Test:** a test of moral character developed in 1932 by Herb Taylor, which requires answering four questions; may be used to assist managers in making decisions.

1. Is it the truth?
2. Is it fair to all concerned?
3. Will it build good will and better friendships?
4. Will it be beneficial to all concerned?[19]

One can see moral values of teleology and the utilitarian component of consequentialism in Taylor's Four-Way Test. Questions 1 and 2 address truth and fairness. The truth is based on the moral value of honesty and fairness, and is itself a moral value. Question 3 addresses good will, which equates to the moral value beneficence and, in part, altruism. Question 4 addresses benefits to all concerned, which is related to utilitarianism in that it calls for acting in a way that provides the most amount of good (benefits) to the most amount of people (all concerned).

The Role of Athletic Directors in the Professional Advancement of Their Coaches

One of the more common ways for an athletic director to support the professional advancement of coaches is to write positive letters of recommendation on their behalf. The decisions related to making such recommendations can be fraught with ethical questions.

"To Bless or not to Bless"

Sue has worked for Mr. Blessing, the head sports information director (SID), for the past two years and has recently been invited to apply for a head SID position at a larger school. Excited beyond belief that she may have the opportunity to be the head SID at a reputable school with a strong athletic program, Sue enthusiastically asks Mr. Blessing if she can include him as a phone reference. Mr. Blessing smiles and says, "Of course, I would be happy to support your professional advancement." Even the thought of Sue leaving, however, discomforts Mr. Blessing because Sue assumes a tremendous burden of the workload in the office. The thought of having to spend endless hours replacing and then training someone to take Sue's place is overwhelming for Mr. Blessing—so much so that he is considering not giving a positive recommendation for Sue. When the athletic director of Sue's prospective new place of employment calls, Mr. Blessing believes it would be okay to say that Sue definitely needs another year of experience before she is ready to become a head SID. This way, Sue probably will not be hired for the new position and Mr. Blessing can at least get through football season and will have time to find a new assistant.

Questions
1. Should Mr. Blessing support Sue? Explain.
2. Discuss loyalty and whether Sue or Mr. Blessing is being disloyal to the other party.
3. Using deontological moral reasoning, if you were Mr. Blessing, what action would you take regarding Sue's request to help her advance professionally?

Coaches frequently attempt to improve their professional positions by applying for jobs while they are already actively employed as a coach in an athletic department. In such cases, it is common for these coaches to request letters of recommendation from their athletic directors. What stance should athletic directors assume when a superb coach asks for a letter of recommendation? Does the athletic director have a professional obligation to write the letter on behalf of the coach, or is this decision more complex than it appears?

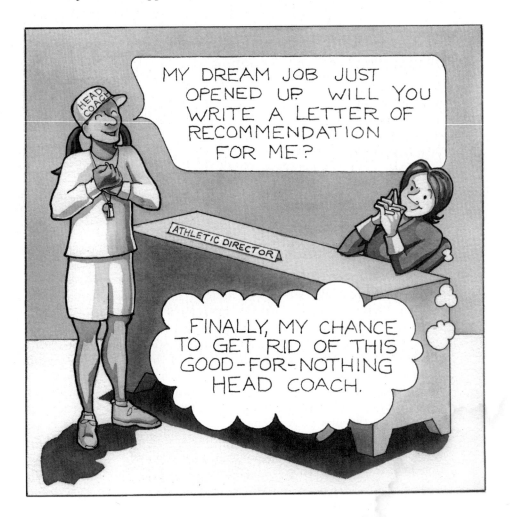

When deciding whether to write a letter of recommendation, the athletic director should consider the effects his or her decision may have on various parties. Three individuals or groups who may have different perspectives on the matter are the coach, the educational institution, and the community. A utilitarianism approach might consider the best interests of the parties involved. In whose best interest is it that the athletic director support or not support the coach's professional advancement? The perspectives held by athletic directors concerning appropriate methods of supporting coaches' professional advancement, including writing letters of recommendation, are likely to vary.

The high demand and low supply of major college head coaching jobs allow colleges and universities the luxury of being selective in making their choices for new hires. Without strong recommendations from reputable fellow coaches, one's chances of obtaining a head coaching position are reduced from extremely low to nearly none. The career of University of Illinois' head basketball coach, Bruce Weber, exemplifies how difficult it can be to become a head coach. As an assistant at the University of Illinois for 18 years, Weber— through his own efforts and strong references from fellow coaches who held him in high regard—was finally presented with the opportunity to be a head coach at Southern Illinois University. From Southern Illinois University, Weber returned to the University of Illinois as head coach.[20]

Perspective of the Coach

The coach is clearly interested in entertaining and exploring opportunities to coach elsewhere. This interest is implicit in the coach's request for a letter of support from the athletic director. The coach probably believes that she has worked hard to build or maintain a strong program and, thus, has earned the right to request and receive a letter of recommendation that will help her advance professionally within the coaching ranks. From the coach's perspective, it is in her best interest to obtain a letter of recommendation in her quest to advance professionally.

Perspective of the Athletic Department and Educational Institution

The reputation of the athletic department and the educational institution it represents reflect the quality of employees. Both have an interest in holding on to talented employees who enhance their quality and reputation. Sport teams are also used to promote the educational institutions they represent. Successful sport teams place the school and its athletic department in a more positive light than unsuccessful squads.

Colleges and universities aspire to achieve quality in their athletic departments and, to do so, make strong attempts to retain their best employees. Retaining quality coaches helps to perpetuate the positive image created by winning teams. Hence, it may be in both the athletic department's and educational institution's best interests to keep the current coach rather than running the risk of hiring a new coach who does not measure up to the current one.

Sometimes, the athletic director may decide to not support the coach for advancement in order to retain the coach instead of having to worry about replacing her. To determine whether this action is appropriate on the part of the athletic director, a few questions are in line. First, if the athletic director were attempting to advance himself professionally, would he want to be held back by one of his bosses who wanted to retain him because of his expertise and skills? If the athletic director sought the support of one of his bosses to advance, he would not want to be held back. Thus, when examining this action from a deontological perspective, it is not supported. Nor is the action supported when examining the value of fairness from a teleological perspective. Holding back the coach to keep her talent in the current department is unfair to the coach, because the norm is to reward good behavior and performance, and in this case, the opposite is taking place. From a strategic perspective, the athletic director may gain in the short term, but it is doubtful that he would gain in the long run. Over time, persons in the athletic department would discover the athletic director's behavior and an atmosphere of distrust would likely pervade the department, leading to larger problems. Furthermore, if an athletic director gains a reputation for stifling the professional advancement of coaches, persons will be less likely to seek employment in that organization.

Perspective of the Community

Although the community may have a variety of interests, the presiding interest seems to be winning, and the probability of winning is increased if a head coach with a proven record of winning is employed. A university community and residential community might advocate doing whatever it takes to keep a successful coach.

Few have established a record of winning that can rival University of Connecticut's head women's basketball coach, Geno Auriemma. To keep Auriemma, the university has provided him with an incentives package that is designed to retain him through at least 2010. Along with his 2006 to 2007 base salary of $250,000 he stands to make $1,250,000 in media and speaking fees. Furthermore, Auriemma is provided with revenue from summer camps, a country club membership, 25 free tickets to games, endorsement contracts, and two months base salary for making the NCAA Final Four.[21]

In Auriemma's case, the likelihood of him leaving to pursue another coaching position is not as high as some coaches employed in less prestigious positions. However, coaches generally are in need of letters of recommendation as they climb the coaching ladder to the top positions, such as the one Auriemma holds. Furthermore, athletic directors might be inclined to consider the winning interests of the community instead of the professional advancement interests of the coach.

How the Athletic Director Will Determine the Coach's Role

After processing the wants and needs of all persons affected by what at first appeared to be a simple letter of recommendation request, the athletic director will be in a better position to make a decision. When making such a decision, it is difficult, if not impossible, to meet the needs of all interested parties. For the athletic director to best serve everyone's interests, it is necessary to make an honest assessment of the possible consequences of the attempt to retain the coach or support his advancement. This approach, which combines utilitarianism and teleology, will help the athletic director decide whose interests should take priority under the circumstances and, ultimately, whether he will write a letter of support.

One must keep in mind that confounding variables may also come into play in such situations. The athletic director might want to consider, for example, whether the coach has completed or has nearly completed her current term of employment. This factor— along with several other factors unique to this, or any, decision—must also be considered by the athletic director if he is to reach a decision in a thorough and fair manner.

Conclusion

The multifaceted jobs of sport managers require myriad decisions that often entail careful thought and moral reasoning. At the more competitive levels, sport managers are expected to win and generate revenue and are also asked to do so in a manner that will keep their organizations safe from ethical misconduct and the sanctions that accompany it. As demonstrated above, the philosophies sport managers adopt and implement concerning ethical standards, and the extent to which they use ethical values and principles in their decision making play an important role in determining (a) how their organizations are perceived, and (b) whether these organizations are able to succeed with integrity. In addition, in looking after their organizations, sport managers who maintain high ethical standards help to improve the contexts of their sporting communities, as well. Thus, sport managers should not underplay the importance of their efforts in regards to ethics. Their work may make a greater difference for sport and society than they realize.

References

1. Conn JH, Gerdes DA. Ethical decision-making: issues and applications to American sport. *Physical Educator*. 1998;55:121–126.
2. Jordan JS, Greenwell TC, Geist AL, Pastore DL, Mahony DF. Coaches' perceptions of conference code of ethics. *Physical Educator*. 2004;61:131–145.
3. Wolverton B. Morality play. *Chronicle of Higher Education*. 2006;52(48):42.
4. Committee on College and University Teaching, Research, and Publication. The faculty role in the reform of intercollegiate athletics. *Academe*. 2003;89(1):64–70.
5. Schneider RC, Stier WF. Recommended educational experiences for high school athletic directors (ADs). *Physical Educator*. 2001;58(4):211–221.
6. Rudd A. Which "character" should sport develop? *Physical Educator*. 2005;62(4):205–211.
7. Oliver CR. Bringing employees on board with ethics. *BizEd*. 2006;5(6):60–61.
8. Division I college head basketball coaches summit convenes in Chicago. NCAA Web site. October 15, 2003. Available at: http://www.ncaa.org/champadmin/basketball/ 2003-04/NABCoctoberSummit/pressRelease.html. Accessed September 28, 2006.

9. Bowley SB. Keeping coaches not so easy. *Connecticut Post* Web site. September 30, 2005. Available at: http://www.connpost.com/. Accessed October 2, 2006.

10. Education requirements for athletic coaches. NASBE Web site. *Policy Information Clearinghouse.* March 2003;11(4). Available at: http://www.nasbe.org/new_resources_ section/policy_updates/PU_Education_Requirement_for_Athletic_Coaches_03.03.pdf. Accessed April 24, 2008..

11. General University Policy Regarding Academic Employees: Termination for Incompetent Performance. February 24, 2000. Available at: http://www.ucop.edu/acadadv/acad-pers/apm/apm-075.pdf. Accessed October 15, 2006.

12. Waxman S. You've read the gossip; still want to see the movie? *New York Times.* 2005;154(53258):E1,E8.

13. Corbin J, May J. What to do about gossip in the workplace? Municipal Research and Services Center of Washington Web site. May 2005. Available at: http://www.mrsc.org/focus/ hradvisor/hra0505.aspx. Accessed September 29th, 2006.

14. Gossip and rumors and hearsay, oh why? Available at: www.management-info.biz/arti-cle/gossip-and-rumors-and-hearsay-5608.html. Accessed: September 29, 2006.

15. Mitrano C. Sportsmanship and ethical programs and policies inquiry. NCAA Web site. March 24, 2005. Available at: http://www1.ncaa.org/membership/governance/division_III/ management_council/2005-4/sup_9_attachmentc.htm. Accessed September 28, 2006.

16. Fish M. Texas tea fills Cowboys' coffers. ESPN Web site. January 11, 2006. Available at: http://sports.espn.go.com/ncf/news/story?id=2285520. Accessed September 30, 2006.

17. Ko M. WIAA to ask what prep coaches earn. *The Seattle Times* Web site. September 26, 2006. Available at: http://seattletimes.nwsource.com/html/highschoolsports/2003275653_ wiaa26.html. Accessed October 3, 2006.

18. Goral T. At all costs. *University Business.* 2004:7(5);40–51.

19. Rotary Global History Fellowship. Available at: http://www.rotaryfirst100.org/presi-dents/1954taylor/taylor/index.htm. Accessed October 10, 2006.

20. Brennan C. Illinois' loyal, patient Weber is tonight's best coaching story. *USA Today* Web site. April 4, 2005. Available at: http://www.usatoday.com/sports/columnist/bren-nan/2005-04-03-brennan-weber_x.htm. Accessed September 29, 2006.

21. Spigel S. Athletic coach salaries. OLR Research Report. February 25, 2005. Available at: http://www.cga.ct.gov/2005/rpt/2005-R-0245.htm. Accessed October 2, 2006.

Gossiping at the Workplace

Sam is a part-time teacher recently hired to the city school district whose job responsibilities are split between two schools. Each of the schools has an administrator who assumes the dual role of athletic director and physical education (PE) supervisor. Although the administrators appear to be nearly identical on paper, they differ significantly in their management approaches and overall goals.

One of the schools is Expectations High School, the location of Sam's first teaching assignment, which is taking place under the most demanding PE supervisor in the district, Ms. Sternberger. Sam is learning from the experience and accepts and respects Ms. Sternberger's disciplined ways. Sam's other school, Easy High School, has a physical education program with significantly fewer demands and rigor. Easy High's administrator, Mr. Laidback, has succeeded in creating a low-pressure, enjoyable work environment for his PE teachers. Unfortunately, Mr. Laidback's area of expertise is that of an athletic director and, in Sam's view, he is incompetent as a PE supervisor.

At Expectations High, Sam is used to handing in lesson plans and getting very critical and detailed feedback from Ms. Sternberger. Although sometimes difficult, it is always a learning experience and helps Sam grow as a teacher. Ms. Sternberger is very close with the director of the district's PE department, knows his expectations, and works her hardest to make sure all her teachers follow these rigorous standards.

At Easy High, things move at a relaxed pace. Mr. Laidback expects no lesson plans, and Sam has begun to realize that many teachers at Easy High are not even teaching. Some of the underachieving teachers began to tease Sam because of his serious approach to teaching, which includes such basics as writing lesson plans and setting high expectations for his students. Finding himself frustrated by the notion that he was being ridiculed for doing his job, Sam made some offhanded comments to his coworkers and Ms. Sternberger at Expectations High. The comments were related to how difficult it was to work at two different schools in the same district with diametrically opposed standards and expectations. This is where the trouble began.

Shortly thereafter, Ms. Sternberger started to ask a lot of questions about Mr. Laidback's PE program at Easy High. Sam answered Ms. Sternberger's questions honestly, because he considered Ms. Sternberger a friend and believed that they shared similar goals in relation to the importance of physical education.

Two weeks later, Mr. Laidback called Sam into his office. He told Sam that it had come to the attention of the Director of Physical Education of the district that Mr. Laidback was not doing his job. This information, Mr. Laidback explained, had been brought up in a meeting with Ms. Sternberger. After hearing those words, Sam became nervous about his job.

Critical Thinking: Finding Common-Sense Solutions

1. Given that Sam was a new employee and possibly naïve to the political workings of school systems, do you believe it was right for Ms. Sternberger to solicit negative information from Sam regarding Mr. Laidback's management at Easy High School? Why or why not?

2. If you were Sam, would you be equally loyal to both administrators (Ms. Sternberger and Mr. Laidback), even though both have very different

philosophical approaches to their programs and Mr. Laidback's style does not align well with yours? Why or why not?

3. If you were Sam, would you ask the advice of another coworker in deciding whether you should take further action regarding Mr. Laidback's perceived incompetence? Can you justify basing your actions on the advice of another? Explain.

4. If you were Sam, would you consider circumventing the administrative chain of command and discussing the situation at Easy High School directly with the Director of Physical Education in the district? Justify your response.

5. If you were Sam, would you be more loyal to yourself and your job or to the overall goals of the district? Could you be loyal to everyone and everything? Explain.

6. If you were the Director of Physical Education of the district, to what extent, if any, would you base your actions on gossip that you heard from Ms. Sternberger regarding the PE program directed by Mr. Laidback at Easy High?

Critical Thinking: Moral Theory-Based Decision Making

7. If you were Sam and were basing your actions on the *consequentialist moral theory*, would you continue to openly discuss your disapproval of Mr. Laidback's management style and philosophy of Easy High School? Why or why not?

8. In your opinion, who carries the burden of *responsibility* and who should be held accountable for good teaching at Easy High School and Expectations High School? Justify your response.

9. Based on a line of reasoning that considers *your own good* versus *the good of others*, explain how you would respond as Mr. Laidback when you found out that your school's PE program was perceived as one lacking standards and a sound work ethic? What changes, if any, would you consider making in the future and why?

Retiring Without Notice

After playing in the Global Football League (GFL) for 3 years, all-star running back Manny Magnificent was traded from the Mintville Miners to the Fishtown Fins for a first and second round draft pick in the following year's draft. Last season, his first in Fort Lauderdale, Manny broke nine team records and ran for over

1,500 yards. Although the Fins lost in the first round of the playoffs, the organization and its coaches, players, and fans knew the groundwork had been laid for future success. All looked forward to the upcoming season with great anticipation, and a great deal of their renewed confidence could be attributed to their new star running back.

Then, just before training camp was to commence, the unthinkable happened. Manny called a press conference and announced that he was retiring from football. The decision left Fins' fans, players, and management in stunned disbelief. How could a player in the prime of his career walk away from the game he said he loved, a week before he was supposed to join his teammates in their quest for a GFL championship? Manny's teammates felt as if he had betrayed them. Fans were furious and even called the Fins' front office to request refunds for season tickets they had purchased when they thought Manny would be leading their team. The Fins' management was outraged. They had given up a lot for Manny and never would have relinquished high draft picks for him if they had thought he would retire after 1 year. Ultimately, the team decided to file a multimillion-dollar lawsuit against Manny for breach of contract, stating that he owed them for retiring 5 years before his contract was fulfilled.

Further clouding the situation, were rumors that Manny retired because he tested positive for marijuana use for the second time in his career. If this was true, he would have been suspended for half of the upcoming season according to the GFL's stringent drug policy. At a second press conference, Manny denied failing the test and asserted that he was retiring from football because the sport had become too violent. As a deeply spiritual person, Manny believed it was no longer the right thing for him to keep playing a sport that promoted violent hitting and the dehumanization of athletes.

Critical Thinking: Finding Common-Sense Solutions

1. Should Manny have retired right before training camp? Why or why not?

2. Is it ethical for professional leagues to test players for the use of recreational drugs such as marijuana? Justify you answer.

Critical Thinking: Moral Theory-Based Decision Making

3. Would Manny have chosen to retire if he was reasoning as (a) a consequentialist, (b) a deontologist, or (c) a teleologist? Why or why not?

4. Was the Fins' management justified in suing Manny? Justify your answer using moral values and/or principles in your reasoning.

5. Is it ethical for athletes to participate in violent sports such as football? Justify your answer using moral values and/or principles in your reasoning.

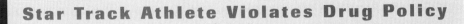

Star Track Athlete Violates Drug Policy

Coach Dilemma is the coach of the track team and a teacher at a high school. Since moving into the community several years ago, he has developed several close relationships and is comfortable in the community. Over the years, he has taught and coached several of his friends' children. One the families he has become particularly close with has a son, Ricky, who is on his track team.

Prior to the beginning of the season, Coach Dilemma held his annual parents' meeting, where he explained his rules and regulations to the parents of his athletes. A point of emphasis this year was the fact that all athletes must sign a code of conduct agreeing to abide by the rules and regulations of their coach as well as the substance abuse policy of the school. The policy specifically states that an athlete is in violation of the substance abuse policy when he or she consumes, uses, or possesses, any alcoholic beverage, tobacco, or illegal drug. The possession of drug paraphernalia while participating on a sports team is also a direct violation of the school's substance abuse policy. All coaches, on knowing of a student-athlete's involvement in substance abuse, are required to notify school officials. The school principal then assumes the responsibility of enforcing the punishment specific to the infraction.

Coach Dilemma's track team is having an outstanding season, and Ricky has become his best 800-meter runner. As the league championship meet approaches, Coach Dilemma received a phone call from Ricky's dad, Harry, who wants to meet with him about Ricky.

The next day, when Harry arrives at Coach Dilemma's office, he gets right to the point and tells him that he has found marijuana in Ricky's room and confronted him and that Ricky has admitted to smoking marijuana almost every day for the past 6 months. Fully aware that his son has breeched the substance abuse policy, Harry confides to the coach that he has come to him with this information because he is the only one he can trust to help Ricky. He also tells the coach that he knows he can trust him and asks him not to tell the school officials. Harry repeats to Coach Dilemma that if the school officials find out, he fears that Ricky will be removed from the team, which could ultimately lead to an increase in his drug use.

Critical Thinking: Finding Common-Sense Solutions

1. If you were Ricky's coach, would you tell the school officials the information that Ricky's father confided in you about Ricky's drug use? Why or why not? To what extent, if any, would your friendship with Ricky's father influence your decision?

2. As Ricky's coach, do you agree with Harry's assertion that Ricky's drug use will worsen if the school officials are notified of his current drug use? Why or why not?

Critical Thinking: Moral Theory-Based Decision Making

3. Using *strategic reasoning* as the basis for your decision, if you were Ricky's coach, how would you have handled this situation?

4. Basing your decision on the *effect it may have on others*, what decision would you make concerning how to deal with the information Ricky's dad has confided in you? Provide the rationale for your decision.

5. If you were Ricky's coach and were attempting to arrive at a decision using the *teleological theory* as your basis, identify and describe the values you would incorporate into your process of moral reasoning.

Questionable Fundraising Practices at Safire High

Safire Falls High School is one of the nation's premier football programs and is located in the heart of football country. As well known for winning games as producing elite professional players, Safire High holds nothing back in its efforts to maintain its storied football reputation. One look at the football program's excessive landscape and facilities is all it takes to understand the year-to-year success of Safire's football program.

Across from the illuminated state-of-the-art turf of the varsity football field and the field house, the softball team struggles for recognition as well as resources. Unlike the glamorized football program, the softball team barely gets by with a playing and practice surface that resembles an unmown field more than a softball diamond. The fans who show up to attend softball games bring their own lawn chairs because there are no bleachers for spectators. Although nearly 10,000 die-hard football fanatics and family members grace the stadium every Friday night in the fall to watch Safire Falls High, fewer than 200 supporters will make up the softball team's total home attendance.

The gender inequities at Safire Falls High go far beyond the gap between the football and softball teams. Last year, the boys' varsity basketball team was able to budget for a new team locker room with a television and sofa along with new uniforms and warm-up jackets. On the other hand, the girls' varsity basketball team was barely able to buy new uniforms for the first time in 2 years.

Safire High's booster club calls for close examination when attempting to understand reasons for the gender-biased manner in which the administration distributes funds to its sports teams. Through the booster club, specific sports have proven to have more earning power when soliciting gifts from outside donors.

In the area of fundraising, certain sports have proven to be significantly more effective than others. Football at Safire High easily outdistances the other sports in fundraising. Gary Greenback is just one former Safire High star who is currently playing professional football and is part of the Safire football revenue-generating machine. As a result of Greenback's professional status, he has the ability to generate large sums of money for his alma mater. Given Greenback's enthusiasm and widespread popularity, he has assisted the booster club in raising nearly $35,000 for top-grade football equipment.

Because of the tremendous interest in football at Safire High, distribution of the funds over all athletic teams was not, in anyway, considered. The view that, because football generates more money than the other sports, it should, therefore, be funded accordingly has been dominant for quite some time now. Even though the stated mission of the booster club is to assist all athletic teams equally, regardless of gender, the decision to earmark the $35,000 for football was made without hesitation.

Mr. Johnson, who has been the athletic director at Safire High School for 15 years, happens to also be a football alumnus of the school and to have a daughter who plays on the girls' softball team. Rarely does a day go by when Mr. Johnson does not hear complaints from his daughter and her teammates about how the boys and their sports teams are unfairly provided with more than the girls and their teams. Even though Mr. Johnson is aware of and sympathetic to these gender inequities, he has not spoken out against them for fear of losing the support of boosters who donate large sums of money.

In light of these obvious monetary gender inequities, many of the school's faculty and peers have begun to question Mr. Johnson's role as athletic director and his lack of leadership. The message he has sent through his inaction is blatantly clear: girls' sports are not as important as boys' sports at Safire Falls High School.

Critical Thinking: Finding Common-Sense Solutions

1. Based on how booster funds are allocated, what message do you believe Mr. Johnson and the athletic department are sending to the girls who participate in athletics at Safire High School?

2. If you were Mr. Johnson, would you be influenced if your favorite sport was football and your political support came from Safire High's football fans? Why or why not? Given the same circumstances of this situation, would you be influenced to act differently if your favorite sport was basketball? If so, how?

3. Is it ethical to allocate more money to football because of its fan interest and ability to produce significant amounts of revenue? Why or why not?

4. If the booster club uses a resource such as a professional football player to facilitate funds, does that give them the right to earmark all of the money

raised for football? Or, should the money go into a general athletic fund? Justify your response.

Critical Thinking: Moral Theory-Based Decision Making

5. If you were Mr. Johnson and decided to base your actions regarding this gender equity dilemma on strategic *reasoning*, what actions would you take and how would you arrive at those actions?

6. Using *deontological moral theory* to guide your reasoning, explain how you would respond to the above gender inequities if you were Mr. Johnson.

7. If you were in Mr. Johnson's role as athletic director, what *moral values* would drive your actions? Why would you emphasize the values you've chosen over others?

Key Terms

circumvent hiring policies—to not follow the established guidelines when hiring an employee.

ethically grounded management philosophy—an approach in which sport management is based on a foundation of moral values.

gossip—either fact-based idle talk or rumor, especially about the private affairs of others.

half-truths—a partially true statement intended to deceive or mislead.

job description—a written statement describing an occupation and listing its required and preferred qualifications.

rumors—a statement or opinion widely circulated from person to person, though unconfirmed by facts or evidence.

Taylor's Four-Way Test—a test of moral character developed in 1932 by Herb Taylor, which requires answering four questions; may be used to assist managers in making decisions.

INDEX